LASERS
(Medical and Cosmetic Photonics)

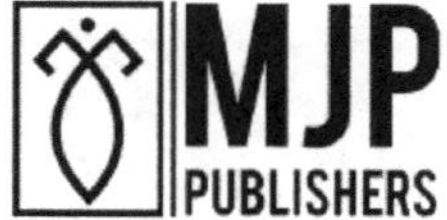

MJP
PUBLISHERS

LASERS
(Medical and Cosmetic Photonics)

S. MOHAN, Ph.D., D.Sc.,

Dean-Research, Vel Tech University, Chennai 600 062
Former Vice-Chancellor, PRIST University, Thanjavur
Former Senior Professor of Materials Science, Asian Institute of Medicine,
Science and Technology University, Malaysia.

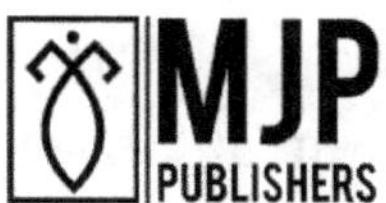

Chennai   New Delhi   Tirunelveli

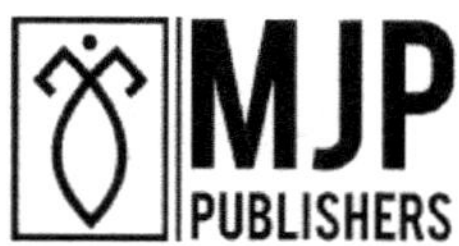

ISBN 978-81-8094-405-5   **MJP Publishers**

All rights reserved   No. 44, Nallathambi Street,
Triplicane, Chennai- 600 005

MJP 281   © Publishers, 2018

Publisher :   C. Janarthanan

Project Editor: C. Ambica

Preface

Prof. Albert Einstein's concept on stimulated emission in 1918 became a reality in 1960 with the advent of masers and lasers. Subsequently, scientific community found many applications of lasers in various fields of science. The laser is very useful to mankind for its invaluable contribution to medical field. The lasers were used in laser medicine and surgery from 1962 onwards. Now it is very popular in all branches of medical field due to the advent of new types of lasers as well as cost reduction in the manufacture of lasers. Diode-pumped solid-state lasers, which will replace gas and ion lasers in future, are commercially available at lower cost. Further, fast healing and painless treatment attracted patients towards laser therapy. Added to this, cosmetic lasers have also become very popular since miracles are possible in beauty treatment.

Although, laser is a non-ionizing radiation, its power and energy may cause severe injuries if it is used carelessly at operation theatres, beauty parlours and in our daily life. Hence, laser knowledge is of utmost importance to those personnel who are in the medical as well as cosmetic profession. Even common man should understand the importance, pros and cons of laser as he may come across laser exposure one day or other. That is, everyone should be aware of laser safety and laser precautions.

The present book has been prepared keeping all these aspects in mind. Since laser is spreading in all walks of life, we need laser personnel for hospitals and other places. At present, we do not have much laser scientists, laser engineers or laser specialists for our needs. We believe that this book will be helpful to know about lasers, its role on tissues, its applications and finally safety of lasers.

The book consists of five chapters. The basics of laser, its principle and some technical aspects are explained in Chapter 1. Chapter 2 deals with most of the lasers starting from solid-state lasers, gas lasers, semiconductor lasers and diode-pumped lasers with emphasis on medical lasers. Laser light–tissue interactions are discussed in Chapter 3 so that it will be easier to follow Chapter 4. In this chapter, various effects of the laser beam on the biological tissues are discussed with relevant examples. Five basic types of laser–tissue interactions, namely photo-thermal, photo-disruptive, photo-chemical, photo-mechanical and biostimulation are discussed in good depth as these interactions are important in using lasers on humans or animals. Chapter 4 deals with medical applications and cosmetic applications in two different sections. Most of the medical areas are covered in this chapter with technical aspects. Section 2 of this chapter explains state-of-art in cosmetic photonics. The final Chapter 5 is devoted to possible laser hazards, safety precautions and safety measures. This chapter gives a guideline to laser safety officers, surgeons, medical and para-medical professionals on the use of lasers and safety measures. It is not the aim of the authors to threaten the medical community by briefing the laser hazards but to caution all those who are exposed to or use lasers in their profession.

We thank our colleagues whose comments and discussions have contributed a lot for the present form of this book. We are also thankful to several learned professors, doctors and laser personnel who were kind enough to offer their valuable criticisms for the improvement of this book. Many Doctors and Professors have given support through their lecture notes and advice then and there. One of the authors (S.M) affectionately thanks his grand daughter P. Mithra for showing a new life to him as well as stimulating him to take up this venture. Last but not the least, our interaction with students in the last three decades and Prof. S. Mohan's service at Asian Institute of Medicine, Science and Technology University, Malaysia were also useful while preparing the manuscript of this book.

Pondicherry   **S. Mohan**

Acknowledgements

We are very grateful to learned Professors from all the Universities and in particular to Professors B.D. Ratner, Engineer, University of Washington, Nick Mamalis, Utah, Derek Grey, Valey Marinor, Lionel C. Kimerling, B.J. Van Zeghbroeck, Neil R. Thomson, John L. Bahr, Saad B.H. Farid, Ahmad Safari, R.K. Panda, V.J. Janes, S.D. Hutagalung, D. Mohankumar, P.A. Tresco, G.L. Kulcinski, J.H. Reibenspies, Y. Ranga Reddy, Druce Dunne, Perry Sprawts and Yao Wang for their informative class notes which were useful in designing this book. Several Professors were kind enough to offer their valuable suggestions and advice for improving the manuscript. We are also thankful to the several well-known websites, including Wikipedia which provided a good amount of information on various topics and it is gratefully acknowledged.

S. Mohan

Contents

Chapter 1

Basics of Laser

INTRODUCTION

What is light? Light is a form of energy. It is a transverse electromagnetic energy. These are the spontaneous answers that one can expect. Visible light which is a small part of the electromagnetic spectrum ranges between 400 to 700 nanometers. The optical portion of the spectrum consists of the infrared, the visible region and the ultraviolet. These are polychromatic and diverging radiations. The photonics technology is concerned with wavelength between 10 microns and 100 nanometres Photonics is nothing but the generation and harnessing of laser radiations.

Laser is a device that generates a very intense beam of light. It usually converts one form of energy into optical energy. The word LASER is an acronym for Light Amplification by Stimulated Emission of Radiation. That is, laser is a light-emitting device with continuous feedback arrangement. It is a process of amplification and laser is a special form of light. It possesses several wavelengths ranging from ultraviolet to infrared. Hence, it is also called UVLASER, IRLASER, free electron lasers, etc. Further it cannot be compared with the ionizing radiations such as X-rays and gamma rays. The different materials such as solids, liquids and gases produce characteristic wavelengths (colours) of light and hence we have different lasers with characteristic wavelengths. In addition to the intensity, several special features make lasers a unique source from the conventional light sources. As all the light rays in the beam are of the same colour, the light is purely monochromatic. Perfectly monochromatic light cannot be produced even by a laser, but laser light is many times more monochromatic than the light from any other source. They are extremely well-collimated. That is, it spreads out very very little as it travels (high directionality). Laser has a high degree of coherence. Laser radiations are characterized by a high degree of ordering of the light (photons) than any other sources. The stimulated emission gives multiphoton of precisely the same wavelength whose wave patterns are perfectly in phase. This special kind of unique radiation is known as coherent radiation. Coherence is the most fundamental property of laser light and distinguishes it from other light sources. Thus, a laser may be defined as a source of coherent light.

LASER RADIATION

In general, laser is named after its active medium. To understand the laser emission, we should know something about energy levels. We know that most of the atoms (or molecules) are available in the ground state at room temperature. Yet, a very few atoms are also available in the higher energy state. The most important requirement for a laser action is that the medium should possess a large number of atoms in the higher energy state than in the ground state. This situation is known as population inversion.

Suppose we supply energy to a medium, the atoms in the ground state absorb the energy and go to the higher energy state. This phenomneon is known as absorption. Ordinarily the atoms in the higher energy state spontaneously decay into ground state by emitting photons. These photons are out-of-phase with one another and this process is entirely random. Hence the emitted light contains many different colours. That is, an incoherent light is emitted in this process. Example of such light are the radiations received from the sun, light bulbs and the fire. On the other hand if the electron in the higher energy state can be stimulated by another photon of precisely the same wavelength as the incident photon, we get a stimulated radiation. Here the atom must be stimulated before it emits its stored energy (light). The induced and inducing photons have the same energy and they have identical direction of their momenta and identical polarization. That is, the secondary photon finds itself in the same state as the primary photon.

Prof. Albert Einstein conceived the idea of stimulated emission in as early as 1900 during his research on photovoltaic mechanism and proposed the new radiation in 1918. Based on Einstein's theories, Schawlow and Townes proposed the maser (microwave amplification by stimulated emission of radiation) emission around 1950. But it was Maiman who created the first laser in 1960 in a ruby rod. Hence, it is appropriate to recognize Dr. Albert Einstein as the father of laser (Figure 1.1).

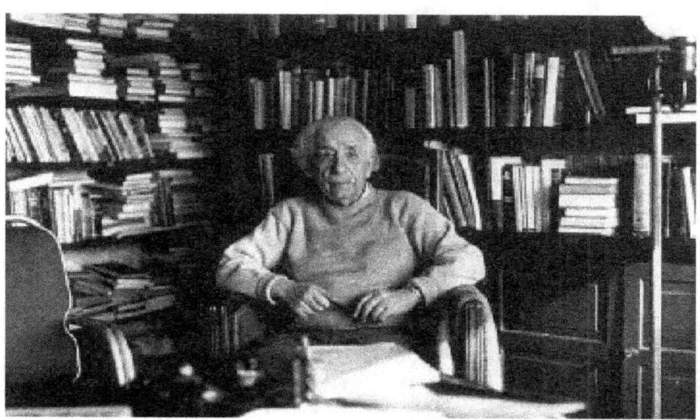

Figure 1.1 Albert Einstein

Leon Goldman has done pioneering work in introducing laser technology in the field of medicine and he was responsible for promoting medical laser applications. Hence Leon Goldman is the father of lasers in medicine.

LASER COMPONENTS

The next question comes in our mind is, how does a laser work? In general, all lasers consist of four components.

1. Active medium

2. Excitation mechanism

3. Feedback mechanism

4. Output coupler

Active Medium

The active medium is the main component of a laser. It may be a solid, liquid, gas or a semiconductor. Ruby, glass, alexandrite, neodymium: yttrium aluminium garnet (Nd:YAG) and holmium: yttrium aluminium garnet (Ho : YAG) are a few mediums for solid-state lasers. For electronic medium, semiconductors are used for producing diode lasers. For gas lasers, carbon dioxide, argon, krypton, helium–neon, helium–cadmium and rare earth halides (excited dimers) are used as medium. Various kinds of dyes are used as medium for liquid lasers.

Excitation Mechanism

As a second step, we need energy source (power supply) to pump the active medium to achieve population inversion. Is it possible for the input energy to cause population inversion of atoms or molecules? We all know that thermal energy can be used just to heat the atoms or molecules. Hence, it is not possible to achieve population inversion by this method.

Therefore one has to explore the other possibilities. One such possibility is just to remove some atoms out of the ground state energy level so that the ground state has less population than the higher energy level. Using this principle, the ammonia maser was built. Ammonia molecules were selectively filtered using electric field so that the remaining molecule exhibited population inversion. Unfortunately this method was not successful with optical masers (lasers).

The second possibility is electrical pumping. This can be achieved by keeping the laser medium in the electron beam so that the electrons create a population inversion by transferring the energy to the atoms or molecules under collision. This technique is adopted in most of the high-power gas lasers. The direct discharge is another technique of electrical pumping. As in the fluorescent lamp, electrical discharge can be effected in a tube containing the gaseous laser medium. A population inversion is created in the ions or atoms of the discharge when they absorb energy from the electrical current. Electrical discharge is used in common gas lasers such as carbon dioxide, argon, krypton, He–Ne and He–Cd lasers. This method of energizing the active medium is known as direct current method.

One more method of creating population inversion is by using radio frequency energy. Carbon dioxide lasers are partially energized by this technique. A sealed electrode tube of the gas is excited by an intense radio frequency field, creating a population inversion. These are known as sealed tube lasers. They do not require external gas sources. It is self-contained within the laser resonator. Sometimes a small gas reservoir is also attached to the tube for the laser's longer life. Ion lasers such as argon and krypton utilize an attached reservoir from which the tube must be periodically recharged manually. Carbon dioxide lasers are designed for flowing gas sys tems to several types of sealed systems.

Free space flowing gas systems are open glass tubes, with mirrors at each end. When a high-voltage DC electricity is applied, it energizes the gas in the tube through the electrodes. After the emission of light radiation, the carbon dioxide molecule dissociates and contaminants are formed at the electrodes.

Therefore, to sustain laser action, new gas must be continuously pumped which can be achieved by a vacuum system.

On the other hand if we use a gas cylinder, it can last only for a few hours. Further, since there would be escape of gas mixtures, it is very expensive when the gas is pumped through, the system is not a sealed tube. The microflow system has evolved with advancement in science, which minimizes gas consumption. The main advantage in the gas flow system is that it operates indefinitely due to continuous fresh gas supply.

The most efficient carbon dioxide laser came into existence with the invention of radio frequency waveguide lasers. These are sealed tube lasers which do not require costly gas tanks and are very quiet in operation. In these lasers, transverse radio frequency (high-frequency electricity) signal across the tube is used to excite the gas instead of direct electrical excitation. One of the advantages of a high-powered RF system is that high-energy pulses may be developed in the super pulse mode on the laser which is much greater than that attainable by direct electrical excitation. This produces higher average powers.

The next generation of carbon dioxide laser is free space-sealed tube lasers. They have the main advantage of low operating costs due to the absence of external gas. These lasers use DC excitation just as the flowing systems. The difference is that they have a gas reservoir built right into the tube and use a special gas mixture. The large reservoir and catalysts reassociate the carbon dioxide molecules after it breaks apart so that it is continuously usable. These tubes will also have to be recharged after several thousand hours or three to five years or so.

Electrical pumping also creates a population inversion in semiconductor diode lasers—an important member in the laser family. When a current passes through the interface between p and n-type semiconductors, it creates mobile charge carriers. If they are enough, it is possible to produce population inversion.

The third possibility is optical pumping. In solid-state lasers like chromium-doped ruby and neodymium-doped YAG, the lasing atoms are embedded in a solid material. It is not possible to pump these lasers by an electrical current or an electron beam. Hence, they are optically pumped. The laser material is bombarded with photons whose energy corresponds to the energy difference between the ground level and the pump levels. The atoms in the ground state absorb energy from the pump photon and are excited to the pump bands.

The fourth possibility is chemical energy. Lasers that use chemical energy are known as chemical lasers in which two or more materials react, liberating energy and forming a new material. These new materials are treated with a built-in population inversion because many of its atoms or molecules have been excited by chemical energy. Chemical lasers are capable of high powers but they are not very common. These lasers were developed in the past by the military for weapons, but today we have various types of lasers that are more appropriate for weapons.

For the sake of completeness, let us look into the fifth possibility of attaining population inversion— using nuclear particles. Lasers have been pumped by nuclear particles, usually from nuclear bombs. The energy in the particles creates a population inversion in the laser medium and a pulse of laser output is obtained before the shock wave and other energy from the bombs destroys the laser. Such lasers may be useful to military applications alone.

Recently, we have a new family of lasers known as diode-pumped solid-state lasers which are commonly known as DPSSL. Here, semiconductor laser radiation is used as pump source for solid-state lasers. Combining non-linear crystals with this arrangement, it is possible to produce IR and deep UV lasers. It is also realized that this technology may very soon replace ion and gas lasers. Further, these lasers are very cost-effective.

Lastly, free electron lasers are pumped by high-energy electrons. The output of a free electron laser is produced from electrons that are free. That is, the physics of a free electron laser is much different from other lasers. There are no fixed energy levels for free electrons. Hence, laser wavelengths can be tuned. Although free electron lasers are promising for future application, they are still in the experimental stage and are in operation only in a few laboratories worldwide.

Feedback Mechanism

The next important aspect of lasers is the feedback mechanism (laser mirrors). The optical resonator is the device to amplify the light produced from stimulated emission. This device provides the necessary feedback for the laser to function. Optical resonator is nothing but a chamber or a laser tube (glass or quartz) that permits a series of reflection of light waves back and forth at the velocity of light between the two ends. Therefore the optical resonator essentially consists of a system of mirrors and the active medium. So, photons are reflected back and forth several times through the chamber stimulating more and more emission on each turn. Hence, the resonance builds in intensity and the light comes out through a partially transmissive mirror. The mirrors used at each end of the tube to form this resonator should be gently curved so that they tend to keep this light concentrated inside the resonator. One of the mirrors in the resonator is 100% reflective while the other mirror is partially reflective. By taking advantage of the partial reflective mirror, laser light emerges from the resonator. This is known as laser amplification which is used for optical gain. The process of stimulated emission starts amplification but the resonator plays an important role in increasing the intensity to a high level. The emerging light from the partially coated mirror is the output beam from the laser. The partial reflective mirror varies from one type of laser to another but is usually somewhere between 1% and 50% reflectivity.

Some lasers can produce easily 10 photons in a single pass and thus possess enormous gain. These super-radiant lasers do not need resonators. Nitrogen lasers sometimes operate this way. Lasers using heavy metal vapours such as copper and gold vapour also have such a high initial gain and hence they lase without mirrors. The mirror alignments which affect power output are much less critical in these type of systems.

Some examples of optical resonators are 1) Simple linear resonator, 2) Coupled linear resonator and 3) Ring resonator. Various types of resonators are shown in Figure 1.2.

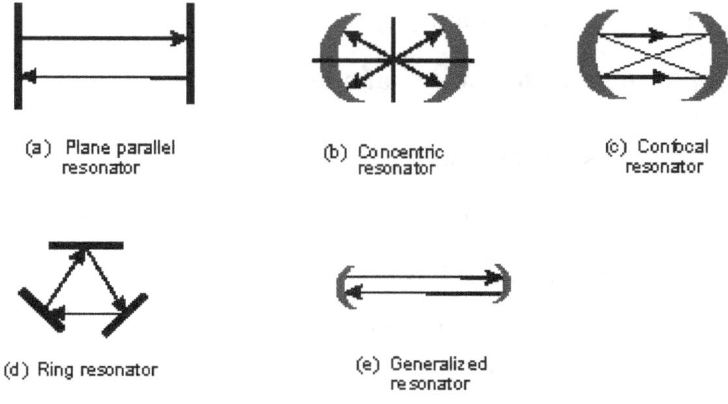

Figure 1.2 Various types of laser resonators

Resonators used in lasers belong to the class of open resonators. They are considerably different from the cavity resonators used in the super high frequency (SHF) band. Fundamentally, an open resonator differs from a cavity resonator in two main aspects.

1. The conducting side walls are removed but the end face reflectors are retained. The end mirrors fix the resonator axis in space.

2. The dimensions of the resonator should be larger than the radiation wavelength.

The quality factor or Q factor of the resonator is defined as (assuming that only one mode exists) the ratio of energy stored in the cavity to the energy loss per radiation.

The smaller the losses in a resonator, the higher its Q. Further, the Q factor of a resonator is inversely proportional to the rate of decrease of field energy in the resonator.

Laser mirrors are coated with dielectric (cerium oxide) or metal layers. The manufacturing of laser mirrors are very complicated. Solid-state laser mirrors are formed on the specially prepared end faces of the active medium. In the case of gas lasers, resonator mirrors are usually mounted at both ends of the gas discharge tube with bellows.

Optical resonators give the direction for the emission of radiation. The process of stimulated emission just compensates for absorption only in this direction. That is, the resonator picks out a direction in space for which the losses are minimized and the condition for generation is satisfied.

It is also possible to add additional optical elements within the optical resonator to maintain selectively for photon states. A prism inside the resonator enables this selection of energy using the concept of dispersion of light.

The laser medium can be enclosed in a variety of resonator configurations.

1. Fabry–Perot configuration
2. Long radii mirror configuration
3. Concentric mirror configuration
4. Confocal configuration
5. Hemispherical configuration

The resonators listed above are stable resonators wherein the beam is usually trapped inside and losses are only due to diffraction. That is, the light is concentrated near the axis of the resonator. If one traces the path of the ray of light between the mirrors of a stable resonator, the ray is eventually reflected back and forth towards the resonator axis by the mirrors. If at all the ray wants to escape, it has to pass through one of the mirrors. Hence, by saying "stable" we mean the trapping of rays between the mirrors. It is nothing to do with resonators sensitivity to malalignment.

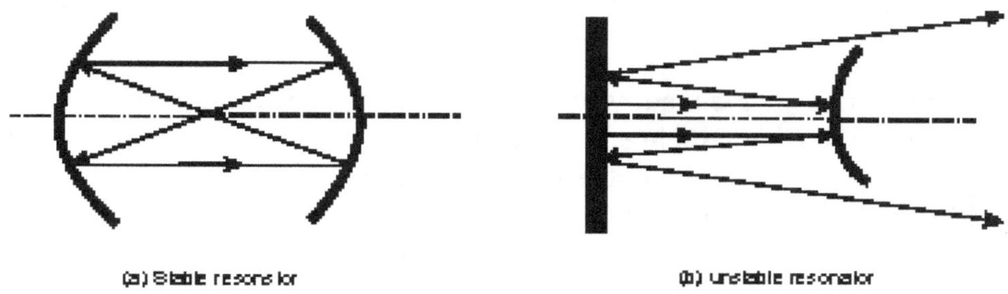

Figure 1.3 (a) Stable and (b) unstable resonators

On the other hand, in the unstable resonator, the light rays keep on moving away from the resonator axis until they miss the small convex mirror completely. The output beam from this resonator will have a doughnut-like shape with a hole in the middle caused by the shadow of the small mirror. It is also possible to construct unstable resonators without a hole in the central beam. The advantage of the unstable resonators is that they usually produce a large beam volume inside the gain medium so that the beam can interact with more of the population inversion and thereby produce more output power. Unstable resonators are usually used only with high-power, pulsed gas and solid-state lasers. There are a number of important laser applications where the large diffraction losses in the unstable region are acceptable or even desirable. The stable and unstable resonators are shown in Figure 1.3.

Output Coupler

An output coupler is a partially reflective mirror used in lasers to extract a portion of the laser beam from the optical resonator. The output coupler usually has reflectance in the range 40% to 70%. There are two important properties of the output coupler. They are:

i.   **Radii of curvature**   The output coupler may be either flat or curved, depending on the design of the optical cavity. In order to optimize power and spatial profile of the laser beam, the output coupler and end mirror have optical surfaces with well-defined radii of curvature. The face of the output coupler facing into the cavity is the side with the applied partially reflective coating. This is the side which partially determines the laser modal properties. If this inner surface is curved then so must be the outer surface can be designed to give a collimated laser output. This outer surface generally has an anti-reflection coating applied to maximise the output power.

ii.   **Reflectivity**   Depending on the gain of the medium, the amount of light the output coupler needs to reflect back can vary widely. Helium–neon lasers require around a 99% reflective mirror to lase, while nitrogen lasers have an extremely high gain (they are "superradiant" and do not require any output coupler (0% reflective). The reflectivity of any output coupler may vary with wavelength. A particular mirror may have a tuning range as low as 10 nm or so.

BASIC MODES OF LASER OPERATION

Laser oscillation can be broadly classified under three categories.

1.   Continuous oscillation,

2.   Pulsed oscillation and

3.   Pulsed mode with controlled losses (Q-switching lasers).

Gas lasers give a continuous mode while pulsed modes are mostly seen in solid lasers. In continuous wave lasers, the light beam is emitted with constant power. That means, this mode requires a continuous steady state pumping of the active medium. This can be achieved by continuously operating optical pumping or by a steady state discharge in a gas. The cross section of the laser beam in these lasers is always lesser than the cross section of the resonator.

In pulsed free oscillation, the radiation comes out in the form of periodic light pulses, 1 to 10 sec. long, at a frequency of 10 Hz to 10 kHz. The pulsed laser is due to the pulsed operation of the pumping system, viz., a flash lamp. In solid-state lasers, the laser beam cross section is equal to the cross section of the active medium. In pulsed mode oscillation, we achieve a considerable concentration of light energy. In these lasers we get a substantial power output within short time intervals. The concentration of light energy reaches a maximum in the giant pulse mode of oscillation.

Continuous wave (CW) generally refers to a steady state power output from the laser. Although medical lasers offer a choice of operating modes to include continuous and pulsed mode, most medical lasers work in the CW mode.

In a pulsed laser, a true laser pulse can compress the power output of the laser tube and deliver a very high peak power of energy during the pulse but cannot maintain these high powers in a steady state. It delivers peak powers which are generally not attainable when operating with a CW beam. Pulsing includes Q-switching, mode-locking, superpulsing and flash lamp pulsing techniques. With the exception of superpulse, most pulsing is designed into the laser.

Some lasers deliver their energy solely as pulsed energy and many CO_2 lasers additionally offer a superpulse mode. Timer on the CW beam is most commonly referred to as gated pulse and it is common on CO_2 lasers.

True laser pulses, which are different, may also be emitted in this timed fashion. Most of the CO_2 lasers offer an option for a repeat pulse which is a very useful feature on CO_2 lasers.

Ultrashort Pulses

Ultrashort pulses, tunable from the visible to mid-infrared, are useful for many applications such as pulse propagation in optical fibres, carrier dynamic studies in semiconductors, in time-resolved relaxation dynamics and the observation of transient chemical species. This is achieved due to the concept of mode locking in the last four decades. Widely tunable ultrashort pulse laser sources are also available for the investigation of optical properties (including second-and third-order non-linear properties) of both organic and inorganic materials. Several techniques exist to generate tunable picosecond pulses. Synchronously mode-locked continuous-wave colour centre lasers directly generate picosecond pulses in the infrared but their tunability (for a given centre type and host material) is limited and these systems generally suffer from a photo bleaching effect which results in fading and poor reliability. On the other hand, synchronously mode-locked dye lasers are reliable and tunable sources. The recent progress in the development of efficient infrared dyes has extended the laser wavelengths coverage to about 1.3 fm.

In recent years, enormous advances have been made in the generation of ultrashort pulses. It is possible to carry out a wide range of measurements within the time scale of 10^{-10} s (pico second) and 10^{-15} s (femto second). In order to derive the ultrashort pulse from a laser, the fluorescence or gain bandwidth of the amplifier must be sufficiently broad to support the pulse. Mode-locking techniques have been used in the last two decades to generate ultrashort pulses. During that time, various refinements to the technique have led to the development of laser systems capable of operating in the femtosecond range.

Giant Pulse Lasers

Q-switching is another common term technically used to represent giant pulses. In fact Q-switching is due to modulation of losses. This term describes the pulsing technique that produces peak powers of the order of 10 watts. These pulses have a duration of only a few nanoseconds. Due to the short pulse width, the total energy of light emitted per pulse is very low—of the order of 3–10 millijoules. Q-switching can be easily understood as storing up energy inside the laser and suddenly letting it out in a giant pulse. That is, the energy is stored in the population inversion until it reaches a certain level. Then it is released very quickly in a giant pulse. This can be easily compared with storing water in a tank and then releasing the water suddenly. Is it possible to achieve this in laser? How can one prevent the energy from draining out of the population inversion as fast as it goes in ?

The answer is simple for these questions. By some technique, the laser is prevented from lasing. This can be achieved either by eliminating population inversion or the feedback.

The elimination of population inversion is not possible as the energy is stored in the population inversion. The other possibility can be attempted. One can eliminate feedback to prevent lasing and hence all the extra energy can be stored in the population inversion by blocking one of the laser mirrors. That is, by eliminating feedback, energy builds up in the population inversion until the feedback is restored. Therefore all the energy comes out in a single giant pulse (Figure 1.4).

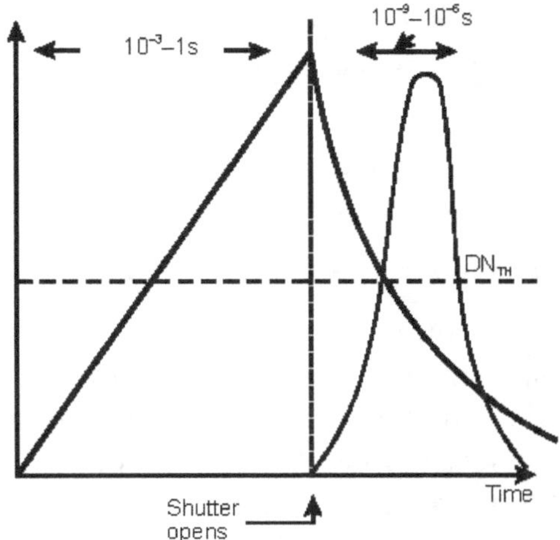

Figure 1.4 Giant pulse Laser

Why is it called *Q-switching* or *Q-spoiling*?

"Q" stands for the quality or quality factor of the resonator. A high-quality (high Q) resonator has low loss. Obviously, a resonator with an obstructed mirror is not a very high-quality resonator. But, when the mirror is suddenly unblocked, the Q is switched from low to high. Thus a Q-switched laser is one whose resonator can be switched from low quality to high quality and back again. Therefore giant pulse lasers can be realized by controlling losses in the resonator. If these losses are sufficiently increased by some technique for a certain time, oscillation cannot develop. Consequently, the system of pumping builds a considerable overpopulation of the upper lasing level in active centres. If the losses are sharply brought down, the process of stimulated emission by the favoured photon states develops in a sudden manner and gives rise to a short light pulse with very high peak power.

All the lasers cannot be Q-switched. The lifetime of the upper laser level must be long enough so that energy does not leak out by spontaneous emission before the resonator Q is switched up, to stimulate a pulse. This is not the case for many types of lasers including ion lasers anddye lasers. Solid-state lasers such as YAG, glass or ruby can be made as Q-switched lasers.

In order to control the losses in a resonator, four types of Q-switching are used in lasers.

1. Mechanical Q-switches—move a mirror to switch the resonator Q.

2. Acousto-optic Q-switches—diffraction reduces feedback from a resonator mirror.

3. Electro-optic Q-switches—polarization prevents light from returning from a mirror.

4. Dye Q-switches—absorbs the light and bleaches the dye.

The giant pulse is generated directly after a drop in losses occurs. The emission of giant pulse is meaningful only if the drop in losses is very sharp. Hence, it is clear that the switches based on mechanical motion are not suitable for Q-switches. Active (electro-optic, acousto-optic) and passive (saturable absorber dyes) Q-switches without moving parts are more effective in producing more giant pulses.

If the Q-switching occurs rapidly for emission of multiple pulses, the peak power of each pulse is less than that of a single pulse of lower frequency but is still much higher than a gated pulse. The potassium titanyl phosphate crystal for instance will Q-switch the laser beam at over 25,000 times per second.

Superpulse is found on many carbon dioxide lasers and they are usually called as superpulse, varipulse or megapulse. This pulse on CO_2 lasers usually produces a train of pulses from 250 to 500 watts with a maximum peak power perpulse at a rate of 300-1000 times per second. This rate is so fast that it appears to be continuous but the pulse can be picked up as an audible sound as and when the focused beam hits the target. Further, the total delivered energy is not as high as the 500 watt pulse but it comes to only 75 millijoules per pulse. This is the average power of the CO_2 lasers. The maximum average power in a superpulse will always be substantially lower than the maximum power available in continuous mode. Most lasers produce approximately one-third of the high power in superpulse in comparison with a continuous wave mode. High-power lasers, such as those with a power of 80–100 watts, allow for superpulsing approximately 25–35 watts average power. Lower-power lasers often produce maximum superpulsing of only 10–20 watts average power. These lower energies per pulse and average powers are useful for cutting but they are insufficient for vaporizing large areas. Hence, the higher powers of a continuous wave mode are useful for vaporization.

An exception is the superpulse mode on some RF-excited CO_2 lasers which are known as ultrapulse. These lasers produce such high energies per pulse so that the average power is not sacrificed. In fact, it can produce average ultra-pulse powers as high as the maximum CW power on the laser.

CAVITY DUMPING

We have seen that Q-switching technique will not work with lasers whose upper-state lifetime is too short to store appreciable energy. Hence, another technique, viz., cavity dumping is used to get pulses from these lasers. The word cavity represents a resonator. A simple cavity-dumped laser can be explained as follows.

Consider two mirrors of maximum (100%) reflectance. In between the mirror, we have an active medium and an electro-optic Q-switch comprising of a Pockel's cell and a polarizer. The basic question arising in our mind is regarding the laser emission. How does a laser escape when both the end mirrors are maximum reflectors?

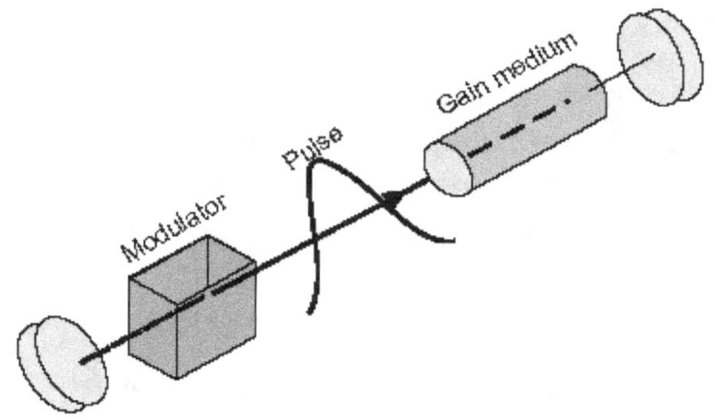

Figure 1.5 Cavity-dumped laser

When the lamp flashes, the electro-optic Q-switch is in its transmission mode. Therefore, light passes through Pockel's cell without any polarization rotation. When the round-trip gain becomes equal to the round-trip loss, the laser begins lasing. The photons start bouncing back and forth between the mirrors. Due to 100% reflectance mirror, the circulating power increases to a very high level. When the maximum intracavity circulating power has been obtained, a voltage is applied to the Pockels cell. The cell rotates the polarization of light passing through it and the polarizer ejects all the light in a cavity-dumped pulse. Cavity dumping is a general technique that can be used with advantage whether the laser be mode-locked, CW or Q-switched. For pulsed, mode-locked lasers, cavity dumping is usually carried out at the time when the intracavity mode-locked pulse reaches its maximum value. In this way, a single ultrashort pulse of high intensity comes out of the laser cavity.

A cavity-dumped laser (Figure 1.5) is a different type of Q-switched laser in the sense, the cavity Q-switches from high to low instead of from low to high. Hence, cavity dumping is also known as pulsed transmission mode Q-switching. The duration of the cavity pumped pulse from the laser depends on the resonator length. The difference between a cavity-dumped laser and a Q-switched laser is that the energy is stored in the population inversion in the Q-switched laser while it is stored in the optical resonator in the cavity-dumped laser.

A solid-state laser that is flash-pumped but not cavity-dumped or Q-switched is known as normal mode laser. Hence, the output contains several spikes and they are not repeatable from one pulse to the next. This type of laser can be used in industrial applications (crude energy) where refinements such as Q-switch or cavity-dumper are not required.

Let as consider ion lasers. They have too short lifetime in the upper state to allow enough energy storage for Q-switching. If one wants a pulsed output from ion lasers such as argon or krypton ion lasers, one must cavity-dump it. An acousto-optic cavity dumper is used for the purpose. Figure 1.6 shows cavity-dumped argon laser.

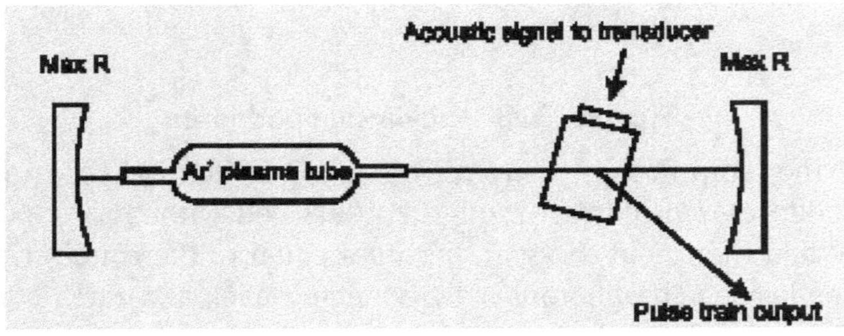

Figure 1.6   Cavity-dumped Argon Ion Laser

MODE-LOCKING

The highest pulse frequency and the shortest pulse are obtained by mode-locking a laser. The lasers which use Q-switching or cavity dumping can also be mode-locked. In short, some lasers are simultaneously Q-switched, cavity-dumped and mode-locked. The shortest pulse of light that has ever been generated come from mode-locked lasers. The duration of a Q-switched laser pulse varies from several hundred nanoseconds to several nanoseconds depending on the laser parameters. The cavity-dumped laser pulse is shorter than nanoseconds. But a mode-locked pulse from a dye laser can be shorter than a pico second. Mode-locked lasers can be operated either with a pulsed or CW pump. Figure 1.7 shows the mode-locking of a laser and semiconductor mode-locked laser.

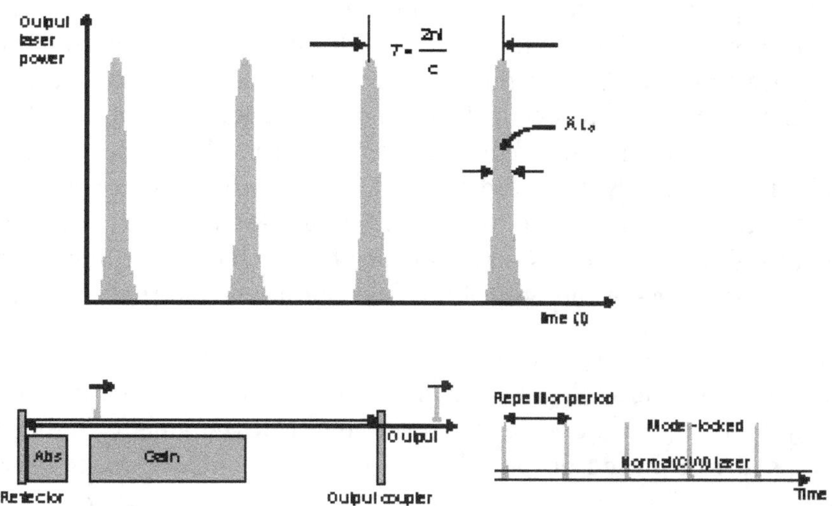

Figure 1.7 Mode Locking and Semiconductor Mode Locking

In a mode-locked laser, the optical energy between the mirrors has been compressed to a very short pulse that is shorter than the resonator itself. In a Q-switched or acavity-dumped laser, the whole resonator is filled with energy. But in a mode-locked laser the energy is compacted into pulse that bounces back and forth between the mirrors. When this pulse reaches the partially transmitted mirror, an output emerges from it. The output of a mode-locked laser is a train of very short pulses. The time separation between the pulse is $2L/c$ where L is the optical distance between the mirrors. Hence, the frequency of the mode-locked pulse is $c/2L$. For example, a laser whose mirrors are separated by 30 cm will produce a mode-locked pulse train at 500 megahertz (MHz), That is, 500 million pulses of light per second.

The duration of the mode-locked pulse depends on various factors including the laser's gain bandwidth and its modulation depth. When the laser's bandwidth is greater, the mode-locked pulse is shorter. As we know, the dye lasers have enormous bandwidths. This produces shortest mode-locked pulses approaching 100 femtoseconds. On the contrary, Nd:YAG lasers. possess narrow bandwidths and hence produce mode-locked pulses of 30 to 60 picoseconds duration.

Electro-optic modulators, acousto-optic modulators and dye cells are used to mode-lock lasers. In a pulsed laser, active mode-locking is commonly achieved either by means of a Pockels cell, electro-optic modulator or an acousto-optic modulator. Passive mode-locking in pulsed lasers is usually achieved by fast saturable absorbers. When a slow saturable absorber is used with a slow gain material, passive Q-switching with a single-mode selection rather than mode-locking will tend to occur. In case of mode-locking with a CW pump, the output beam consists of a continuous train of mode-locked pulses. Active mode-locking is usually achieved by Pockels cell modulator or by an acousto-optic modulator. An acousto-optic modulator used for mode-locking differs from that used for Q-switching since the face to which the transducer is bonded and the opposite face of the optical material should be parallel to each other.

Passive mode-locking with CW lasers can be achieved, under special circumstances, using slow absorbers combined with fast laser gain media. Just like cavity-dumping, mode-locking is a very descriptive name for the process of obtaining shortest pulsed output from a laser. Now one can raise a few questions such as 1) What modes are locked? 2) What does it mean to lock modes? This can be understood as follows.

The longitudinal modes of the resonator are locked together in phase when one mode-locks a laser. Hence, they are also referred to as phase locking. The longitudinal waves travelling in the medium interfere constructively and destructively at some places in the resonator. The constructive interference at certain places in the resonator creates the mode-locked pulse. In a free-running laser, the mode does not stay in phase with each other. Further, due to resonator perturbations some modes stop oscillation. When they start once again, they will have different phase. Hence, it is necessary to lock them together in phase to produce a mode-locked pulse. This is achieved by mode-locking the modulator in mode-locked lasers.

Mode-locked lasers do not usually have very high peak power. They are used when very short pulses are needed. One such application is in communication. They are used in experimental systems developed by the military for communication among spacecrafts and with submarines. Ranging is another application of mode-locked lasers. Although Q-switched lasers are also used in ranging, mode-locked lasers give greater accuracy. Mode-locked lasers are also used as spectroscopic tools to investigate very fast phenomena. The short pulse from a mode-locked laser is one of the few probes that can be used to investigate veryfast chemical or physical reactions. The most commonly used mode-locked lasers are are given in Table 1.1.

Table 1.1 Active media, modulator and pulse width of common mode-locked lasers

Active medium	Modulator	Mode- Locking operation	Pulse width
Gas lasers			
He–Ne	Quartz–AM	CW	1 ns
He–Ne	Neon cell–SA	CW	350 ps
Ar	Quartz–AM	CW	150 ps
CO_2 (low pressure)	SF–SA	CW	10–20 ns
CO_2	Ge–AM	CW	10–20 ns
CO_2 (TEA)	Ge–AM	Pulsed	1ns
CO_2 (TEA)	SF–SA	Pulsed	1 ns
Solid-state lasers			
Nd : YAG	Quartz–AM	CW	100 ps
Nd : YAG	LinBO–EOM	Pulsed	40 ps
Nd : glass	Kodak-9860 SA	Pulsed	5 ps
GaAs	SA	CW	5 ps
Liquid (Dye lasers)			
Rhodamine 6G	DODCI–SA	Flash-pumped	1 ps
Rhodamine 6G	Sync. pump	CW, Ar-pumped	0.5 ps

AM–Acousto-optic modulator, SA-Saturable absorber
EOM– Electro–optic modulator, DODCI-, 3,3–Diethyloxydicarbo cyanine iodide

ENERGY CONCEPTS

Laser power is expressed in milliwatts (mW) to megawatts (MW) to gigawatts (GW). There is a considerable difference between small m and capital M. This indicates whether the laser is a low-power laser or a high-power laser. Power in watts is a measure of the rate of energy delivery in joules second. To determine peak power of a laser pulse, energy delivered is divided by the required time. For example, if 200 millijoules is delivered in 200 microseconds, the peak power is 1000 watts.

Power density is the most important factor in the effective operation of any laser. It is synonymous with irradiance. It determines the laser's ability to vaporize, excise and coagulate various tissues of the body. It describes the intensity of light in terms of power per unit area. Power density is expressed in watts/cm. The surface area of the spot (spot size controlled by the surgeon) and the total power of the laser in watts determine the power density. If the spot radius is in millimetres, then power density helps in determining the rate of tissue removal and create the perception of eye-hand coordination of the physician. A common misconception is that power alone determines the coordination required to avoid perforations or shredding of tissue with the laser. Power density over a spot determines the rate of tissue removal within that spot. One can effectively change the size of the spot with which one is working, without changing the overall rate of tissue removal (power density) within the spot by varying spot size and power. The larger the spot, the greater is the power required to maintain the same power density. At extremes, a very low-power density is very easy to be controlled by the surgeon but it burns tissue excessively. On the contrary, a very high-power density produces a very clean tissue effect but it is very hard to be controlled by the surgeon. When vaporizing or debulking tissue, spot sizes are made easier so that the total time required to burn the tissue can be considerably reduced.

The total light energy is described by the unit Joule. Laser pulses are measured in joules (1 Joule = 1 watt second). Therefore the total energy delivered depends upon the power and the duration of the laser source. That is, longer the light delivered or higher the power, more is the total energy delivered. Joules describes the total energy delivered but does not indicate how concentrated this light dose is. For example, surgical Nd:YAG and ophthalmic lasers have joules read out while carbon dioxide lasers do not have joules read out. The rate of energy delivery is described by flux. For example, 100 joules can be delivered in 1 second by 100 watts or in 100 seconds by one watt. 100 watts per second is a higher flux.

Combining the concept of rate of delivery with that of power density leads to the concept of 'fluence'. The unit of fluence is joules/cm. Fluence is also known as radiant exposure. Fluence is an energy concept which considers both radiant pressure and power density from the surface and exposure from all other directions. In short, high energy delivery in quicker phase is represented by fluence. When the fluence is very high, it has very precise thermal effect on tissues. Due to very high peak power, laser pulse with short period of exposure, minimizes or eliminates any unwanted heat conduction to adjacent tissues. Due to this, superpulsing CO_2 laser gives a clear-cut effect. Pulsed laser of this type is also used to make birth marks and similar lesions which minimize any unwanted burning effects of the laser. The high fluence pulsed laser energy creates non-linear effects. These are generally acoustical shock waves not associated with direct tissue heating. A Nd : YAG pulsed laser of tens of millions of watts within a few nanoseconds can create the cold cutting sparks used inside the eye to cut membranes. A little lesser power than the above laser is a pulsed dye laser which has high fluence can create shock waves. In combination with fibre the shock waves destroy the kidney stones.

Even when a low-power laser is left in a place for a considerable time, the thermal conduction of adjacent tissues is very extensive. It is very important to visualize this spread of heat during any laser procedure. The excess tissue damage is proportional to the time the beam is applied. It does not depend on the total power. That is why surgeons should choose the high-power density laser. Further they can control the time of exposure to perform the jobs quietly and restrict the spread of damage.

This principle applies only where power density is greater than 1000 watts/cm at the tissue. Let us not be under the impression that significantly high power densities, achieved by using very small spots with low-power lasers will achieve satisfactory surgical results for vaporization. In order to debulk or vaporize large volume of tissues, the spot must be broad, approximately the size of a pencil eraser. This allows for more uniform, smooth vaporization of tissues but requires higher total power to compensate for the dilution of power density. If one tries to debulk a mass with a pinpoint spot size and high power densities, it will create uneven ridges, furrows, bleeding and the process is generally unsatisfactory. An elegant technical solution to the problems is to use a random electronic scanner with these focused beams. The speed of the scan eliminates the problems of high-power density spots while retaining the clean tissue effects. This is one way of achieving high fluence with a CW beam. This gives a char-free clean tissue vaporization. While selecting a laser apparatus, one has to pay attention to the power density which is an important parameter. Hence, the higher the power capabilities of the laser, the greater are its applications and future flexibility.

For example, CO_2 laser with power range of 50–60 watts is more versatile for all specialists. Although the higher powers of CO_2 lasers are available, they are very costly and may not find much applications. One aspect of 50–60 watts CO_2 laser is its potential limitations which may pose on pulsed average power such as superpulse. The other advantage of high-power CO_2 lasers ranging from 60 watts to 100 watts is that the average power of the superpulse is also in the useful range. In the recent years, CO_2 lasers have become out-dated and in their place DPSSL (Nd:YAG, KTP lasers) play an important role in surgery.

IMPACT SIZE AND SPOT SIZE

The actual size of the incision width made by the laser on the object is known as **impact size.** When the laser beam is focused with the help of a lens, it is known as spot size. Spot size of the laser is an important factor which controls the power density.

The spot size depends on:

1. *Focal length of the lens* Short focal length of the lens produces smaller spots.

2. *Diameter of the incident beam into the lens*   When the beam is larger, the spot size is smaller. This is inherent in the laser design.

3. *Wavelength of the light*   When wavelengths of the laser beam are shorter, the spot sizes are smaller.

4. *TEM of the beam*   Transverse electromagnetic mode TEM_{00} mode produces the smallest spots.

5. *Delivery system*   Fibres control spot size in a manner different from focused beams. Spot diverges continuously from the fibre.

Lenses are interchangeable and therefore spot size can be controlled. The smaller the focal length of the laser lens, the smaller will be the spot and hence higher the power density. For example, in a CO_2 laser unit, 400 mm lens gives

0.8 mm spot size; 300 mm lens gives 0.6 mm spot size; 200 mm lens gives 0.4 mm spot size and 125 mm lens gives 0.2 mm spot size.

The spot size of the focused beam is determined by the size, shape and colour of the beam as it enters a lens. The spot size of a laser is an aspect entirely different from the impact size.

The spot size is a mathematical measurement whereas the impact size relates the active size of the crater (or incision width) left by the laser. Keeping spot size the same, the impact size will increase when the beam is applied longer to the site. The edges of the beam are longer to create an effect which increases its width.

The wavelength of the light also determines how small the spot may be focused. That is, when the wavelength is smaller, the spot size is smaller keeping all things equal. For example, an argon ion laser produces a much smaller spot than a carbon dioxide laser. However, the laser is chosen for its specific effects on tissues and delivery mechanism rather than for its spot size abilities. The mode refers to the distortion of power over the spot size area and determines the precision of the operative spot. The term used to describe this is transverse electromagnetic mode (TEM). The fundamental mode TEM shows an even power distribution over the spot so that most of the power is at the centre and there are no hot or cold spots. A look at the power distribution reveals a cone-shaped pattern. The spot is brightest in the centre and faded towards the edges. This mode can produce very fine spots.

Because the impact size of the beam on the tissue is a function of tissue heating, time is very important as spot size determines the actual impact size. The longer the beam is on, the more the heat that builds up around the blurred fizzy edges of the spot and wider the impact. When the light is not distributed in this fundamental manner, it is said to be in multimode distribution. This can occur in many different patterns. But common mode in some older surgical lasers is the TEM_{01} mode. It has a cold spot in the centre and it is also known as doughnut mode. It is not possible to focus this mode to a fine spot as TEM_{00} mode.

For example, a 400 mm lens and TEM_{00} beam would focus to 0.8 mm spot while the same lens with TEM_{01} would focus to 2.00 mm spot. High-power output of carbon dioxide laser changes the mode structure at the beginning of lasing. A high-power setting, viz., 80–100 watts used in timed pulses of around 0.1 sec. tends to create multimode beams and one sees the resulting beam in doughnut shape.

Review Questions

1.   Distinguish between spontaneous emission and stimulated emision.

2.   What is Photonics?

3.   Can laser produce a monochromatic radiation? if not why?

4.   What is coherence? what is its importance?

5.   Explain population inversion.

6.   Why is two level laser not possible?

7.   What are the four laser components?

8.   Explain the various excitation mechanisms to produce population inversion.

9.   What is a feedback mechanism?

10.   What is the role of a resonator in laser generation?

11.   Describe various types of lasers resonators?

12.   What is meant by Q factor?

13.   How will you produce a giant pulse?

14.   Explain mode-locking and its importance.

15.   What is fluence and explain its use.

16.   Discuss on positive mode-locking.

17.   Mention the factors on which laser spot size depend.

18.   What is cavity dumping?

19.   Discuss on electro-optic and acousto-optic modulators.

20.   What is the advantage of unstable resonator?

Chapter 2

Types of Lasers

INTRODUCTION

So far we have seen the various principles employed in lasers. But we have not mentioned the laser types. Today, we are familiar with lasers such as helium–neon and diode lasers, which are used in bar code reader in shops and super-markets, in home CD players, in laser printers and in hundreds of alignment tasks. The various laser systems in use today differ in their active medium and in the pumping methods. A brief list of lasers used in medical applications is listed in Table 2.1.

Table 2.1 Lasers used in Medical Applications

Lasers	Wavelength (nm)	Applications
Solid -State Lasers		
HOLMIUM:YAG Ho:YAG	2100 (mid-IR)	General laparoscopic use, primary use in orthopaedic surgery
Neodymium:YAG Nd:YAG	1318 (mid-IR)	Tissue welding (fusion)
Neodymium:YAG Nd:YAG	1064 (near IR)	General laparoscopic use With contact fibers and devices, photocoagulation hysteroscopy, ophthalmology
Ruby	694	Tattoo and hair removal

Lasers	Wavelength (nm)	Applications
Diode lasers	Variable with system	Dentistry
Erbium YAG Er:YAG	2940 (mid-IR)	Bone cutting and drilling
KTP (Potassium Titanyl phosphate)	1064	A frequency-Doubled YAG includes a Nd:YAG in the same machine
Gas Lasers		
Carbon dioxide	10600 (far-IR)	Best laser for cervical, vulvar, vaginal use; general surgery, general laparoscopic use
Hydrogen fluoride	2040 (mid-IR)	Bone cutting and drilling
Krypton	647 568 531	Opthalmology and photocoagulation
Helium–Neon (He–Ne)	632	Defining target alignment, low-power photochemical interactions (non-thermal)
Gold vapour	632	Dermatological and photodynamic uses
Copper vapour	577 510	Dermatological uses
Argon	488, 515	Photo-coagulation, ophthalmology, microsurgery
Excimer	UV region	
ArF	193	Ophthalmology
KrCl	222	Cardiovascular
KrF	248	Orthopaedics
XeCl	308	Eye surgery LASIK and to treat a variety of dermatological conditions including psoriasis, vitiligo, atopic dermatitis, alopecia areata and leukoderma.

Lasers	Wavelength (nm)	Applications
XeF	351	Surgery (particularly eye surgery) and for dermatological treatment
LIQUID LASERS		
Tunable dye lasers		Cardiology, dermatology and laser treatment of vascular lesions, laser angioplasty, laser cancer phototherapy (photodynamic therapy or PDT) and urology.
	632	Dermatology
	577	Photodynamic action
	504	

We will examine the above types of lasers in the following sections.

SOLID-STATE LASERS

Solid-state lasers are made of a crystal or glass with small amount of doping such that the upper laser level is optically pumped by a suitable light source. There is another class of lasers which use a solid as the active medium and which are becoming more and more important. These are the semiconductor crystals, usually with one or more junctions, and pumping is achieved by injecting a current in the crystal. The solid-state laser (SSL), also known as Optical Maser, was the first laser operated in 1960 by Maiman. He obtained laser action in a ruby crystal (Cr^{3+}: Al_2O_3), excited by a pulsed flash lamp. Today SSLs are still the most important class of lasers, both in industrial and medical applications. In industrial applications the only competitor for the SSL in average power is the CO_2 laser. In medical applications, the possibility to transport the laser beam by a thin optical fibre opens the possibility of easy surgery.

In recent years the pumping mechanism is done not by flash lamps but by semiconductor lasers. Hence, we have a new class of lasers pumped by diodes. They are known as Diode-Pumped solid lasers.

DIODE-PUMPED SOLID-STATE LASERS (DPSSL)

In the history of lasers, 1980 is a remarkable year. It was in 1980 that an efficient, powerful room temperature AlGaAs semiconductor laser revolutionized the field of solid-state lasers. Replacement of conventional flash lamps paved a path for diode-pumped solid-state lasers. Many Nd^+-doped laser crystals such as $Nd+:+LiYF_4$ and $Nd:YVO_4$ have emerged. As you know, Erbium-doped fibre amplifier (EDFA) needed 980 nm laser to make a revolution in amplifying optical signals. Luckily, InGaAs laser diodes with 980 nm were developed. This laser was used as diode-pumped laser for Yb:YAG laser which was discarded as inefficient laser during the 1960s. Hence, Ytterbium-doped (Yb^{3+}-doped) solid-state laser (Yb:YAG) pumped with InGaAs laser diodes have been intensively and successfully developed. A search is in progress for novel Yb-doped crystals possessing properties superior to known Yb laser with new capabilities. Several such materials have been identified and characterized recently. This sub-heading concerns such new laser materials for diode-pumped solid-state lasers and its potential use in cosmetic, medical and veterinary photonics.

Photonics is the technology of generating and harnessing light and other forms of radiant energy whose quantum unit is the photon. The present century is portrayed as the photonics era. Basic physics provides insights into how we can use Photonics Technology to understand and change the world around us. The range of applications of photonics extends from energy generation to communication, information processing and a variety of tasks beneficial to the society. In recent years, great interest has been shown in photonics for medical applications because of their useful emission wavelength. Initially, use of lasers in medicine was initiated mostly by natural scientific curiosity and it was hoped that the laser could become a super-tool. Today the situation has completely changed. More delicate and precise lasers are available at present for skilled surgeons to perform even complicated and delicate operations. Lasers have now shifted to the hands of plastic surgeons and beauticians. Such types of lasers are widely known as cosmetic lasers.

DEVELOPMENTS IN DIODE-PUMPED SOLID-STATE LASERS

The recent advances in diode-pumped solid-state lasers (DPSSL) have made a revolution in laser physics. DPSS lasers in many ways approach the ideal output power, beam quality and repeatability of gas lasers but their efficiency and size are more like those of semiconductor diode lasers. Although the initial cost of a DPSSL and an ion laser are comparable,the annual operating cost of the DPSS system is significantly less because of its operating lifetime of nearly 10,000 hours. With modern InGaAs diode pumps, Yb:YAG lasers have been intensively developed and today we have successful Yb:DPSSLs. Yb-based lasers are said to operate in a "quasi three level" laser scheme. Beyond Yb:YAG, attempts have been made to achieve Yb-doped crystals with highly favourable spectroscopic properties. The nomenclature for new Yb-doped laser materials are given in Table 2.2.

Table 2.2   Nomenclature for new YB-doped laser materials

DPSSL	Diode-pumped solid-state laser
YAG	Y3Al3O12
FAP	Ca5(PO4)3F
S-FAP	Sr5(PO4)3F
KGW	KGd(WO4)2
KYW	KY(WO4)2
BCBF	BaCaBO3F
CAS	Ca2Al2SiO7
LNB	LiNbO3
LTA	LiTaO3
YCOB	YCa4O(BO3)3

Subsequently materials science research yielded several Yb-doped crystals including hosts, which are as follows:

- $LiNbO$—LNB)
- $Ca_2Al_2SiO_7$—CAS)
- $BaCaBO_3F$—(CBF)
- $SrLGaO_4$
- $SrLaa_3O_7$
- $KY(WO_4)$—KYW)
- $KGa(WO_4)_2$— KGW)

- $CGaS_2$
- $AgaSe_2$
- $AGaS_2$
- LiTaO—LTA)
- $YCa_4O(BO_3)_3$—(YCOB)

Yb-doped crystal DPSSLs continue to advance in performance using well-developed Yb:YAG crystal and developing Yb-doped fluoroapatite crystals. Yb-doped double tungstates (KYW and KGW) provide a new opportunity for design of practical Yb-based DPSSLs. A continued research is necessary for Yb-based laser crystals amenable to channel waveguide formation and possessing more favourable laser spectroscopic values.

The novel self-frequency doubling of Yb:YCOB and Yb:GdCOB crystals seem destined for practical use in visible DPSSL applications. A 10 W Q-switched ultraviolet DPSSL sets a new record in operating at 355 nm.

Diode-pumped solid-state laser sources started replacing gas and ion laser sources for commercial and laboratory applications and the trend is accelerating because of progress in two areas.

First, more powerful, reliable laser diodes are available at lower cost, making diode pumping not only attractive but also practical.

Secondly, advances in manufacturing have improved the quality while reducing the volume pricing for laser crystals such as Nd:YAG and Nd:YVO$_4$, and nonlinear optical crystals such as (β-BaB$_2$O$_4$ (BBO), LiB$_3$O$_5$ (LBO) and KTiOPO$_4$ (KTP). To meet requirements of expanding laser applications, important progress has occurred in searching for new crystals that can cover broader spectral applications.

Non-Linear Optical Crystals

The nonlinear optical crystals are important because the fundamental output wavelength of Nd:YAG and Nd:YVO$_4$ is 1064 nm in the near infrared, a wavelength that is extremely useful for many applications. However, if these lasers are to replace gas and ion lasers that emit in the visible and ultraviolet portions of the spectrum, they need some type of device that can shorten the wavelengths by doubling or tripling their frequencies. As the most powerful laser frequency conversion devices, nonlinear optical crystals are playing an increasingly important role in advanced laser technologies. The development of new crystals has combined with other laser technologies (diode pumping, ultra fast technologies and optical parametric processes) to greatly accelerate the creation of all solid-state lasers. Because of these changes, recently introduced laser sources have much shorter wavelengths (down to 187 nm), faster laser pulses (down to less than 10 fs), much wider tuning ranges (from 187 nm –10 μ m) and higher powers and yet are considerably smaller than the predecessors. Several low power (10–400 mW) diode-pumped solid-state green lasers with performances similar to the air-cooled argon-ion lasers are available at present and they are typically used in graphics and diagnostic medical applications. The high-power pulsed lasers are used in micro machining, marking and trimming applications.

For UV generations (third, fourth and fifth harmonics of Nd:YAG and Nd:Y-VO$_4$ lasers), output power has reached 1–2.5 W. BBO and LBO have proved to be the only candidates that could generate high power over a considerable period. BBO will continue to be the most important crystal for deep-UV generation.

Meanwhile, there is an increasing demand for all solid-state, high-power, deep-UV laser sources for fibre Bragg grating fabrication, laser drilling of polymers and other industrial applications. Super-BBO (S-BBO) crystal is for rescue, which offers high transmission at 266 nm, low scattering and good optical homogeneity.

The most promising non-linear crystals are :

1. For the far-ultraviolet, $Sr_2Be_2B_2O_7$ (SBBO), $KBe_2BO_3F_2$ (KBBF).
2. For the infrared, $KTiOAsO_4$ (KTA), $ZnGeP_2$, $AgGaSe_2/AgGaS_2$.
3. Periodically pooled nonlinear crystals such as $LiNbO_3$ (PPLN) and KTP (PPKTP) have demonstrated very low operating thresholds and high efficiencies for optical parametric and harmonic operations. The compact size of the system due to nonlinear crystals has made many applications possible.

In general materials for laser operation must possess sharp fluorescent lines, strong absorption bands, and reasonably high quantum efficiency for the fluorescent transition of interest. These characteristics are often shown by solids such as crystals and glasses. A very small quantity of doping elements—the rare earth (lanthanide) and the actinide series—in them causes optical transitions between states of inner incomplete electron shells. The sharp fluorescence lines in the spectra of crystal doped with these elements result from the fact that the electrons involved in transition in the optical regime are shielded by the outer shells from the surrounding crystals lattices. The corresponding transitions are similar to those of the free ions. In addition to a sharp fluorescence emission line, a laser material suitable for optical pumping should possess broad-band pump transitions, i.e., incandescent lamps, CW arc lamps, or flash lamps are used as pump sources for pumping solid-state lasers. The gain in solid state lasers is achieved through

i.   The host material with macroscopic (mechanical, thermal and optical) and microscopic (lattice) properties,

ii. The active ions with their distinctive charge states and free-ion electronic configurations and

iii. The optical pump source with particular configuration, spectral irradiance, and duration.

These elements are interactive and their proper selection yields a high-performance laser.

Solid-state host materials may be broadly grouped into crystalline solids and glasses. The host must have good optical, mechanical and thermal properties to withstand the severe operating conditions of lasers. The desirable properties of the host material include hardness, chemical inertness, absence of internal strain and refractive index variation, resistance to radiation-induced colour centres and ease of fabrication. Several interactions between the host crystal and the active ion restrict the number of useful material combinations. These include size, disparity, valence and spectroscopic properties. Ideally the size and valence of the additive ion should match that of the host ion which it replaces.

Glasses

Glasses are an important class of host materials for some of the rare earths, particularly Nd and very recently Yb. The outstanding practical advantage compared to crystalline materials is the tremendous size capability for high-energy applications. Rods up to one metre length and over 10 cm diameter and discs up to 90 cm diameter and several cm thickness are currently available for laser hosts. The optical quality is excellent and the beam divergence approaching the diffraction limit can be achieved in glasses. Glass can be easily fabricated and yields a good optical finish. Laser ions placed in glass generally show a large fluorescent line-width than in crystals, because of the lack of a unique and well-defined crystalline surrounding for the individual active atom. Therefore, the laser threshold for glass lasers have been found to run higher than their crystalline counterparts. Further, glass has a much lower thermal conductivity than most crystalline hosts. The latter factor leads to thermally induced birefringence and optical distortion in glass rods when they are operated at high average powers. For these reasons, glass media are used mainly in high-energy laser systems with low repetition rate. In addition to the Nd:glass, another important glass laser medium is Er:glass. Glass doped with erbium is of special importance because its radiation 1.55 μm does not penetrate the lens of the human eye, and therefore cannot destroy the retina. Due to the three-level behaviour of erbium and its characteristic small absorption of pump light, multiple doping with neodymium and ytterbium is necessary to obtain satisfactory system efficiency. Ho : glass is another laser medium which attracted the medical profession for medical lasers.

Crystals

A large number of crystalline host materials have been investigated since the discovery of the ruby laser. Crystalline laser hosts are advantageous over glasses due to their higher thermal conductivity, narrower fluorescence line-widths and in many cases, greater hardness. For all these reasons, they are used for high average power, CW or repetitively pulsed lasers.

However, the optical quality and doping homogeneity of crystalline hosts are often poorer and the absorption lines are generally narrower. Therefore let us review briefly two typical crystals mainly used as laser hosts.

Sapphire   Sapphire (Al_2O_3) was used as a host in ruby laser. Sapphire is a hard material and has high thermal conductivity. The transition metals can readily be substituted for the Al. But the Al site is too small for rare earth and it is not possible to incorporate appreciable concentrations of these impurities into sapphire. Besides, ruby and Ti-doped sapphire have gained significance as tunable laser material.

Garnets Some of the most useful laser hosts are the synthetic garnets such as yttrium aluminium garnet or $Y_3Al_5O_{12}$ (YAG), gadolinium gallium garnet or $Gd_3Ga_5O_{12}$ (GGG) and gadolinium scandium gallium garnet or $Gd_3Sc_2Ga_3O_{12}$ (GSGG). These garnets have many desirable properties for use as laser host material. They are stable, hard, optically isotopic and have good thermal conductivities which permit laser operation at high-average power levels. In particular, yttrium aluminium garnet doped with neodymium (Nd:YAG) has achieved a high status among solid-state laser materials. In recent days Ytterbium-doped yttrium aluminium garnet is becoming popular due to the ytterbium's quasi three level. YAG is a very hard, isotropic crystal which can be grown and fabricated in a manner that yields rods of high optical quality. Presently, it is the best commercially available crystalline laser host for Nd^{3+}, (although several new host materials are available at present) offering low threshold and high gain. The most important ions used in crystal doping for SSLs can be divided into two main classes, viz., transition metal ions and rare earth ions. The most important members of the transition metal family are Cr^{3+} and $Ti^{3+.}$ The former was the first to show laser action, using sapphire as host crystal (ruby : Cr^{3+}: Al_2O_3). Titanium used in sapphire shows a very broad tunable emission range which is useful for spectroscopic applications. The rare earth ions are the natural candidates to serve as active ions in solid-state laser materials because they exhibit a wealth of sharp fluorescent transitions representing almost every region of the visible and near-infrared portions of the electromagnetic spectrum.

These lines are very sharp, even in the presence of the strong local crystal fields. The other rare earth ions have also shown laser action in many different crystals. Out of the several rare earth ions, Nd^{3+} was used as a common dopant for many crystals as well as for glasses. Nd^{3+}, Er^{3+}, Ho^{3+} and Yb^{3+} are becoming more and more popular due to their eye- safe emission wavelength.

Neodymium

Nd^{3+} was the first trivalent rare earth ions to be used in a laser and it remains the most important element in this group. Stimulated emission has been obtained with this ion by incorporating it with several host materials. Further, a high power level has been obtained from Nd lasers than from any other four-level material. The principal host materials are YAG and glass. In these hosts, stimulated emission is obtained at a number of frequencies within three different groups of transitions centred at 0.9, 1.06, and 1.35 μm

Erbium

Numerous studies of the absorption and fluorescence properties of erbium in various host materials have been conducted to determine its potential as an active laser ion. Laser oscillation was observed most frequently in the wavelength region 1.53 to 1.66 μm Stimulated emission around 1.6 μm is of interest to ophthalmologists because the eye is subjected to less retinal damage by laser radiation at 1.6 μm . The reduced transmissivity of the ocular media is the reason for selecting this wavelength.

LASER CRYSTALS

Among the many crystals used as the active media of the solid-state lasers, a few have gained great prominence. The first is ruby (Cr^{3+} in sapphire), both for historical reasons (it was the first laser to be used in surgery) as well as for some unique properties. Next comes the Nd :YAG and all the other Nd-based materials. Recently a new class of materials, viz., Alexandrite and Ti:Sapphire, has become popular and they can be used as the tunable laser crystals.

Ruby

The ruby laser, although a three-level system, still remains in use today for many applications. From an application point of view, ruby is attractive because its output lies in the visible range, in contrast to most rare earth four-level lasers, whose outputs are in the near-infrared region. Photodetectors and photographic emulsions are much more sensitive at the ruby wavelength than in the infrared. Spectroscopically, ruby possesses an unusually favourable combination of a relatively narrow line-width, long fluorescent lifetime, a high quantum efficiency, and broad and well-located pump absorption bands which make unusually efficient use of the pump radiation emitted by available flash lamps.

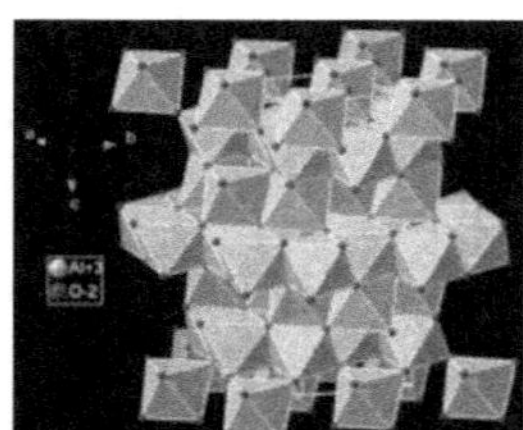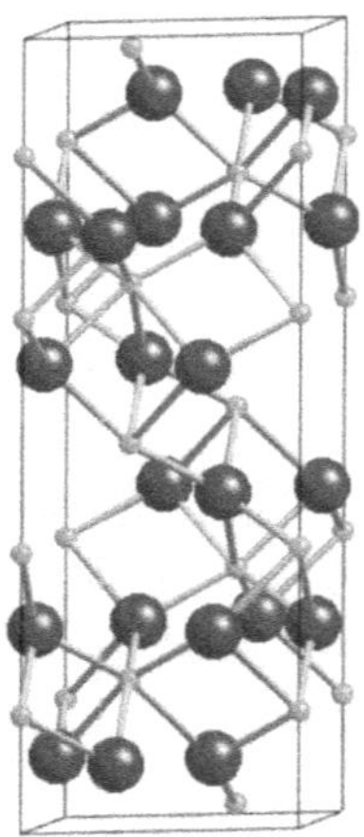

Figure 2.1   (Structure of Al_2O_3 (sapphire/corundum) [a=b= 4.767 A°;c = 12.9947 A°; $\alpha = \beta = 90°$, $\lambda = 120°$)

Ruby chemically consists of sapphire (Al_2O_3) in which a small percentage of the Al^{3+} has been replaced by Cr^{3+}. This is done by adding small amounts of Cr_2O_3 to the melt of highly purified Al_2O_3. The pure single host crystal is uniaxial and possesses a rhombohedral or hexagonal unit cell as shown in Figure 2.1.

The crystal has an axis of symmetry, namely c axis, which forms the major diagonal of the unit cell. Since the crystal is uniaxial, it has two indices of refraction, the ordinary ray having the E vector perpendicular to the c (optic) axis, and the extraordinary ray having the E vector parallel to the c axis. As a laser host crystal, sapphire has many desirable physical and chemical properties. The crystal is a refractory material, hard and durable. It has a good thermal conductivity, chemical stability, and is capable of being grown by the Czochralski method to very high quality. In this procedure the solid crystal is slowly pulled from a liquid melt by initiation of growth on high-quality seed material. Iridium crucibles and radio frequency heating are used to contain the melt and control the melt temperature, respectively. The crystal boles can be grown in the 0°, 60° or 90° configuration, where the term refers to the angle between the growth axis and the crystallographic 'c' axis. For laser grade, 60° ruby type is commonly used. Ruby can be grown in relatively larger boules with high optical quality. The boules are cut into smaller cylindrical sections. Core-free cylindrical rods up to 30 cm length and 2.5 cm diameter can be obtained. Typical commercially available rods with flat ends are fabricated to the following specifications.

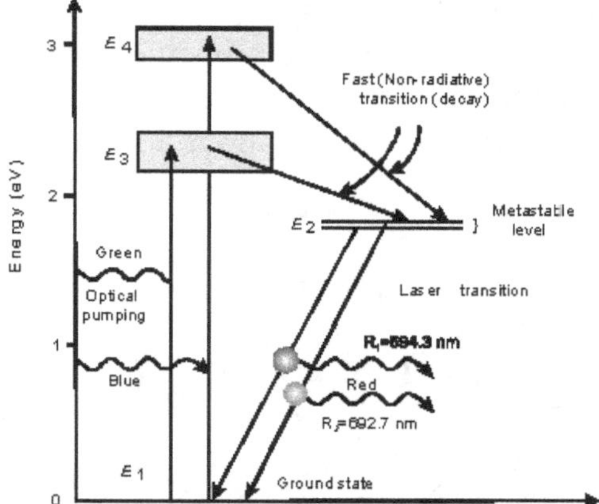

Figure 2.2   Energy level diagram of a ruby laser

- Ends flat to 1/10,

- Ends parallel to growth axis (0°, 60°, 90°) to +5.

- Common rod geometries may be plane parallel, wedged surfaces, Brewster angle, or prismatic.

- The best way to inspect a laser rod is by means of interferometers which show optical inhomogeneities, strain and distortion, etc., as fringes. Scattering centres of regions of high defects in a laser rod are revealed by illuminating the crystal from the side with a He–Ne gas laser. The energy level diagram of ruby is shown in Figure 2.2. The optical and laser properties of ruby at room temperature are given in Table 2.3.

Ruby is a synthetic crystal of aluminium oxide (Al_2O_3) and is more familiar in daily life as a precious stone used in jewellery. The chemical structure of ruby is that of Al_2O_3 (which is called sapphire), with 0.05% (by weight) impurity of chromium ions (Cr^{3+}). The active ion is Cr^{3+}, which replaces Al atom in the crystal. This ion is responsible for the red colour of the crystal. The impurity ion of Cr^{3+} is responsible for the energy levels which participate in the process of lasing. This system is a three-level laser with lasing transitions between E_2 and E_1. The excitation of the chromium ions is done by light pulses from flash lamps (usually xenon).

The chromium ions absorb light at wavelengths around 545 nm. As a result, the ions are transferred to the excited energy level E_3. From this level, the ions are going down to the metastable energy level, E_2, in a non-radiative transition. The energy released in this non-radiative transition is transferred to the crystal vibrations and changed into heat that must be removed away from the system. The lifetime of the metastable level E_2 is about 5 msec.

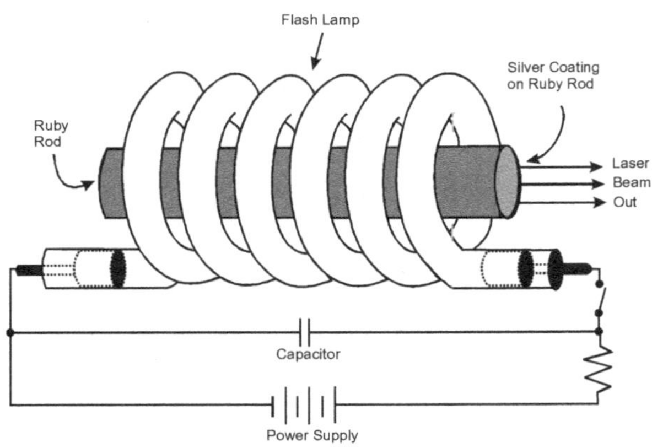

Figure 2.3 Schematic diagram of the first ruby laser

Ruby laser has another absorption band which can be used for pumping, in the spectral range of 350–450 nm. It is difficult to achieve continuous operation of a ruby laser since it is a three-level laser. However, in 1962, by using a very intensive pump and an arc lamp with high-pressure mercury vapour, a continuous-wave ruby laser was built. The energy gap between the upper lasing level and the ground level in a ruby laser is 1.789 eV. The wavelength of the emitted light out of a ruby laser is 694.3 nm. A schematic diagram of the first ruby laser is shown in Figure 2.3.

Table 2.3 Optical and laser properties of ruby at room temperature

Property	Values
Cr_3O_2 doping	0.05 wt. %
Cr concentration	1.58×10^{19} ions. Cm^{-3}
Output wavelengths, 25°C	694.3 and 692.6 nm
Fluorescent lifetime (g)	3.0 ms at 300 K
Photon energy (hv)	2.86×10^{19} Ws
Quantum efficiency	0.7

Property	Values
Separation of R_1 and R_2 lines	29 cm
Major pump bands	Blue (4040), Green (5540)
Refractive index (n) at 694.3 nm	1.763 ordinary ray; 1.755 extraordinary ray
Brewster angle	60° 37' at 694.3 nm
Maximum extractable energy	2.35 J/cm (complete inversion)
Maximum upper-state energy density	4.52 J/cm (complete inversion)
Upper-state energy at threshold	2.18/cm
Density	3.98 g/cc
Melting point	2040°C
Young's modulus	345 Gpa
Hardness	9 Mhos, 2000 Knoop
Birefringence	0.008

Nd-Doped Materials

From the large number of Nd-doped materials, only few have prominence. Nd:YAG laser is the most important solid-state laser for scientific, medical, industrial and military application due to its high gain, good thermal and mechanical properties. Nd:glass is important for laser fusion drivers because it can be produced in large sizes. Very recently, Nd:Cr:GSGG have received considerable attention because of the good spectral match between the flash lamp emission and the absorption of the Cr ions. An efficient energy transfer between the Cr and Nd ions results in a highly efficient Nd laser. Nd:YLF is a good candidate for certain specialized applications because the output is polarized and the crystal exhibits lower thermal birefringence. Nd:YLF has a higher energy storage capability due to its lower gain coefficient compared to Nd:YAG. Further, its output wavelength matches that of phosphate Nd:glass. Hence mode-locked and Q-switched Nd:YLF lasers have become the standard oscillators for large glass lasers employed in fusion research.

Nd:YAG

The Nd:YAG laser is the most commonly used solid-state laser. Neodymium-doped yttrium aluminium garnet (Nd:YAG) possesses a combination of properties uniquely favourable for laser operation. The YAG host is hard and possesses good optical quality and a high thermal conductivity. Furthermore, the cubic structure of YAG favours a narrow fluorescent line-width which results in high gain and low threshold for laser operation. In Nd:YAG, trivalent neodymium substitutes for trivalent yttrium, so charge compensation is not required. By improving the quality of the material and the pumping techniques, CW power can be obtained to several hundred watts from a single laser rod. On the other hand, in single-crystal Nd:YAG fibre lasers, threshold was achieved with absorbed pump powers as small as 1 mW. Today, more than thirty years after its first operation, the Nd:YAG laser has emerged as the most versatile solid-state system. In addition to the very favourable spectral and lasing characteristics displayed by Nd:YAG, the host lattice is noteworthy for its unique physical, chemical, and mechanical properties. The Nd:YAG laser and its energy level diagram are shown in Figures 2.4 and 2.5 respectively.

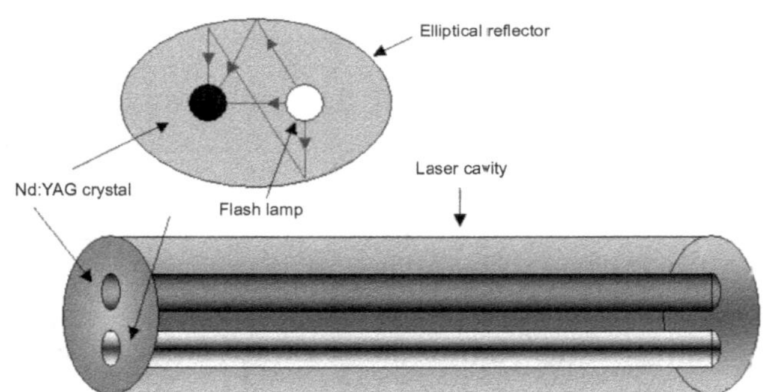

Figure 2.4 Nd: YAG laser

The YAG structure is stable from the lowest temperature to the melting point and no transformations have been reported in the solid phase. The strength and hardness of YAG are lower than ruby but still high enough, so that normal fabrication procedures do not produce any serious breakage problems. Pure $Y_3Al_5O_{12}$ is a colourless, optically isotropic crystal which possesses a cubic structure characteristic of garnets. In Nd:YAG, about 1% of Y^{3+} is substituted by Nd^{3+}. The radii of the two rare ions differ by 3%. Therefore, with the addition of large amounts of neodymium, strained crystals are obtained, indicating that either the solubility limit of neodymium is exceeded or that the lattice of YAG is seriousy distorted by the inclusion of neodymium.

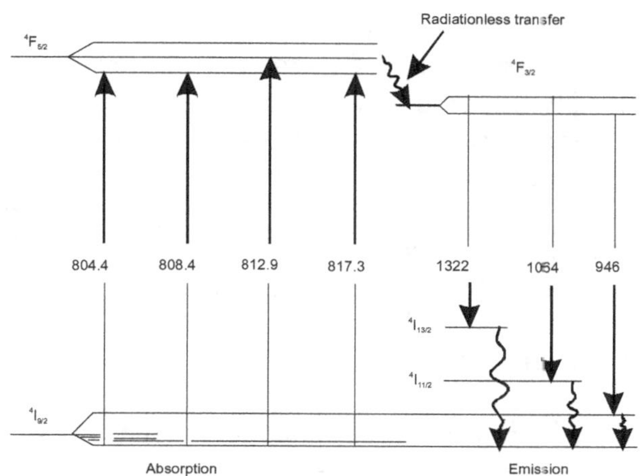

Figure 2.5   Energy level diagram of Nd:YAG

Commercially available laser crystals are grown exclusively by the Czochralski method. The high manufacturing costs of Nd:YAG are mainly due to the very slow growth rate of Nd:YAG which is of the order of 0.5 mm/h. Typical boules of 10–15 cm length require a growth run of several weeks. However, all Nd:YAG crystals grown by Czochralski techniques show a bright core running along the length of the crystals. The cores originate from the presence of facets on the growth interface which have a different distribution coefficient for neodymium than the surrounding growth surface. That is, in order to provide rods of a given diameter, the crystal must be grown with a diameter that is some what more than twice as large. The boules are processed by quartering into sections. At present times, rods can be fabricated with maximum diameters of about 10 mm and lengths up to 150 mm. The optical quality of such rods is normally quite good and comparable to the best quality of Czochralski ruby or optical glass. For example, 6×100 mm rods cut from the outer sections of 20×150 mm boules typically may show only 1 to 2 fringes in a Twyman–Green interferometer.

Neodymium concentration in YAG has been limited to 0.1 to 1.5%. Higher doping levels tend to shorten the fluorescent lifetime, broaden the line-width, and cause strain in the crystal, resulting in poor optical quality. In specifying

Nd:YAG rods, the emphasis is on size, dimensional tolerance, doping level, and passive optical tests of rod quality. In a particular application, the performance of a Nd:YAG laser can be somewhat improved by the choice of the optimum Nd concentration. As a general guideline, it can be said that a high doping concentration (approximately 1.2%) is desirable for Q-switch operation because this will lead to high-energy storage. For CW operation, a low doping concentration (0.6 to 0.8%) is usually chosen to obtain beam quality. It is worth noting that in contrast to a liquid or a glass, a crystal host is not amenable to uniform dopant concentration. This problem arises as a result of the crystal-growth mechanism. In the substitution of the larger Nd^{3+} for a Y^{3+} in $Y_3Al_5O_{12}$, the neodymium is preferentially retained in the melt. The increase in concentration of Nd from the seed to the final stage of a 20-cm-long boule is about 20 to 25%. For a laser rod 3 to 8 cm long, this end-to-end variation may be 0.05 to 0.10% of Nd_2O_3 by weight. The physical and optical properties of Nd:YAG are given in Table 2.4.

Table 2.4 Physical and optical properties of Nd:YAG

Properties	Values
Chemical formula	$Nd:Y_3Al_5O_{12}$
Crystal structure	Cubic
Lattice constants	12.01
Concentration	$\sim 1.2 \times 1020$ cm^{-3}
Melting point	1970°C
Density	4.56 g/cm^3
Hardness	8.5 Mohs
Refractive index	1.82
Thermal expansion coefficient	7.8×10^{-6} /K [111], 0–250°C
Thermal conductivity	14 W/m /K at 20°C, 10.5 W/m/K at 100°C.
Lasing wavelength	1064 nm
Stimulated emission cross section	$2.8 \times 10-19cm^{-2}$
Relaxation time of terminal lasing level	30 ns
Radiative lifetime	550 ms
Spontaneous fluorescence	230 ms
Loss coefficient	0.003 cm^{-1} at 1064 nm

Properties	Values
Effective emission cross section	$2.8 \times 10{-}19$ cm^2
Pump wavelength	807.5 nm
Absorption band at pump wavelength	1 nm
Linewidth	0.6 nm
Polarized emission	Unpolarized
Thermal birefringence	High

ND:GLASS

There are several characteristics which distinguish glass from other solid-state laser host materials. Its properties are isotropic. It can be doped at very high concentrations with excellent uniformity and it can be made into large pieces of diffraction-limited optical quality. In addition, glass lasers have been made in a variety of shapes and sizes, from fibres, rods and discs. There is wide variety of Nd-doped laser glasses depending on the compositions of the glass network and the ions. Among various laser glasses, only silicates and phosphates are commercially available at present with sufficient optical, mechanical and chemical properties.

There are two important differences between glass and crystal lasers. First, the thermal conductivity of glass is considerably lower than that of most crystal hosts. Secondly, the emission and absorption lines of ions in glasses are inherently broader than in crystals. A wider line increases the laser threshold value of amplification. Neverth less, this broadening has an advantage. A broader line offers the possibility of obtaining and amplifying shorter light pulses and in addition, it permits the storage of larger amounts of energy in the amplifying medium for the same linear amplification coefficient. Thus, glass and crystalline lasers complement each other. For continuous or very high repetition rate operation, crystalline lasers provide higher gain and greater thermal conductivity. Glasses are more suitable for high-energy pulsed operation because of their large size, flexibility in their physical parameters and the broadened fluorescent line. Unlike many crystals, the concentration of the active ions can be very high in glass. The practical limit is determined from the fact that the fluorescent lifetime and therefore the efficiency of stimulated emission decreases with higher concentrations. In silicate glass, this decrease becomes noticeable at a concentration of

5% Nd_2O_3. The main constituents of glasses are non-metal oxides such as SiO_2, B_2O_3, and P_2O_5. Different metal oxides alter the structure in various ways and make it possible to obtain a large variety of properties. The components are mixed before melting with the laser activators. The mixture is heated in a heat-resistant crucible. The principal laser glass manufacturers use either platinum or ceramic crucibles, clay pots or ceramic continuous tanks to contain the melt. When the melt has reached a high viscosity, it is cast into a mould. Finally, the glass in the mould is placed into an annealing furnace where it is very slowly cooled. Nd-doped phosphate glass has been widely used in high-average power solid-state lasers, laser material processing, range finder and other industrial and scientific applications.

Glass laser rods are fabricated in a large variety of sizes. Typical rod sizes are 10–50 cm length, with 1 to 3 cm diameter. However, rods up to 1 m length and 10 cm diameter are commercially available. Standard rod end configurations are the same as those mentioned for ruby and Nd:YAG rods. Besides Nd:YAG and Nd:glass, a lot of Nd-doped laser crystals have been doped. Some important ones are the following.

- Nd:YLiF$_4$ (YLF) for low thermal lensing
- Nd:YAlO$_4$ (YALO or YAP) for polarized output,
- Cr,Nd:Gd$_3$(Sc,Ga)$_5$O$_{12}$ (GSGG) for high efficiency, and
- Cr,Nd: Y$_3$(Sc,Ga)$_5$O$_{12}$ (YSGG) for high efficiency.

The physical and optical properties of Nd^{3+}-doped glasses are given in Table 2.5.

Table 2.5 Properties of Nd^{3+}-doped phosphate glass

Properties	Values
Nd_2O_3 (wt%)	2.2
Nd^{3+} conc. (10^{20}ions/cm^3)	2.68
Cross section for stimulated emission (10^{-20}cm^2)	3.40 ± 0.3
Fluorescence half-line width at 290 K(Å)	240
Center lasing wavelength (nm)	1053
Non-linear refractive index coefficient.n$_2$ ($\times 10^{-13}$e.s.u)	

Properties	Values
n (1053 nm)	1.3 ± 0.1
n_d	1.5652
n_F	1.5758
n_c	1.5731
Abbe value	1.5820
Coefficient of linear thermal expansion $(10^{-6}/°C)$ $(20\sim100°C)$	65.3
Thermal coeff. of optical path length $(10^{-6}/°C)$ $(20\sim100°C)$	11.0 1.9
Transformation temp. (°C)	500
Softening temp. (°C)	530
Coefficient of linear thermal expansion $(10-6/°C)$ $(100\sim Tg°C)$	12.0 5.53
Thermal conductivity (25°C) $(10-3W/cm°C)$	0.75
Specific heat (25°C) $(J/cm3°C)$	
Knoop hardness $(kg/cm2\ 650\ Density(g/cm3))$	650
Young's modulus $(kgf/mm2)$	3.40
Poisson's ratio	5640
	0.27

ND,CR:GSGG

Soon after the invention of the Nd:YAG laser, attempts were made to increase the efficiency of transferring radiation from the pump source to the laser crystal using a second dopant called a "sensitizer". A particularly attractive sensitizer is Cr^{3+} because the broad absorption bands of chromium can efficiently absorb light throughout the whole visible region of the spectrum.

The higher pump efficiency of Nd,Cr:GSGG does not automatically translate into better system performance because Nd,Cr:GSGG does exhibit much stronger thermal focusing and stress birefringence, compared to Nd:YAG. The absorption efficiency and the heat-deposition rate for the Nd,Cr:GSGG rod is almost three times at of Nd:YAG. Hence thermal focusing power as a function of lamp input power is several times larger in Nd,Cr:GSGG than in Nd:YAG. Therefore, if beam brightness is the criteria, rather than output energy, some of the advantage of GSGG is offset, particularly at high-average powers. Tunability of the emission in solid-state lasers is achieved when the stimulated emission of photons is intimately coupled to the emission of vibrational quanta (phonons) in a crystal lattice. In these "vibronic" lasers, the total energy of the lasing transition is fixed but can be partitioned between photons and phonons in a continuous fashion. This results in broad wavelength tunability of the laser output. In other words, the existence of tunable solid-state lasers is due to the subtle interplay between the Coulomb field of the lasing ion, the crystals field of the host lattice, and electron–phonon coupling permitting broadband absorption and emission. Therefore, the gain in vibronic lasers depends on transitions between coupled vibrational and electronic states. That is, a phonon is either emitted or absorbed with each electronic transition. The best known and most used vibronic lasers now available are the Alexandrite and Ti:sapphire lasers.

Alexandrite   Alexandrite is a colour changing variety of the mineral chrysoberyl. The chemical composition of chrysoberyl is $BeAl_2O_4$ and it occurs in granitic pegmatite and mica schist. This is a rare oxide mineral that has two very rare varieties. The first is the colour-changing alexandrite and the second is the cat's eye chrysoberyl. Alexandrite is the best characterized commercially developed vibronic laser. Alexandrite is the common name for chromium-doped chrysoberyl, with four units of $BeAl_2O_4$ forming an orthorhombic structure. The crystal is grown in large boules by Czochralski method much like ruby and YAG. The main problem is handling the very toxic beryllium oxide. In any case, laser rods up to 1cm in diameter and 10 cm long with a nominal 2-fringe total optical distortion are commercially available. The chromium concentration of alexandrite is expressed in terms of the percentage of aluminium ions in the crystal which have been replaced by chromium ions. The Cr^{3+} dopant concentration, occupying the Al^{3+} sites, can be as high as 0.4 atomic per cent and still yield crystals of good optical quality. In Alexandrite, concentration of 0.1 atomic per cent represents 3.51×10^{10} chromium ions per cubic centimetre. Alexandrite shows the typical absorption spectrum of Cr-doped materials (Figure 2.6).

Absorption spectrum of Alexandrite has chromium lines in the red (doublet plus two other lines), a broad band in the yellow–green and two narrow bands in the blue. The most dramatic feature of alexandrite is the colour change. This effect is caused by a combination of factors. The presence of the chromium in combination with the fact that alexandrite is doubly refractive and bi-axial allows alexandrite to possess three different refractive indexes in its three different optical directions. Each of these has a strongly different absorption spectrum, causing different colours to be seen. Daylight contains high proportions of blue light, so the stones appear green. Incandescent light contains a higher portion of red light, so the stones appear red. Many variances of the shades of colours seem to occur because each alexandrite can absorb light of different wavelengths many different ways.

It is optically and mechanically similar to ruby and possesses many of the physical and chemical properties of a good laser host. Alexandrite possesses hardness, strength, chemical stability and high thermal conductivity equal to two-thirds that of ruby and twice that of YAG.

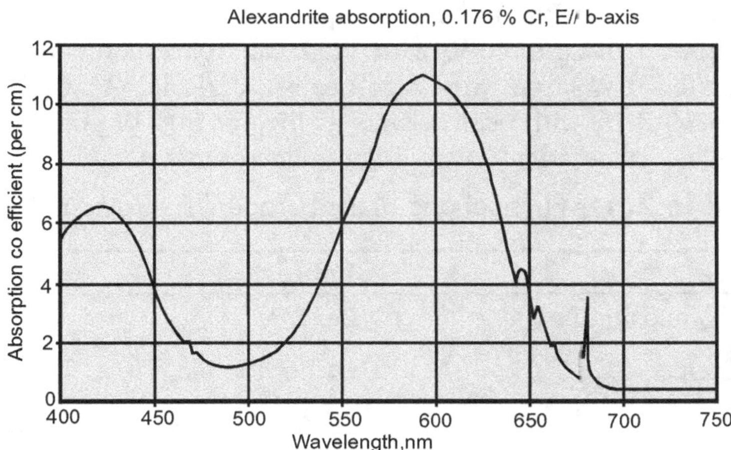

Figure 2.6 Absorption spectrum of alexandrite (a strong doublet at 680.5 and 678.5 nm and weak lines at 665, 655 and 645 nm).

This enables alexandrite rods to be pumped at high average powers without thermal fracture. Alexandrite has a thermal fracture limit which is 60% that of ruby and five times higher than YAG. Surface damage tests using focused 750 nm radiation indicate that alexandrite is at least as resistant as ruby.

The development of the alexandrite laser has reached maturity after nearly 10 years of efforts. Its current high-average power performance is 100 W if operated at 100 Hz. Overall efficiency is close to 0.5%. Tunability over the range of approximately 700 to 818 nm has been demonstrated with tuning accomplished in a manner similar to dye 21–a combination of etalons and birefringement filters. With these standard spectral control devices, 0.5 cm line widths and tunability over 150 nm has been achieved. Alexandrite has been lased in pulsed and CW modes. It can also be *Q*-switched and mode-locked.

When a rod 10 cm long and 0.63 cm in diameter is *Q*-switched in a stable resonator, it gives long pulses (5J), with pulse duration less than 30 ns. The reason for such high output energies is that alexandrite is a low-gain medium ($g = 0.04$ cm $-$ 0.1 cm) at room temperature.

Commercially available alexandrite lasers feature continuous, automatic tuning and a minimum 100 mJ of *Q*-switched output with 0.3 nm bandwidth over the wavelength range of 730–780 nm. Because of alexandrite's physical strength and thermal properties, CW operation is possible at room temperature. The bulk of the experimentation to date has been with CW xenon arc lamps. CW operation with arc lamp pumping has proved difficult to achieve, yet output powers of up to 40 W with good transverse-mode quality are now being generated. CW lasers were also acousto-optically Q-switched at rates greater than 10 KHz, with peak powers as high as 300 W and pulsewidth of 1 fs.

Table 2.6   Physical and optical properties of alexandrite

Properties	Values
Chemical composition	$BeAl_2O_4$
Crystal system	Orthorhombic
Habit	Tabular or prismatic; also trillings (repeated twinning producing
Pseudo-hexagoncal or cyclic crystals	
Cleavage	Distinct (prismatic)
Fracture	Conchoidal to uneven 1053
Hardness	8.5 mohs
Toughness	8

Properties	Values
Specific gravity	3.72
Lustre	Vitreous
Refractive index	1.746–1.755
Double refraction and optic sign	0.008 – 0.010, positive
Dispersion	low (0.015)
Pleochroism	Strong in alexandrite (green, yellowish, pink—in daylight; red, orange-yellow, Green— in filament light).
Luminescence	Red fluorescence in LW UV. Weak red in SW UV

Ti:sapphire   The $Ti:Al_2O_3$ laser is one of the more promising tunable solid-state systems, combining a broad tuning range (800 nm peak, 300 nm bandwidth) with a relatively large-gain cross-section (50% of Nd:YAG's value at its peak). One of the greatest advantages is the material properties of the sapphire host itself, namely very high thermal conductivity, exceptional chemical inertness and mechanical rigidity. Titanium sapphire is presently available from commercial vendors in sizes of 3.5 cm diameter and 15 cm length optical quality, due to the well-developed growth technology for sapphire. The absorption and emission spectra for $Ti:Al_2O_3$ are shown in Figure 2.7.

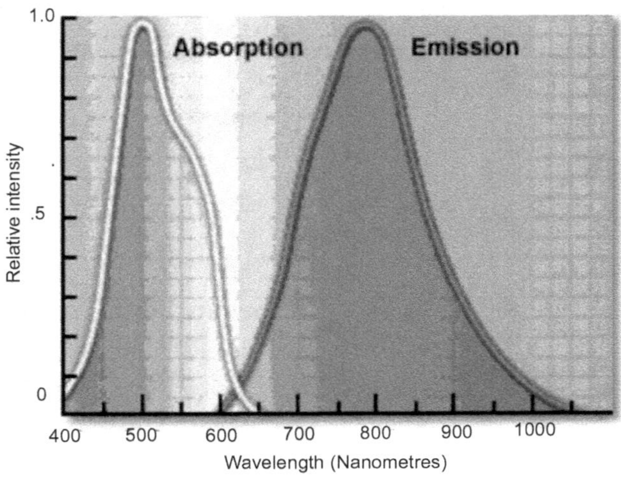

Figure 2.7 Absorption and emission spectra of Ti:Sapphire

The broad, widely separated absorption and fluorescence bands are caused by the strong coupling between the ion and host lattice, and they are the key to broadly tunable laser operation.

Development of Ti:Al_2O_3 laser has been confined mainly to optical pumping due to short spontaneous-emission lifetime (3.2 μs) of the material. Flash-lamp pumping of titanium sapphire causes serious technological problem in terms of the lifetime of the flash lamp. It was not possible earlier to get the short pulse duration needed for driving the crystals above threshold from the flash lamp. Only recently did the development of a special flash lamp allow the construction of Ti:Al_2O_3 laser with high power and reasonable flash lamp lifetime, in excess of 1 millions shots.

PUMPING

Many different light sources have been used for the optical excitation of solid-state lasers. They can be divided into two broad classes, viz., the standard incoherent sources and the coherent sources. The incoherent sources are used for pumping until now, because of their lower cost and easy availability. The maximum average power available from lamp-pumped solid-state lasers is also of the order of magnitude higher than that available from laser-pumped systems. This situation is now evolving, because of the recent availability of relatively high-power semiconductor lasers, but their high cost limit the average power level in the watt range. On the other hand, lamp-pumped systems are commercially available in the kW range. The incoherent light sources used for solid-state laser pumping are

1. *Noble-gas arc and flash lamps*   They are the most common sources, and come in many different shapes and technology according to the application of the laser.

2. *Metal vapour arc lamps*   They are different from the previous lamps due to the narrow emission spectrum which sometimes leads to a higher efficiency. The main drawbacks of metal vapour arc lamps are the low power capabilities and the CW operation.

3. *Filament lamps*   They are made by the same tungsten halogen technology used for illumination and hence are very cheap and the power supply is very simple. Due to their well-known drawbacks, such as the limited available average power, the low transfer efficiency at CW operation and the broadband blackbody emission spectrum, they are confined to low-power and inexpensive Nd:YAG systems.

4. *Sun*   There are several examples of solid-state lasers pumped by the solar radiation, using mirrors to collect the light on the crystals. Of course, they depend on the availability of the sources but they are very interesting for space application. In some cases, for example using a Nd,Cr:GSGG crystal, the overall efficiency competes with that of photovoltaic solar cells.

5. *Chemical reactions*   They are mainly single-shot devices because the chemicals used for the reaction must be replaced after each shot. The most common of these sources is the flash-bulb similar to that used in old photographic flash-lights.

6. *Light-emitting diodes*   (LEDs) These are similar to diode lasers in concept but their broader emission bands and especially their wide emission angle give a lower coupling efficiency.

The flash lamps are gas discharge devices generally filled with xenon or krypton gases which give pulsed radiation. But the arc lamps are basically the same gas discharge devices but designed and optimized to produce continuous radiation. The most common shape of both flash and arc lamps is linear. Other shapes are also available . In the early stage of ruby lasers, the helical lamps, and U-shaped and point lamps were employed. Linear lamps are now preferred for laser pumping since they are much easier to cool by means of a coaxial water flow confined by a transparent tube. In addition a cylindrical emitter can be more easily coupled to a laser rod. Since almost 50% of the lamp input power is dissipated as heat, the lamp body needs cooling.For small power systems,namely, low-energy, low-repetition rate pulsed lasers, static or forced gas cooling can be used. For higher power systems, liquid cooling can be used.

Although liquid cooling of flash lamps and D.C. krypton arc lamps is occasionally performed using coolants other than water, deionized purified water continues to be the most popular liquid coolant. The purity of the water must be high to prevent the etching of quartz and the attachment of dark deposits to the outside surface of the lamp envelope. In systems where electrical connections and the coolant are in contact with one another, the water must be deionized to prevent the shorting or weakening of the starting pulse and to minimize erosion of electrical contacts due to electrolysis. Water resistivity greater than 0.2 megohms is highly recommended. All cooling systems component materials should be plastic, stainless steel, or nickel-plated metal.

The flow velocity of the coolant around the flash lamp must be high in such a way that the heat exchange between the lamp walls and the liquid is maximum.

PUMPING CAVITIES

Since lamps and most other incoherent sources emit light diffusely in any direction, an optical system is used to collect the light into the laser-active medium. This is usually done with a reflector surrounding the lamp and the laser crystals.

The most widely used pump cavity is a highly reflective elliptical cylinder with the laser rod and pump lamp at each focus. The elliptical configuration is based on the geometrical theorem that rays originating from one focus of an ellipse are reflected into the other focus. Therefore an elliptical configuration transfers energy from a linear source placed at one focus to a linear absorber placed along the second focus. The elliptical configuration is closed by two plane-parallel and highly reflecting end plates. Optically this makes the elliptical cylinder infinitely long.

A single elliptical cylinder can have a cross section with a large or small eccentricity. In one case, the laser rod and lamp are separated by a fairly large distance while in the second case they are close together. If the elliptical cylinder closely surrounds the lamp and rod, the configuration is known as close-coupled elliptical geometry. This geometry usually results in the most efficient cavity. This cavity has further advantage in that it minimizes the weight and size of the laser heads. Such reflectors are made by machining from solid metal blocks usually brass or aluminium. The reflective surface is then optical-grade polished and coated with a suitable reflective film. For Nd:YAG or Nd:glass, the best laser coating is electroplated gold which has a good reflectivity on the main absorption bands of Nd. For crystals requiring blue or ultraviolet pumping (as ruby or Ti:sapphire), vacuum-evaporated aluminium is often used, since it gives higher reflectivity than gold at wavelengths shorter than 500 nm. The other possible technology is to close-coupled, nonfocusing, pump cavity, where the lamp and the rod are placed as close as possible and a reflector closely surrounds them. The various pumping configurations are given in Figure 2.8.

Since all high-average power solid-state lasers are pumped by broadband flash or arc lamps, thermal effects dominate in their operating characteristics. Typically, 5–10% of the power from the exciting flash-lamps is converted to heat within the host material. This heating is due to:

1. energy loss when ions decay from the pump bands to the upper laser level.

2. non-radiative decay of a fraction of the ions in the upper laser level.

3. direct excitation of the host material by the broadband flash-lamp light.

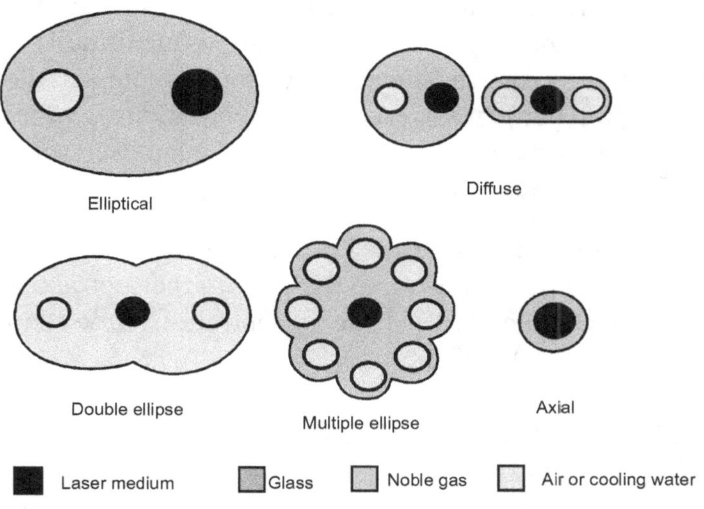

Figure 2.8 Various pumping configurations

The heat is removed by cooling the laser rod. This leads to the development of a near-parabolic temperature profile in the material. The temperature distribution takes between a few seconds (Nd:YAG) or a minute (Nd:glass) to stabilize. The resulting temperature gradients in an operating laser influence optical behaviour. The two mechanisms encountered for this purpose are

1. they lead to variations in refractive index causing lensing and wavefront distortion, and

2. they produce variations of stress within the body of the material inducing birefringence.

At very high flash-lamp powers the induced stress can lead to rupture of the laser rod. There are some possible techniques which can be used to compensate for thermal effects in laser rods. Several of these methods can be incorporated within a resonator design. Birefringence problems can be reduced in crystals by selecting the proper orientation of the crystal axes relative to the cylindrical axis. In commercially grown YAG, the rod is along the (111) direction. However, it has been shown that the (001) direction would be preferable for lower losses if the heat dissipation of the rod is lesser than 50 W. Generally, losses become independent of orientation axis for powers in excess of 50 W. Unfortunately, cutting the (001) direction rod from a (111) grown boule of Nd:YAG limits the size and material waste. Compensation of thermal focusing has been accomplished in many ways, for example, by grinding the ends of the rod to form a negative lens. The cavity mirror selection depends on the negative lens and the rod focal length in the resonator design. It should be noted that each of these passive schemes only provides compensation at one (selected) average pump power. However, many applications require a broad variation of the output power, and a more complicated adaptive resonator should be used (adaptive mirrors and phase conjugation, etc.).

Since heat is concentrated at the central axis of the cylindrical ruby rod in ruby laser, the material can be removed close to the central axis of the ruby rod. In this way we can remove the heat concentration at the centre of the rod. But this gives an annular laser output.

SEMICONDUCTOR LASER PUMPING

The most important alternative to flash-lamp pumping of solid-state lasers is the diode laser. In the last twenty-five years, numerous laboratory devices have been assembled which incorporate single-diode lasers, small laser-diode arrays or LEDs for pumping of Nd:YAG, Nd:glass and a host of other Nd lasers. The low power output, low packaging density and extremely high cost of diode were barriers to any serious applications for laser pumping in the past. The reason for the continued interest in this area stems from the potential dramatic increase in systems efficiency and component lifetime and reduction of thermal load of the solid-state laser material. The latter will not only reduce thermo-optic effects (which lead to better beam quality) but will also increase in pulse repetition frequency. The attractive operating parameters combined with low-voltage operation and the compactness of solid-state laser system have a high potential in applications.

The high pumping efficiency compared to flash lamps stems from the good spectral match between the laser-diode emission and the Nd absorption bands. Actually, flashlamps have higher radiation output to electrical input efficiency (70%) compared to laser diodes (25–50%).

The spectral match between the diode-laser emission and the long-wavelength Nd absorption band reduces the heat deposition in the laser material. Added to this, system lifetime and reliability will be higher in laser-diode-pumped solid-state lasers compared to flash lampbased systems. Laser-diode arrays have exhibited lifetimes of the order of 19,000 hours in CW operation and 10^9 shots in the pulsed mode. Flash lamp life is of the order of 10^7 shots and about 200 hours for CW operation. In addition, the high pump flux combined with a substantial UV content in lamppumped systems cause material degradation in the pump cavity and in the coolant which lead to systems degradation and contribute to maintenance requirements. Such problems are virtually eliminated with laser-diode pump sources. The absence of high-voltage pulses, high temperatures and UV radiation encountered with arc lamps are the special operating features of laser-diode-pumped systems.

In contrast to flash lamps or filament lamps, the emission from laser diode is highly directional and hence requires different pump configurations. The techniques for transferring pump radiation from laser diode arrays to the solid-state laser material are discussed below.

We have to distinguish between optical system employed for end-pumping of a laser crystal, side-pumping of a cylindrical rod, and side-pumping of a rectangular slab.

The focused end-pumping configuration is the most efficient pump-radiation transfer scheme, provided the pump light distribution and resonator mode match (Figure 2.8). Since the pump beam from the diode array is collinear with the optical resonator, the overlap between the pumped volume and the TEM_{00} mode can be very high. In addition, the coupling efficiency is high as long as the absorption length is equal to the crystal length. In its basic form, end pumping involves a collimating lens with a large numerical aperture in order to collect radiation from a large cone angle and a focusing lens to produce a small-diameter spot inside the laser crystal. Since the radiation emitted from a diode array has a high degree of astigmatism, one can introduce prisms or cylindrical optics to transform the beam into a circular shape. The purpose of the coupling optics is to shape the radiation distribution from the diode array such that the pumping volume coincides with the laser's TEM_{00} mode. Radiation from the laser diode array diverges approximately 40 degrees in the plane perpendicular to the active layer. The radiation is collected by a lens. After passing through a pair of prisms, the radiation is focused on the rod by a lens. The resulting divergence inside the Nd:YAG rod is about 6 degrees. In the most common geometry, a plano-concave configuration with high-reflection coating at 1.06 µm at one planar rod surface and anti-reflection coating at 0.81 µm is chosen to allow the pump light to enter the rod. The intra cavity rod surface is anti-reflection-coated at 1.06 µm and an output mirror can be placed either outside the rod or coated directly on the rod itself.

End-pumping of a miniature Nd:YAG laser diode array is an attractive means of obtaining efficient CW lasers. However, at present, the end-pump scheme is useful only for low-power lasers due to the smaller pump area. In order to achieve a somewhat higher output power, two sources can be polarizably coupled to double the pump power, or a double-ended pumping arrangement can be employed.

In side-pumping configuration, the diode arrays are placed along the length of the laser rod and pumped perpendicularly to the direction of propagation of the laser. As more power is required, more diode arrays can be added along and around the laser rod. There are three practical approaches to couple the radiation emitted by the diode lasers to the rod.

1.   Direct coupling

2.   With optics between sources and absorber

3.   Fibre-optics coupling

The direct coupling option does not permit variations other than the position of the diode lasers around the rod. Fibre-optics coupling is very impractical for a large number of diode lasers. Optical coupling can be achieved by using optics such as lenses or elliptical and parabolic mirrors or by non-imaging optics such as reflective or refractive flux concentrators.

The side-pump geometry is not as efficient as the end-pump design. However, it permits scaling of the laser to large power levels. As a matter of fact, the side-pump geometries are normally due to a small absorption length, low pumping density and wasted pump energy due to resonator-mode and pump-distribution mismatch. Large lasers require large rod diameters which increase the pump efficiency. They also require densely packed high-power diode arrays which provide gains over the whole cross section of the rod at sufficient intensity to permit the use of unstable resonators. All these factors contribute to a more efficient utilization of the pump radiation as compared to small systems.

The side-pump geometry is most suitable for slab laser pumping. Side-pumped-slab lasers are usually pumped by 2-D arrays or densely packed linear arrays. In a slab laser, the face of the crystal and the emitting surface of the laser diodes are in close proximity and no optics is employed. The slab can be pumped from one face only. In this case, the opposite face is bonded to a copper heat sink containing a reflective coating to get back the unused pump radiation to the slab for a second pass. An antireflection coating on the pump face is used to reduce coupling losses. Further, liquid cooling is employed to remove heat from the YAG and diode heat sink.

The laser diode-pumped solid-state laser (DPSSL) are employed to perform the applications that are listedin Table 2.7

Table 2.7 Applications of diode-pumped solid-state lasers

Laser power	Application area	Example
< 10 W	Laboratory light source	Spectroscopy, kinetics
	Semiconductor microfabrication	Interferometery, link blowing, thin film triming
	Entertainment Communication	Projection TV
		Communications space-based point to point
		fibre laser repeaters
		Metal cutting and welding etc.
>10 W	Materials Processing	Space-based point to area:
	Semiconductor microfabrication com-munication	Drive for soft X-ray source
>kw	Fusion power	Laser reactor driver

The largest application of solid-state lasers is in military equipment where they are used in range-finders and target designators. Beyond that, solid-state lasers are important in material processing, in medicine and in scientific research that are summarized in Table 2.8

Table 2.8 Application of solid-state lasers

Laser gain medium and type	Operation wavelength(s)	Pump source	Applications
Ruby solid-state laser	694.3 nm	Flash lamp	Holography, tattoo removal. The first type of laser invented, in 1960

Laser gain medium and type	Operation wavelength(s)	Pump source	Applications
Neodymium:YAG Nd:YAG) solid-state laser	$1.064\ \mu m$, ($1.32\ \mu m$)	Flash lamp, laser diode	Material processing, range-finding, laser target designation, surgery, research, pumping other lasers (in combination with frequency doubling). One of the most common high power lasers. Usually pulsed (down to fractions of a nanosecond).
Neodymium:YLF (ND:YLF) solid-state laser	1.047 and $1.053\ \mu m$	Flash lamp, laser diode	Mostly used for pulsed pumping of certain types of pulsed Ti:sapphire lasers, in combination with frequency doubling.
Neodymium:YVO_4 (Nd:YVO) solid-state laser	$1.064\ \mu m$	Laser diode	Mostly used for continuous pumping of mode-locked Ti:sapphire lasers, in combination with frequency doubling
Neodymium:Glass (Nd:Glass) solid-state laser	$\sim 1.062\ \mu m$ (silicate glasses), $\sim 1.054\ \mu m$ (phosphate glasses)	Flash lamp,laser diode	Used in extremely high-power (Terawatt scale),high energy(Megajoules) multiple-beam systems for inertial confinement fusion. Nd:glass lasers are usually frequency-tripled to the third harmonic at 351 nm in laser fusion devices.
Titanium-sapphire (Ti:sapphire) solid-state laser	650–1100 nm	Other laser	Spectroscopy, LIDAR, research. This material is often used in highly-tunable mode-locked infrared lasers to produce ultra-short pulses and in amplifier lasers to produce ultra-short and ultra-intense pulses

Laser gain medium and type	Operation wavelength(s)	Pump source	Applications
Thulium:YAG (Tm:YAG) solid-state laser	2.0 μm	Laser diode	Laser radar
Ytterbium:YAG (Yb:YAG) solid-state laser	1.03 μm	Laser diode, flash lamp	Optical refrigeration, material processing, ultra-short pulse research, multiphoton microscopy, LIDAR
Holmium:YAG (Ho:YAG) solid-state laser	2.1 μm	Laser diode	Tissue ablation, kidney stone removal, dentistry
Cerium-doped lithium strontium (or calcium) aluminium fluoride (Ce :LiSAF, Ce:LiCAF)	~280 to 316 nm	Frequency- quadrupled Nd:YAG laser- pumped, excimer laser pumped, copper vapour laser pumped.	Remote atmospheric sensing, LIDAR, optics research
Promethium-147-doped phosphate glass solid-state laser	933 nm, 1098 nm	Laser diode	Laser material is radioactive, Once demonstrated in use at LLNL in 1987, room temperature 4 level lasing in [147] Pm doped into a lead-indium-phosphate glass etalon.

Laser gain medium and type	Operation wavelength(s)	Pump source	Applications
Chromium-doped chrysoberyl (Alexandrite) solid-state laser	Typically tuned in the range of 700 to 820 nm	Flash lamp, laser diode, mercury arc (for CW mode operation)	Dermatological uses, LIDAR, laser machining.
Erbium-doped fibre laser	1.53–1.56 μm	Laser diode	Optical amplifier for telecommunications over optical fibre.
Uranium-doped calcium fluoride (U:CaF2) solid-state laser	2.5 μm	Flash lamp	First 4-level solid-state laser (1960) developed by Peter Sorokin and Mirek Stevenson, second laser invented overall (after Maiman's ruby laser), liquid helium-cooled, not in use today

GAS LASERS

A gas laser consists of a gas or vapour (active medium) whose atoms or molecules are raised to a higher energy state by excitation and hence there exists an inversion between a certain pair of energy levels in the gas. A gas laser essentially consists of 1) a resonator (a long cylindrical glass tube with required gas) 2) an exciting mechanism to cause discharge in the tube and 3) a set of mirrors facing each other. The important types of gas lasers are

1. Neutral atom lasers (He–Ne laser) and metal vapour (Cu, Au) lasers.

2. Molecular gas lasers (CO, CO_2, N_2 , CHF_3) lasers

3. Ion lasers (Ar, Kr, He–Cd lasers)

4. Excimer lasers (rare earth halide lasers, KrF, XeCl)

Gas lasers can be fabricated in many sizes and configurations. The optical,thin film, vacuum, instrument and electrical technologies are involved in the construction of gas lasers. The four essential parts of gas lasers are the following.

1. Plasma tube and cathodes,

2. Optical components, Brewster windows and dielectric coated mirrors

3. Mechanical mounts and fixtures, etc.

4. Electrical power supply

In addition to the above, vacuum is a very important parameter in gas lasers. This process is essential to remove absorbed gas molecules from the plasma tubes before filling with noble gases or mixtures.The ordinary gas lasers vary in length from 30 to 100 cm. The gas leakage occurs from the walls of the glass tube due to the collision of active gas molecules with the walls. Hence it is impossible to obtain the laser output proportional to the cross sectional area of the tube.

Gas lasers are usually electrically excited by gas discharge using direct current, radio frequency or pulse source. In a few cases, gas dynamic expansion and chemical pumping are also used as excitation mechanisms. The gas lasers are also excited through optical pumping by means of another laser.

The electrical discharge in gas lasers falls under two categories. The first category is due to the excitation by electron impact and can be represented as

$$e+X \rightarrow X+e$$

This is known as collision of the first kind. The second category is due to the excitation by resonant energy transfer and it can be represented as

$$A+B \rightarrow A+B + DE \ (DE < KT)$$

This is known as collision of second kind.

The collision of second kind, the collision between atoms and molecules, collision with walls of container and stimulated and spontaneous emission causes de-excitation of excited levels.

A population inversion between two given levels will occur when the excitation rate R is greater for upper laser level than for lower laser level.

HELIUM–NEON (HE–NE) LASER

The He–Ne laser is an electrically pumped neutral atom laser that usually produces a red beam at 632.8 nm, but there are also infrared lines at 1.5 and 3.39 μm . Normally the laser is designed in such a way that these infrared lines do not oscillate. He–Ne is the first gas as well as the CW laser that was discovered in 1960. A schematic diagram of the He–Ne laser is given in Figure 2.9.

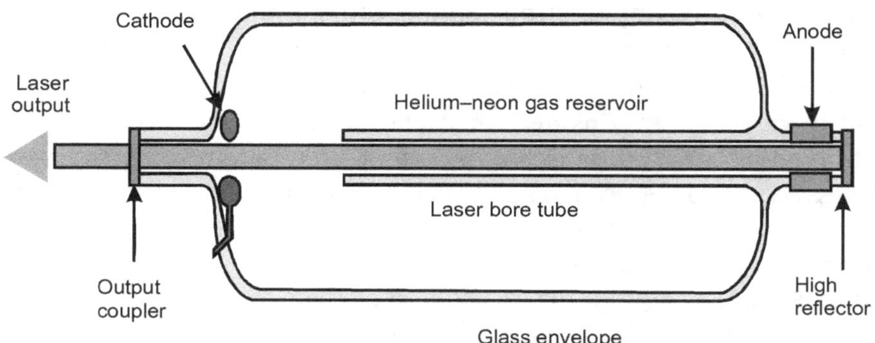

Figure 2.9 Schematic diagram of He–Ne laser tube

A high voltage (in kilovolts) an d low current (in milliamps) discharge between the aluminiumcathode and the anode provides the energy for the population inversion. The discharge is confined to a small inner tube called the bore to keep it concentrated for maximum energy transfer to the tiny beam bouncing back and forth between the mirrors. Even so, the electrical efficiency of this laser is typically low. Energy is transferred from the current when electrons collide with gaseous atoms in the tube.

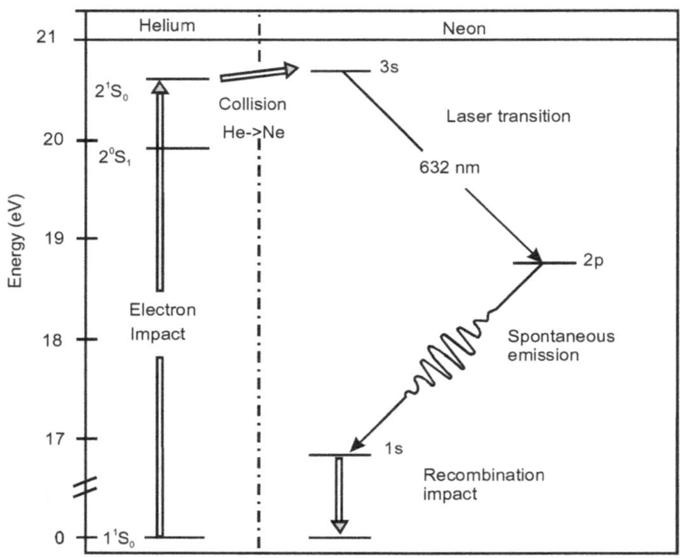

Figure 2.10   Helium and Neon Energy Levels

When a fast moving electron collides with a ground-state atom, a part of the electron's kinetic energy can be transferred to the atom, leaving it in an excited state. But creating a population inversion in a He–Ne laser is not so straightforward and easy as described above. The lasing neon atom absorbs very little energy from the discharge current. Neon atom seems to have a very small cross section to the electron and so a few electrons collide with and transfer energy to the neon atoms. Helium atoms, on the other hand seem to have a large cross section to the electron, and the energy is easily transferred from the discharge current to helium atoms. Fortunately, the excited helium energy levels are quite close to the upper levels in neon, so energy can readily be transferred from an excited helium atom to a ground- state neon atom when the two collide. The laser transition between electronic energy levels of Ne atom is shown in Figure 2.10.

After a helium atom is excited to one of its upper states by collision with an electron, it can collide with a neon atom and transfer its energy to the neon, leaving the neon atom in its upper laser level. Based on the feedback of the resonator, one of the three transitions lase. As we are interested in the visible region, we prefer the laser mirrors with low infrared reflectivity. From its lower laser level, the neon atom decays spontaneously to its ground level. The operation characteristics of He–Ne lasers are as follows.

Gas pressure	mbar
Gas mixture	He : Ne 5:1 to 20 : 1
Discharge	Cold cathode, longitudinal, Dc voltage in kv current in mA
Laser output power (commercial lasers)	<1mW to 50 mW

Most modern He–Ne lasers use internal mirrors that are attached directly to the ends of the discharge tube. The earlier and special-purpose lasers had the external mirrors that are separated from the tube. In these lasers, a non-reflecting window, often at Brewster's angle, must be placed at the end of the discharge tube. Because the internal mirror design has greater reliability, it is always preferred. The modern commercial He–Ne lasers have weldlike hard seals between the mirrors and discharge tube and their shelf lives are at least a decade. The ultimate limitation on shelf life now appears to be diffusion of helium through the walls of the tube. The typical data of He–Ne lasers are as follows:

Wavelength (Nm)	Laser transition (MHz)	Gain(%)	Laser power(mW)
543.3 (green)	3s–2p 1750	0.5	1
594.1 (yellow)	3s–2p 1600	0.5	0.5
611.8 (orange)	3s–2p 1550	1.7	1
632.8 (red)	3s–2p 1500	10 to 50	5 (up)
1152.3 (IR)	2s–2p 825	—	1
2323.1 (IR)	2s–2p 625	—	1
3391.3 (IR)	3s–3p 280	104	10

The operating lifetime of most commercial He–Ne lasers is about 15,000 or 20,000 hours and the most common failure mechanism is cathode decay. In a longer tube,the output power is maximized and in a short bore tube, power is decreased.

METAL VAPOUR LASERS

Metals such as copper, gold, tin, lead, zinc, cadmium and selenium have been used in vapour form to produce metal vapour lasers. These lasers are also known as neutral-atom metal vapour lasers. Cadmium vapour produces strong continuous-wave laser action in the ultraviolet region at the wavelengths λ = 441 nm and 325 nm. Copper and gold vapour lasers are self-terminating pulsed-operation lasers. The pumping mechanisms for metal vapour lasers are different from ion gas lasers. Penning ionization and charge transfer ionization are the two processes through which the pumping process is carried out in metal vapour lasers. The low current density and electrical power per unit length are required for metal vapour lasers when compared to ion gas lasers. Penning ionization is a non-resonant process while charge transfer ionization is a resonant process. In its construction, a metal vapour laser is not very different from a gas laser. We will discuss the construction and operation characteristics of metal vapour lasers such as gold, copper and He–Cd lasers.

The laser transitions between electronic energy levels of copper are shown in Figure 2.11

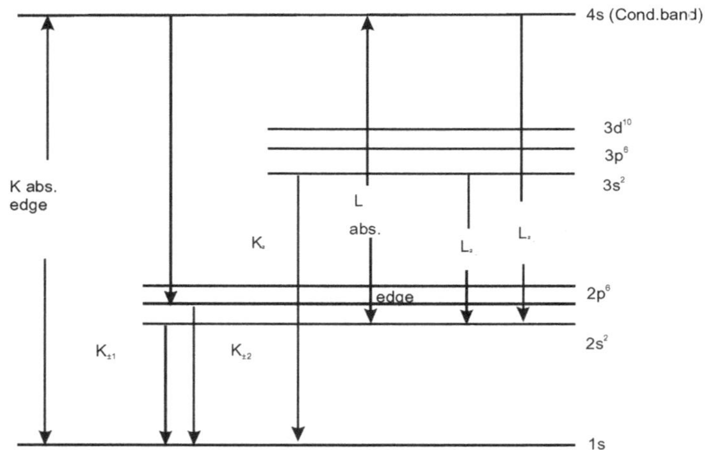

Figure 2.11   Relevant Energy Levels of Copper

One such possible configuration for copper vapour lasers is shown in Figure.2.12

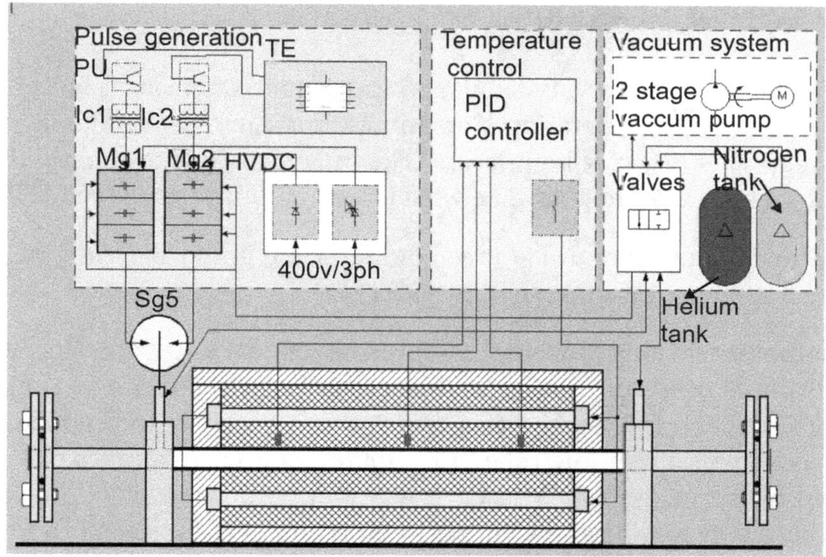

Figure 2.12 Schematic Diagram of Copper Vapour Laser

The refractory ceramic tube which has gold or copper metal is surrounded by insulation. The entire set-up is in the vacuum envelop. Just as in gas lasers, it has mirrors and windows. The operational temperature for copper is 1480°C–1530°C while it is 1590°C–1640°C for gold. Neon is used as buffer gas in this set-up. The total efficiency of the laser comes to 1%. The gain of these lasers are 10 times higher than for Ar ion laser. The typical data for copper and gold vapour lasers are as follows:

Parameters	Copper laser	Gold laser
Wave lengths (nm)	510.6/578.2	627.8
Average power (W)	60	9
Pulse energy (m)	10	1.5
Pulse duration (ns)	15–60	15–60
Peak power (kW)	300	60
Repetition rate (KH$_z$)	5–15	6–8
Beam diameter (mm)	42	42
Bean divergence (mrad)	0.6	0.6

GOLD VAPOUR LASER

The gold vapour laser is very similar to the copper vapor laser both in structure and principles of operation. Sometimes, the same system (laser tube and power supply) is used for both lasers. The only change is to replace the solid copper by a wire of pure gold. The wavelength of gold lasers is red (628 nm).

The main applications of gold vapour laser are in the experimental cancer treatment of photo–dynamic therapy (PDT).

Another interesting laser used in this category is He–Cd and He–Se lasers. In He–Cd laser, the tube has a small reservoir near the anode to contain the metal. This reservoir is heated to a temperature of 250°C to produce the desired vapour pressure in the tube. A cataphoresis discharge takes place in the tube and hence we get a CW laser. It gives an output power of 50–100 mW. Therefore this type of laser lies in between the red He–Ne lasers (a few mW) and Ar laser (a few watts). He–Cd laser emits a blue radiation or an UV beam. This laser is mostly used in facsimile systems, reprographic systems and in Raman and fluorescence experiments.

He-Cd LASERS

The helium–cadmium (He–Cd) laser is one type of gas lasers (metal vapour lasers) using helium in conjunction with a metal which vaporizes at a relatively low temperature. Other examples are the helium–mercury (He–Hg) and helium-selenium (He–Se) lasers. Cadmium is a metal, the lasing action in helium-cadmium laser occurs between energy levels of cadmium ions, so the lasing medium is ionized metal vapour. The He–Cd laser is a gas laser, and the metal cadmium can be transformed into the gas phase by heat. The excitation to the upper laser level of the cadmium atoms in the gas is similar to the excitation process of the Neon gas in a helium–neon laser. Helium atoms are excited by collisions with accelerated electrons. Then they pass their energies to cadmium atoms by collisions. The transitions in helium–cadmium laser are between energy levels of single-ionized cadmium atoms, and about twelve lines are available. These wavelengths are in the shorter wavelength region, violet and ultraviolet (UV). Thus, the main application of the He–Cd laser is in the optics laboratory, for fabricating holographic gratings. The practical problem in helium–cadmium laser is to maintain homogeneous distribution of the metal vapour inside the electrical discharge tube.

The ions are attracted to the cold windows at the ends of the cavity. In order to prevent coating of the windows with cadmium, cold traps are put before the laser windows.

The typical He–Cd laser produces a high-quality beam at 442 nm (violet-blue) and/or 325 nm (UV) depending on the optics. Typical power output is in the tens to hundreds of milliwatts range. Its wavelengths are highly desirable for some forms of spectroscopy, non-destructive testing and stereo-lithography. But it is not good for laser shows and these lasers are not popular due to the high complexity and cost. The characteristic properties of a typical He–Cd laser is given below.

Property	Values
Output wavelength	325 nm (near UV) and/or 442 nm (violet).
Output power	From 3 to 55 mW (325 nm) or 30 to 130 mW (442 nm)
Operating voltage	2.4 to 2.6 kV DC
Operating current	90 to 120 mA
Starting voltage	10 kV DC
Helium heater voltage	6.5 VAC
Cadmium heater voltage	2 to 3 VAC
Re-melt heater voltage	6 to 7 VAC
Coherence length	10 cm for natural isotopic cadmium; 30 cm for isotopically pure cadmium
Polarization	Random

He–Cd Laser Safety

1. The power output of a He–Cd laser may be 10 s to 100 s of mW continuous at one or both of two wavelengths. The brightness of the 442 nm (violet-blue) is deceptive because of the human eye's low sensitivity to this wavelength–the perceived brightness is only about 1/25th that at 555 nm (green) or about 1/6th that of the common red He–Ne (632.8 nm, actually appears orange-red) laser. However, the potential for damage depends on the optical power, not the perceived brightness! The 325 nm (UV) output is, of course, totally invisible and therefore even more dangerous.

2. The power supply for the He–Cd laser operates at between 700 and 3,000 V DC with 100 mA or more of tube current. This is quite a lethal combination.

3. Portions of the He–Cd laser tube may be hot enough to burn flesh in addition to being electrically live.

4. Cadmium is classified as a toxic heavy metal. This is not a problem with an intact laser tube. However, should the tube be broken, no attempt should be made to salvage anything unless one has the appropriate experience in dealing with these substances.

Figure 2.13 shows a schematic diagram of a helium–cadmium laser

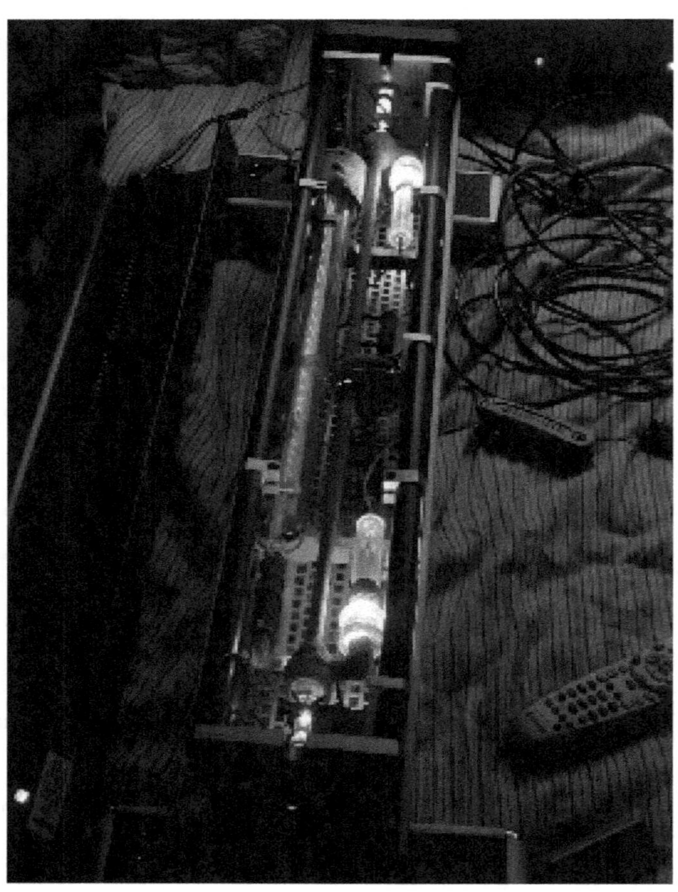

Figure 2.13   Helium–Cadmium Laser

ION LASERS

A laser in which the transition involved in stimulated emission of radiation takes place between two levels of an ion is called an ion laser. It emits spectral lines in the visible and near-visible range. Neon, argon, krypton and xenon are the commonly used gases in the ion laser and such lasers can be called ion gas lasers.

ION GAS LASERS

Ion gas lasers are high-power continuous-wave visible lasers with an output of 20 watts. Neutral noble gases are not useful practically as laser media, except neon gas. When the rest of the gases are used as laser media, they must be ionized by electron collisions. The resulting ion is excited by further electron collisions and an inverted population of the ion energy level occurs. A good example for such a laser is argon laser fluorescing in the singly- ionized argon lines. This is a very widely used ion laser. The argon ion laser and the energy level diagram of singly-ionized argon ion relevant to operation of the argon ion laser are shown in Figures 2.14 and 2.15 respectively.

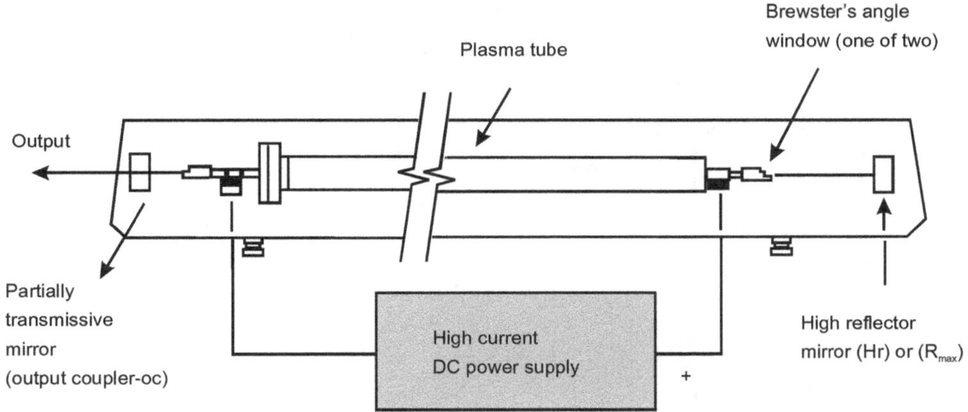

Figure 2.14   Schematic diagram of argon ion laser

Excitation processes are

i.   Ar (3p)—Ar (4p)

ii.   Ar (metastable state)—Ar (4p)

iii. Ar (higher levels)—Ar(4p)

In order to achieve high current densities,a narrow diameter tube is employed in the construction of Ar laser. In addition, an axial magnetic field can be employed to maximize the current density by constraining the electron to move in a spiral path around the magnetic field to avoid collision with the walls of plasma tube. Very high current densities in ion lasers require specialized construction methods for the tube. The oxides of ceramics, i.e., alumina beryllia and magnesia, etc., are all superior to fused silica. The water-cooled fused silica has poor thermal conductivity which sets an upper limit on the power input per unit area of the capillary bore, particularly at the cathode end of the DC arc tubes where a high gas temperature is encountered. Even the ceramics are often strained in manufacture and crack as soon as the first arc is struck. Segmented metal bores or segmented graphite bores can be used as ion laser tubes. The operation characteristics of an argon ion laser are as follows.

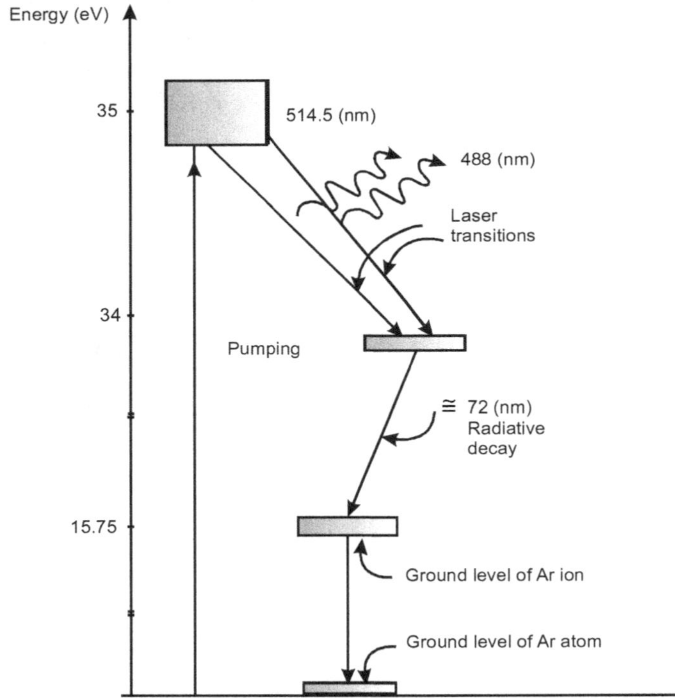

Figure 2.15 Energy-level diagram of a singly-ionized argon ion relevant to operation of the argon ion laser

Parameters	Values
Gas pressure	Mbar
Kind of gas	Pure argon gas
Gas discharge	Hot cathode, longitudinal, DC, high current density (1 kA/cm)
Laser power	Several watts
Total efficiency	0.1%
Special design of laser tubes required	6.5 VAC

Many different wavelengths are available from argon, krypton and xenon lasers as shown in Table 2.9.

Table 2.9 Wavelength (nm) from argon, krypton and xenon ion laser

Neon (Ne)	Argon (Ar)	Krypton (kr)	Xenon (Xe)
332.4	351.1	350.7	460.3
334.5	363.8	356.4	541.9
337.8	418.3	406.7	597.1
339.3	454.5	413.1	627.1
371.3	457.9	415.4	714.9
	472.7	476.2	798.8
	476.5	482.5	871.6
	488.0	520.8	905.6
		530.9	969.9
	496.5	568.2	
	501.7	647.1	1092.3
	514.5	676.4	
	528.7	752.5	
		793.1	
		799.3	

The most common argon wavelengths are the blue line at 488 nm and the green line at 514.5 nm. Krypton's stronger output is the red line at 647.1 nm but it can also provide yellow, green and blue light.

Unlike other gas lasers which operate with low current, high voltage discharges,ion laser discharges are relatively low-voltage and high-current. The high current is necessary to ionize the argon or krypton gas in the plasma tube. This high current density and the resulting power dissipation require careful electrode design and water cooling of all but the lowest power ion laser.

MOLECULAR GAS LASERS

Molecular lasers take the advantage of transition between energy levels of a molecule. Based on the laser transition, we have three different categories of lasers.

1.   *Vibronic lasers*   Vibronic (a contraction from the words vibrational and electronic) laser transition between vibrational levels belonging to different electronic states. In this case emission wavelengths fall from the UV to the visible region.

2.   *Vibrational–rotational lasers*   Vibrational–rotational laser transition between different vibrational and rotational levels of the electronic ground state. These lasers emit radiation in the mid-IR to far-IR (5 – 300 μm For example, CO_2 laser ($\lambda=9 - 11$ μm) and CO_2 ($\lambda=5 - 6$ μm) laser.

3.   *Pure rotational lasers*   Rotational laser transition between different rotational levels within a vibrational state of the electronic ground state. The corresponding emission wavelength is in the far-IR region (25 μm to 1 mm). (For example CH_3F laser ($\lambda= 496$ μm) These lasers are usually optical pumped with CO_2 lasers.

Among the various gas lasers, we will concentrate only on carbon dioxide lasers. Carbon dioxide lasers are widely used molecular gas lasers for several applications in industry and medicine. They are based on vibrational transitions of carbon dioxide molecule. Hence to understand the working of a molecular laser, one has to know the vibrational modes of the concerned molecule. The fundamental modes of vibration of a CO_2 molecule are illustrated in Figure 2.16.

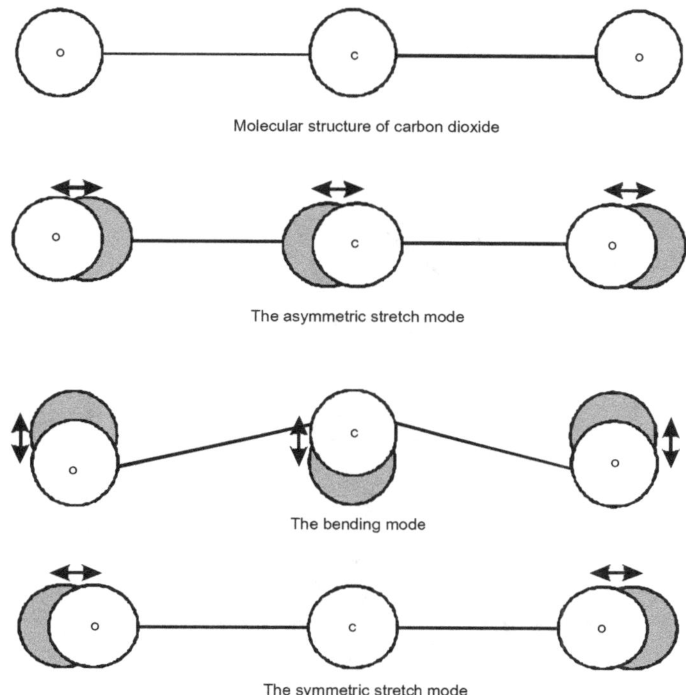

Figure 2.16   Vibrational Modes of a Carbon Dioxide Molecule

The carbon dioxide molecule possesses three different independent modes. They are symmetric stretching mode n_1 (1,0,0), bending mode n_2 (0,1,0) and asymmetric stretching mode n_3 (0,0,1). The simplified energy levels of all three modes in a single energy-level diagram is shown in Figure 2.17. Only the four lowest excited levels are shown in the figure because they are the only ones that take part in the lasing. The energy state of the molecule is represented by the three numbers (i, j, k) which represent the amount of energy or number of energy quanta associated with each mode. The upper laser level is state (001), the lower laser level is provided by state (020) and (100). The transition (001) $\rightarrow$ (100) yields a line at the wavelength $\lambda = 10.6$ μm whereas the (001) $\rightarrow$ (020) gives a line at . States (020) and (100) decay into the ground state mainly by resonant energy transfer to the unexcited CO_2 molecules so that these accumulate in the (010) state. The depopulation of state (010) is the bottleneck of the process. To overcome this, special additives such as helium or water vapour are introduced in the gas mixture. Hence the level degrades due to the collisions with additives.

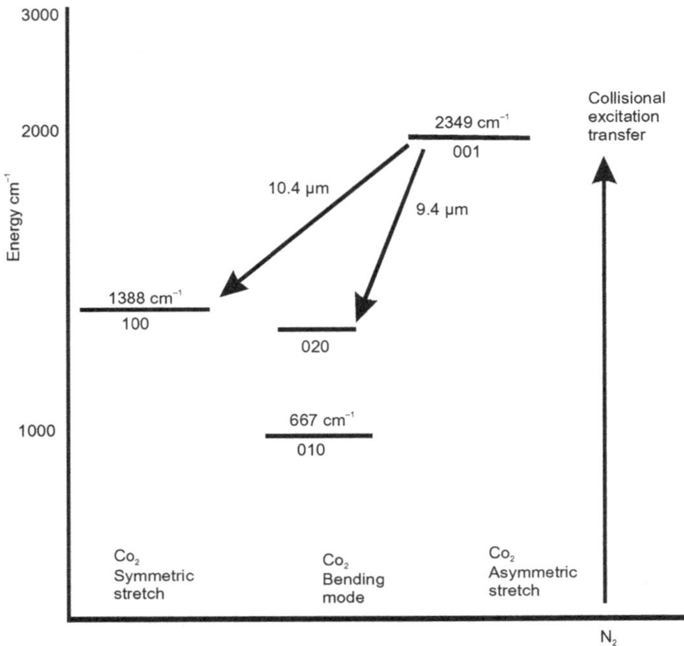

Figure 2.17 Vibrational Energy Levels of Carbon Dioxide

All commercial CO_2 lasers are based on vibrational transition within the ground electronic state process. Most CO_2 lasers require a mixture of three gases, viz., carbon dioxide, molecular nitrogen and diverse additives such as helium. The nitrogen gas provides collisional excitation for carbon dioxide while helium has high thermal conductivity. This property helps to keep the gases cool. The helium efficiently transports heat to the outside of the laser. The nitrogen in the CO_2 discharge takes the role that helium plays in the helium–neon laser.

Carbon dioxide lasers are commercially important because they can generate very high powers with relatively high electrical efficiency. The lasers with average power greater than 20 kW are available and the kilowatt CO_2 lasers are common. The powerful lasers are line tunable and emit radiation in the mid-IR region. They find an extensive application in research, medicine and industry.

Most of the CO_2 lasers are gas-discharge lasers. They are

1. lasers with slow axial gas flow
2. sealed-off lasers

3.   waveguide lasers

4.   lasers with fast axial or transverse flow

5.   transversely excited atmospheric pressure (TEA) laser

6.   continuously tunable high-pressure lasers

7.   gas-dynamic lasers

The operation characteristics of a CO_2 laser are as follows:

Parameters	Values
Gas pressure	Mbar (longitudinal discharage 100 mbar (wave guide lasers >1bar (TEA laser)
Gas mixture	CO2: N2:He 1:1:8
Gas discharge	DC, rf, pulsed, TEA
Laser power	Watts to > 20 kilowatts. Continuous wave–kW to TW pulsed.
Total efficiency	Greater than 10 %

In general, there are five major types of CO_2 lasers. They are 1) sealed or no-flow, 2) slow axial flow, 3) fast axial flow, 4) fast transverse flow and 5) transverse excited atmosphere (TEA).

EXCIMER LASERS

Excimer is a contraction of the term "excited dimer" of excited di-or triatomic complexes which are usually rare gas halides. Dimers are usually considered to be "molecules made up of two identical atoms". However, the term "excimer" has subsequently been extended to include other excited molecules (though usually diatomic). If two systems (atoms or molecules) do not form a strong chemical bond when they are in their ground states but do form a strong chemical bond when one of them is in an excited state, then the bound excited state is called an excimer.

The fact that the excimer dissociates in the ground state has important consequences in a laser system, as this helps to maintain the population inversion necessary for lasing action. The lack of well-defined bonding electron energy levels in the ground state means the excimer lasers usually, have a small tuning range (up to 1 nm). The early development and theory of excimer lasers has been reviewed by Rohodes, Huestis, and Hecht. The energy states of excimer laser is shown in Figure 2.18.

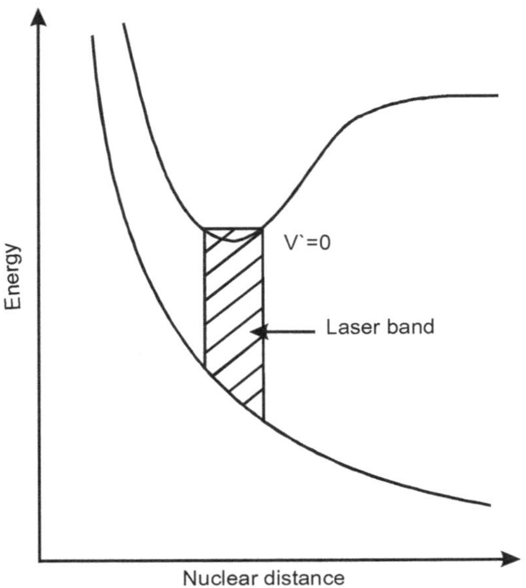

Figure 2.18 Energy states of an excimer laser [Svelto, O. 1989 Principles of Lasers. Plenum Press, New York]

Excimer and their continuous ultraviolet (UV) spectra have been studied since the 1930s. In 1960, it was first proposed by Houtermans that excimers could be introduced for laser emission. However, problems associated with the very high pump energies meant that true stimulated emission was not observed until 1971. Basov *et al.* observed lasing action in condensed xenon (Xe), and a year later stimulated emission was observed from Xe in a gaseous state (a true excimer laser). It was the developments in the production of high-energy electron beams to provide the pump energy, which facilitated the production of stimulated emission from excimer systems.

The first rare gas halide excimer laser was reported in 1975 by Searles and Hart. This was closely followed by a number of reports of other rare gas excimer lasers. Rare gas halide excimer lasers have since evolved into the most efficient and well-developed excimer laser and are used in many applications.

The first suggestions that the excimer laser may be used in corneal surgery were made by Trokel, Srinivasan and Braren in 1983. They used far-ultraviolet light of 139 nm wavelength from an argon-fluoride excimer laser in short intense pulse to make a series of linear excimer laser cuts in bovine eyes. Because of the precise nature of the action of this laser modality, its application for refractive keratoplasty was suggested. The implication of this variety of corneal surgical procedure was that it could be extended to the removal of a shaped area of the cornea to any depth, as done in lamellar keratectomy or to a controlled penetrating corneal incision for corneal transplantation.

Excimer lasers are relatively straightforward to construct. However, the technology to make these lasers work efficiently and with reasonable component and gas lifetime is extremely complex. Excimer lasers usually consist of a large, elongated aluminium box. This box is filled with the appropriate gas mixture. Running the full length of this box are two metal electrodes spaced about 2–3 cm apart. At one end of the box, aligned with the gap between the electrodes, a mirror is mounted and at the other end, a window. The window is usually an uncoated optic. The small amount of reflection that normally occurs from each surface is enough to provide laser action.

Outside the box,there is usually a large bank of capacitors. And these are charged using a high-voltage power supply to several tens of kilovolts. A special switch (thyraton) is used to dump the energy stored in these capacitors across the electrodes inside the box. The electrical discharge through the gas allows the formation of excimer molecules. Lasing action usually occurs within nanoseconds.

Excimer laser can have a ceramic or aluminium head. Ceramic head is manufactured by lamda physics in which case electrodes are ceramic. The advantage of the ceramic head is that the gas life of a single fill is longer, although the cost is double. Aluminium head normally has a single-day gas fill.

Excimer lasers are an important class of molecular lasers offering most intense pulsed ultraviolet radiation. They utilize diatomic molecules as active medium which are bound only in the excited electronic states and unbound or weakly bound in the ground state. The excited dimers also decay with lifetime of the order of tens of nanoseconds. These molecules decay by emitting one photon with energy of few eV. That is, the wavelength ranges from visible to vacuum ultraviolet. These characteristics are extremely interesting when excimers are used as active media for UV lasers. Ultraviolet lasers are important when compared with visible or infrared lasers because

    i.   the absorption of materials increases for UV radiaton,

    ii.   it decreases the minimum divergence of the beam,

iii.   it decreases the minimum cross section,

iv.   it increases the resolution in material processing,

v.   it increases the power density at a given beam power,

vi.   the ablative mechanisms for material change from thermal to non thermal, i.e., photo-ablative process. In this process the chemical bonds are directly broken but there is no increase in temperature and

vii.   the laser radiation can travel in silica fibres which is an important property for medical application.

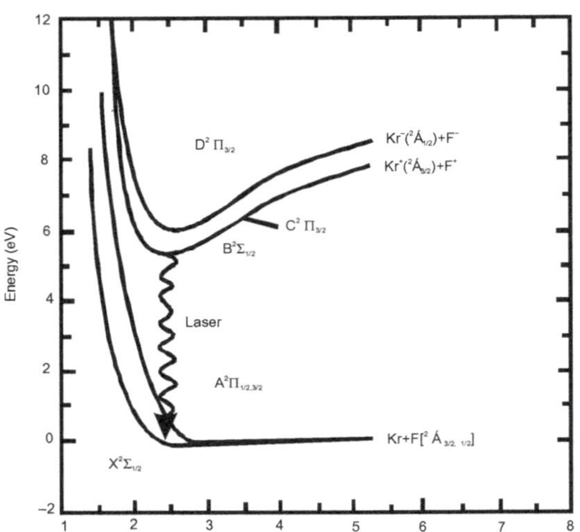

Figure 2.19 Potential energy diagram showing the molecular struc ture of KrF [Svelto,O. *Principles of Lasers*, (1989). Plenum Press, New York.]

The first experimental evidence of laser emission from excimer system was demonstrated in 1970 by Basoy and others. A classification of excimer laser can be done, based on the different active media employed. The first excimer lasers developed use the rare gas dimers [Xe_2 at 172 nm, Ar_2 at 126 nm, and Kr_2 at 146 nm] emitting lasers in the ultraviolet range. The energy level diagram for the laser transition between bound excited electronic state and repulsive electronic ground state is shown in Figure 2.19 for KrF.

Mercury halide such as HgCl, HgBr and HgI present excimer characteristics with laser transitions between an excited bound state and a weakly bound ground state. The laser emission for the mercury halides is in the visible region of the spectrum at 557.6, 501.8 and 441.2 nm.

Rare gas halide excimer lasers are pumped either by a high-pressure transverse gas discharge or by an electron beam. In the former case either electron beam or ultraviolet pre-ionization techniques are used. Two typical construction of excimer lasers involving laser pumping by self-sustained discharge with ultraviolet pre-ionization and electron beam pumping are shown in Figures 2.20 and 2.21.

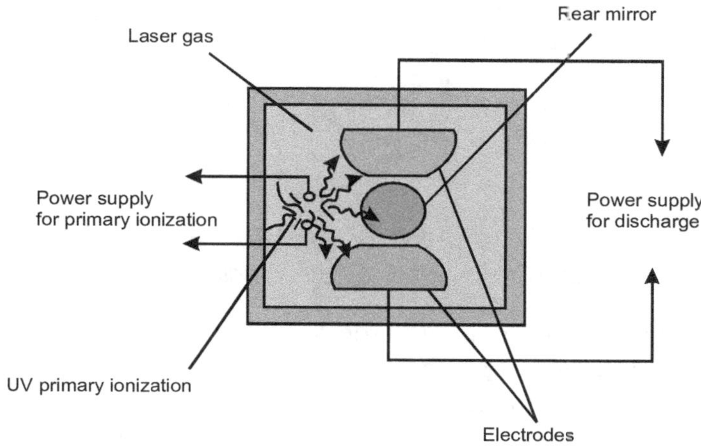

Figure 2.20 Schematic construction of an excimer laser pumped with a gas discharged [Gerhardt, H. *"Fundamentals of laser physics and laser technology." (Lambda Physik)]*

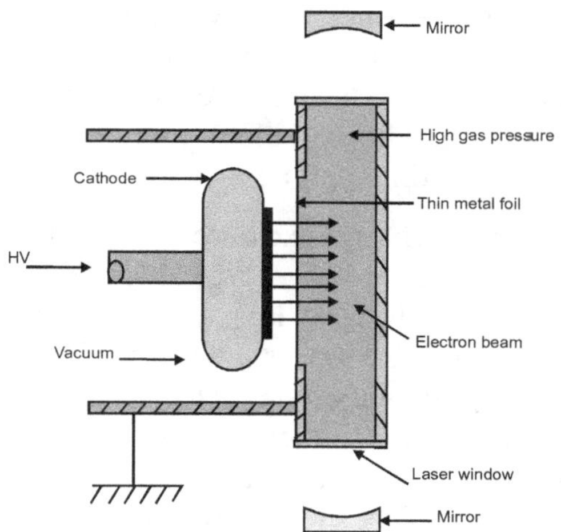

Figure 2.21 Schematic construction of an excimer laser pumped with an electron bea [Gerhardt, H. *"Fundamentals of laser physics and laser technology," (Lambda Physik)]*

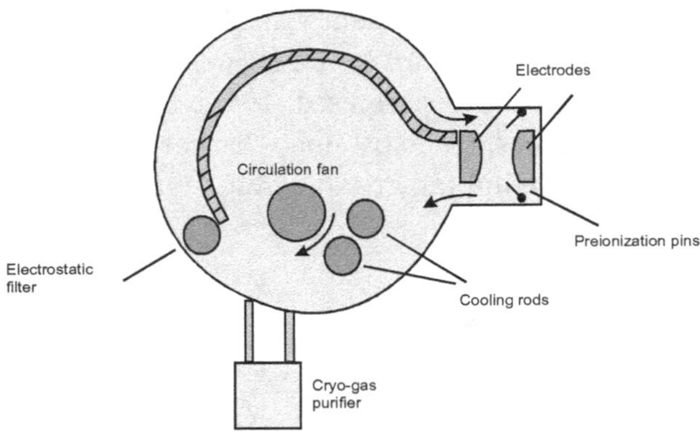

Figure 2.22   Typical construction of a modern excimer laser [Gerhardt, *H. "Fundamentals of laser physics and laser technology." Lambda Physik.]*

In the electron beam pumping process, an electron beam, generated by a suitable accelerator, enters the gas region through a thin window made up of mylar, aluminium and titanium with thickness ranging between 5 and 50 μm. This thickness depends on two factors, viz., 1) the capacity to withstand the gas pressure and 2) the requirement of minimum electron energy losses in crossing the window.

The advantages of this technique are the possibility of easy sealing to systems with large volumes (i.e., high energy per pulse) and the possibility of achieving high pumping density (i.e., high peak power laser pulses). The disadvantages of the system are a) the system is technically complicated b) it causes unforeseen radiation and shielding problems and c) some components such as the window have limited lifetime.

In the self-sustained discharge excitation, the laser chamber consists of two conveniently shaped electrodes. A typical gas mixture with three components — 1) a buffer gas (Ne, Ar, He) at a pressure between 1 bar and 10 bars 2) the reacting gas (Xe, Kr) at a pressure between 10 torr and 100 torr and 3) the reacting halogen gas (F_2, HCl) at a pressure between 1 torr and 10 torr—is kept in between the electrodes. A pulsing ionizing radiation (UV, X-rays and electrons) creates a suitable electron density so that when a charged capacitor is connected to the electrodes, an electric discharge can develop in the conducting gas. The laser chamber can take different shapes, depending on the pre-ionization source. The pre-ionization is carried out using ultraviolet radiation by employing sparks near the discharge origin.

Rare gas	Ar_2	126 nm
	Kr_2	146 nm
	Xe_2	172 nm
Rare gas halides	ArCl	175 nm
	ArF	193 nm
	KrCl	222 nm
	KrF	249 nm
	XeBr	282 nm
	XeCl	308 nm
	XeF	351, 450–550 nm
Triatomic molecules	Kr_2F	390–450 nm
	Xe_2Cl	450–550 nm

In the rare-gas halide (RGH) lasers, the active molecule is formed by a rare gas (Kr, Xe, Ar) and a halogen atom (F, Cl, Br) which after excitation form a diatomic molecule in a excited state. Decay to the unbound ground level occurs with the emission of a photon in the UV spectral region. The RGH lasers are the most important UV sources, for the efficiency and for the high average and peak power. They are currently produced in a commercial scale. The emission wavelengths of rare gas and rare gas halide excimer lasers are as follows:

The typical data of commercial excimer lasers are given below.

Parameter	ArF	KrF	XeCl	XeF
Wavelength (nm)	193	249	308	351
Pulse energy (mJ) at 1 Hz	500	1000	500	500
Pulse duration (ns)	14	15	13	14
Peak power (MW) at 1 Hz	10	15	9	6
Repetition rate Hz	80	100	150	100
Average power	10	20	10	6

The gas lasers find very wide applications. Some of the applications with the specific lasers are given in Tables 2.10 and 2.11.

LIQUID LASERS (DYE LASERS)

When the active medium is liquid solutions of organic dyes or specially pre-pared liquids doped with rare earth ions, the laser is known as liquid laser or dye laser. The special liquids are grouped under two heads, viz., organometallic (chelate) and inorganic (aprotonic) liquids. The laser action is obtained in more than 200 organic dyes. They are classified under eight groups such as xanthenes, polymethines, oxazines, coumarins, anthracenes, acridines, azines and phthalo-zianines. These dyes cover a wide range of wavelengths from 0.3 to 1.5 μm

The active medium of a dye laser consists of an organic dye dissolved in a suitable solvent. The dye molecules are composed of many atoms and have many closely spaced energy levels. These are broadened to form continuous bands of emission and absorption in the dye. Dye lasers may use any of several dozen dye types, each tunable over its own spectral range.

Dye lasers are available in three basic types. CW dye lasers use a dye jet as the active medium. Their excitation mechanisms are the focused beams of argon ion lasers. Wavelength tuning is accomplished with birefringent filters or tuning wedges.

Pulsed dye lasers employ a dye cell and are produced in two types. One is pumped by the short-duration pulse of a nitrogen laser. This laser system pro-duces as many as several hundred pulses per second with pulse durations of a few nanoseconds. Tuning is usually accomplished with a diffraction grating. The dye in a flash lamp-pumped dye laser is excited directly by the flash lamp light. These systems are typically capable of a few pulses per second, with pulse duration of several microseconds. They may be tued by diffraction gratins or birefringent filters.

Table 2.10   Applicatios of Gas Lasers.

Laser gain medium and type	Operation wave-length (s)	Pump Source	Applications
Helium–neon (He–Ne) gas laser	632.8 nm (543.5 nm, 593.9 nm, 611.8 nm, 1.1523 to 3.3913 mm	Electrical discharge	Interferometry holography, spectroscopy, barcode scanning, alignment, optical demonstrations.
Argon ion gas laser	488.0 nm, 514.5 nm, (351 nm) 465.8 nm, 472.7 nm, 528.7 nm)	Electrical discharge	Retinal phototherapy (for diabetes), lithography pumping other lasers.
Krypton ion gas lasers	416 nm, 530.9 nm, 568.2 nm, 647.1 nm, 676.4 nm, 752. nm, 799.3 nm	Electrical discharge	Scientific research mixed with argon for creation of "white-light" lasers, light shows.
Xenon ion gas laser	Many lines throughout entire visible spectrum extending into the UV and IR.	Electrical discharge	Scientific research.
Nitrogen gas laser	337.1 nm	Electrical discharge	Pumping of dye lasers, measurement of air pollution, scientific research, nitrogen lasers are capable of operating super radiantly (without a resonator cavity)

Laser gain medium and type	Operation wave-length (s)	Pump Source	Applications
Hydrogen fluoride laser	2.7 to 2.9 mm for hydrogen fluoride 2.7 to 2.9 mm for deuterium fluoride	Chemical reaction in a burning jet of ethylene and nitrogen tri-fluoride (NF3)	Used in research for laser weaponry, operated in continuous wave mode and capable of extremely high powers in the megawatt range.
Chemical oxygen-iodine laser (COIL)	1.315 mm	Chemical reaction in a jet of single delta oxygen and iodine	Laser weaponry, scientific and materials research laser used in the U.S. military' x airborne laser, operated in continuous wave mode and capable of extremely high power in the megawatt range.
Carbon dioxide laser (CO_2)	10.6 mm (9.4 mm)	Transeverse (high power) or longitudinal (low power) electrical discharge.	Material processing (cutting, welding, etc.), surgery.
Carbon monoxide (CO) gas laser	2.6 mm to 4 mm 4.8 to 8.3 mm	Electrical discharge	Material processing (engraving welding, etc.,), photoacoustic spectroscopy.
Excimer chemical laser	193 nm (ArF), 248 nm (krF), 308 nm (XeCl), 353 nm (XeF)	Excimer recombination via electrical discharge	Ultraviolet lithography for semiconductor manufacturing laser surgery, LASIK.

Table 2.11 Applications of metal vapour lasers

Laser gain medium and type	Operation wavelength (s)	Pump source	Applications
Helium–cadmium He–Cd) metal–vapour laser	440 nm, 325 nm	Electrical discharge in metal vapour mixed with helium buffer gas.	Printing and typesetting applications, fluorescence excitation examination (i.e., in U.S. paper currency printing), scientific research.
Helium–mercury (He–Hg) metal–vapour laser	567 nm, 615 nm	Electrical discharge in metal vapour mixed with helium buffer gas.	Rare, scientific research.
Helium–selenium (He–Se) metal–vapour laser	Up to 24 wavelengths between red and UV	Electrical discharge in metal vapour mixed with helium buffer gas.	Rare, scientific research, amateur laser construction.
Copper vapour laser	510.6 nm, 578.2 nm	Electrical discharge	Dermatological uses, high-speed photography, pump for dye lasers.
Gold vapour laser	627 nm	Electrical discharge	Rare, dermatological and photodynamic therapy uses.

The most important single characteristic of dye lasers is their tunability. This makes them among the most valuable tools available for spectroscopic analysis and photochemistry

Figure 2.23 shows the output powers and wavelengths of several of the most common dyes used in CW dye lasers.

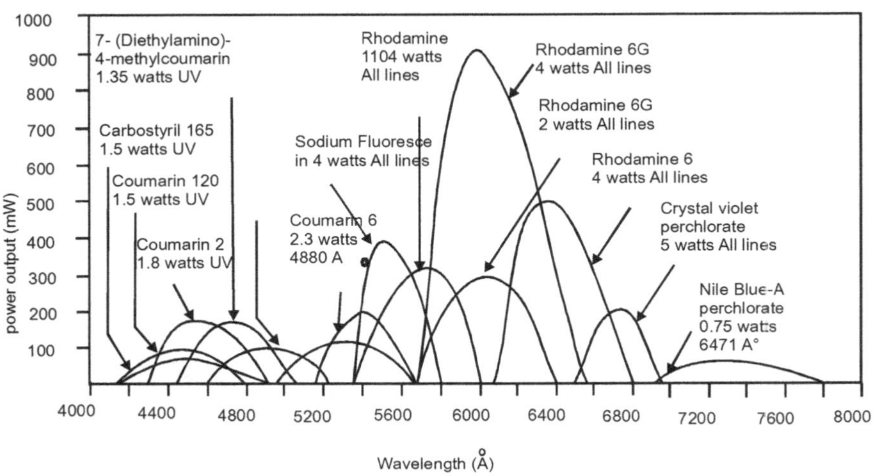

Figure 2.23 Dye laser output curves of some common laser dyes

By selecting a proper dye, one can obtain radiation of any wavelengths. That is, the chemical organic dyes provide a path to wavelength tunability. The organic dye molecules are large and have complicated molecular systems with conjugated double bonds. They show strong absorption bands at visible and UV range of the spectrum. When these dye molecules are excited by light, it emits radiation with large bandwidth of the order of 100 nm in some dyes. The dye lasers were discovered in 1966 by Schafer, Sovoken, Lankara and Stephanoy. They were using dyes for Q-switching of ruby lasers at that time.

The discovery of the dye laser started a revolution in atomic and molecular spectroscopy. The dye lasers are the most important type of laser in scientific research. By virtue of their broad wavelength tunability, wide spectral coverage, and simplicity, organic dye lasers are playing an important role in various fields. The gain of dye lasers can be made extremely high so that lasers with only a few microns of active length can be operated.

These dye lasers are always optically pumped either by a flash lamp or by an auxiliary laser. In the laser pumping, the pump wavelength must be shorter than the output wavelengths. Hence the tunable output of a dye laser has always a longer wavelength than the pump laser.

The complexity of the dye molecule and the factors leading to line splitting produce broad absorption and emission curves as illustrated in Figure 2.24.

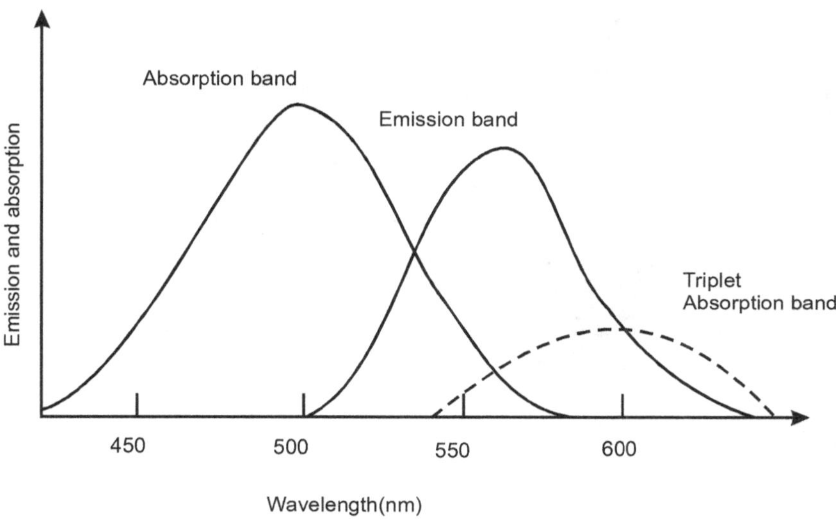

Figure 2.24 Absorption and emission (fluorescence) spectrum of a typical laser dye

A highly simplified energy-level diagram for a typical dye is shown in Figure 2.25.

Rhodamine 6G belongs to xanthene group which absorbs the pumping radiation and fluoresces in the visible region. The structure of Rhodamine 6G, and its absorption and fluorescence spectrum are shown in Figures 2.25 (a–c).

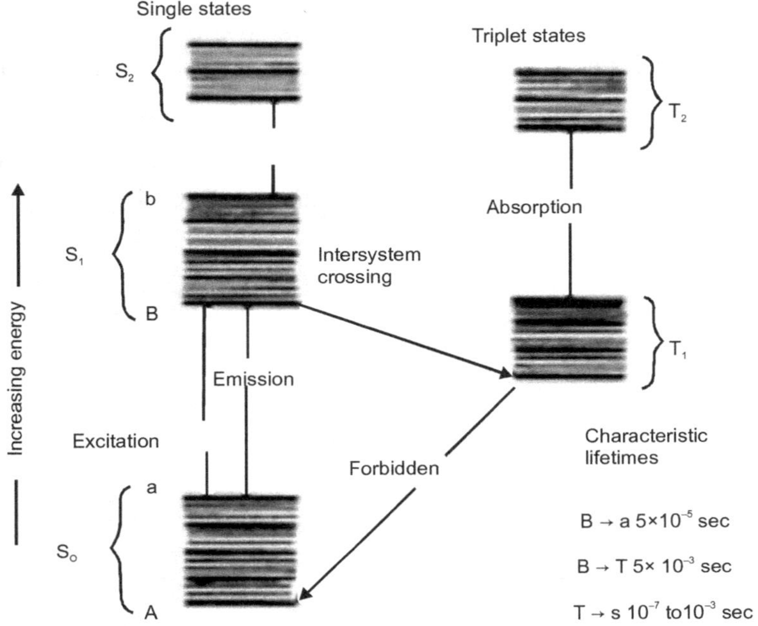

Figure 2.25   Energy-level diagram of a laser dye

(a)

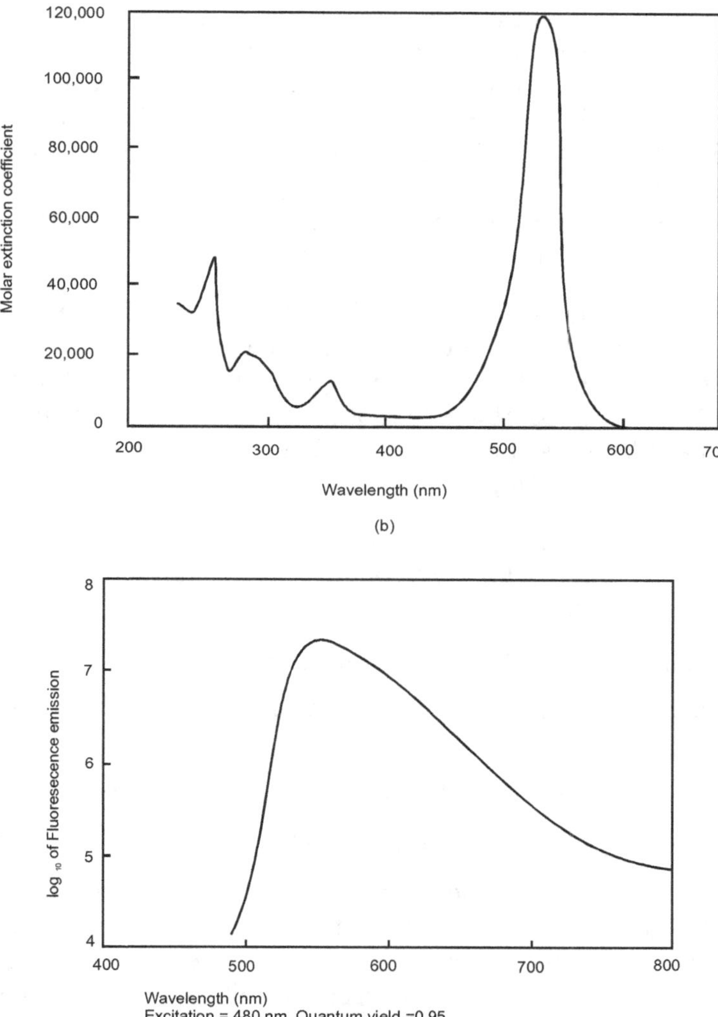

Figure 2.26   (a) Structure (b) Absorption spectra (c) Fluorescence spectra of Rhodamine 6G

The pump laser for the dye laser is a neodymium-doped glass laser or Nd:YAG laser operated in a pulse mode. The pumping beam enters the dye cavity either along the axis or transverse to it. Continuous laser pumping can also be employed to excite dye lasers. In that case argon ion laser is preferred. The dye flow in the cavity not only cools the laser but also removes photo-decay products. That is, the flow systems can be used to carry away excess heat and to cool the active medium as well as the reservoir to any wanted operating temperature even at high average powers. The dye lasers are almost used in research applications in spectroscopy and photochemistry. If laser enrichment of uranium isotopes is possible, then dye laser can be used for this purpose economically. The high-power dye lasers can be used for industrial applications provided the efficiency is high. Unfortunately the efficiency of flash-pumped dye lasers are about 1%. If its efficiency is raised, then the dye lasers become competitive with CO_2 lasers in applications. In that case, the short wavelengths of dye lasers are important.

Flash lamp-pumped dye laser head consists of the dye cuvette, the flash lamp and a pump light reflector or diffuser. The latter serves to concentrate the pumplight emitted from the flash lamp (the extended, uncollimated, broad-band source) onto the absorbing dye solution in the cuvette. A great variety of flash lamps have been used in dye lasers. The simplest possibility is the use of commercial xenon flash lamp.

Fine-tuning and simultaneous attainment of small linewidth can be achieved only by using wavelength-selective resonators. The commonly used four classes of wavelength-selective resonators are

1. resonators including devices for spatial wavelength separation,

2. resonators including devices for interferometric wavelength discrimination,

3. resonators including devices with rotational dispersion and

4. resonators with wavelength-selective distributed feedback.

In this configuration, the grating itself acts as a beam expander of high magnification. Later it was shown that it is more efficient to use a two-prism expander in series with a grating in grazing incidence. These arrangements can be made very compact and are thus especially well-suited for pumping with the short-pulse nitrogen lasers where the cavity round-trip time of the dye laser must be short enough for the spectrally dispersed feedback to reach the dye cell in a state of high inversion.

The important features of good dye lasers are its wavelength stability, reproducibility, amplitude stability and spectral purity. Increasing the efficiency of the flash lamp-pumped dye lasers will bring the average power of dye lasers into the multi-kilowatt region and might make them eligible for specialized industrial applications. The dye lasers which are tunable lasers have a bright future due to their scientific and technological applications listed in Table 2.12

Table 2.12   Applications of Dye Lasers

Laser gain medium and type	Operation wavelength (s)	Pump source	Applications
Dye lasers	390–435 nm (Stilbene), 460–515 nm (Coumarin 102), 570–640 nm (Rhodamine 6G), many others	Other laser, flash lamp	Research, spectroscopy, birthmark removal, isotope separation. The tuning range of the laser depends on the exact dye used.

SEMICONDUCTOR LASERS

At present, nearly 80 per cent of the entire laser market is dominated by semiconductor lasers or laser arrays which are used to pump other solid-state lasers or operate with a coherent output from a two-dimensional array. Output powers in excess of one kilowatt with more than 10 per cent power efficiency should become commercially available. These lasers will provide a major boost for industrial processing and medical applications.

Monolithic diode lasers which operate without an external cavity have spectral linewidths that are typically, 30 MHz at output power levels of about 10 mW. Such spectral linewidths are not useful for a wide range of applications such as radar, optical heterodyne communications and high-resolution spectroscopy.

The source of the spectral broadening in these semiconductor diode lasers is fundamental and quantum in nature and arises from the spontaneous emission noise within the laser. This spontaneous emission noise causes the phase of the electric field vector of the radiation to fluctuate, which in turn leads to a spectral broadening. In addition, damped relaxation oscillators due to the perturbation of the field amplitude by spontaneous emission give rise to side bands. These side bands are typically 1–2 GHz away from the main peak.When such devices are placed into high Q external cavities, the linewidths are significantly reduced. The linewidths of less than 400 Hz have been produced in such lasers. The frequency stability characteristics of free-running external-cavity GaAlAs diode lasers which have already been demonstrated are listed below:

Property	Values
Fundamental width	<1000Hz
Future capability	<10 MHz
Short-term jitter	5 kHz/30 ms
Long-term jitter	7 kHz
Centre frequency drift	5 kHz/h
Locking stability	<10 mHz
Baseband noise	+/–0.5 GHz< 100 dB

Extending the useful frequency range of presently available diode lasers such as GaAlAs can be accomplished by the use of efficient nonlinear frequency conversion. Wide band gap semiconductor diode lasers have been very difficult to operate at wavelengths shorter than 600 nm. The materials of choice would be the II–VI compounds but so far have not proven to operate as diodes because of the inability to fabricate p-type material. Therefore, nonlinear frequency conversion would be one solution for the near-term operation of compact blue diode laser sources.

The **blue laser** is a laser that emits electromagnetic radiation at a wavelength of between 360 and 480 nanometres, which the human eye sees as blue light or else light at the blue end of the spectrum. Diode lasers which emit light at 445 nm are becoming popular as laser pointers. Lasers emitting wavelengths below 445 nm appear violet to the human eye, a distinctly different colour. This is true, for example, of the most commercially common "blue" lasers, the diode lasers used in Blue-ray applications, which emit 405 nm light that is violet. This light causes fluorescence in some chemicals, in the same way that ultraviolet or "black light" does. The class of blue lasers are frequently semiconductor laser diodes based on gallium(III) nitride (violet colour) or indium gallium nitride (often true-blue in colour, but able to produce other colours, as well). Both blue and violet lasers can also be constructed using frequency-doubling of infrared laser wavelengths from diode lasers or diode-pumped lasers. Devices that employ blue laser light have applications in many areas ranging from optoelectronic data storage at high density to medical applications.

Major advances in high-power diode lasers have been made in the world with the development of the graded index-separate confinement heterostructure GaAlAs diode laser. These lasers have produced over one watt of CW power at room temperature with more than 50% power conversion efficiency. One problem with these monolithic devices is the poor spectral output. This may be improved by operation in an external cavity. Because the broadening mechanism in semiconductor lasers leads to a homogeneous gain line, all of the laser output will occur in a single frequency when the devices are operated in a single spatial mode. Such a diode laser has been operated in an external cavity and has produced more than 1.5 watts of continuous power at room temperature in a spectral width of less than 8 GHz and a spatial beam quality which was better than 2–3 times diffraction limited. Because of the energy band properties of quantum-well laser materials, the gain bandwidths can be very broad. A single such laser when operated in an external cavity with a grating has been continuously tuned from 790 to 860 nm at room temperature. Two such lasers have covered the range from 720 to 870 nm. Frequency-doubling of such high-power devices would produce useful radiation from 360–435 nm with additional tuning over the entire visible range possible by parametric conversion.

The use of efficient diode lasers and diode laser arrays are now in widespread use as efficient pump sources for solid-state lasers to provide all solid state, compact, reliable and efficient lasers which are able to produce output from a few mW to 100 W. Such lasers would find numerous applications where the disadvantages of lamp pumping are obvious. The most common material that has been pumped by diode lasers is Nd:YAG which has its main output lines at 1.06 and 1.32 μm.

Laser Diodes

A laser diode is a laser where the active medium is a semiconductor similar to that found in a light-emitting diode. The most common and practical type of laser diode is formed from a *p*-n junction and powered by injected electric current. These devices are sometimes referred to as injection laser diodes to distinguish them from (optically) pumped laser diodes.

A laser diode, like many other semiconductor devices, is formed by doping a very thin layer on the surface of a crystal wafer. The crystal is doped to produce an *n*-type region and a *p*-type region, one above the other, resulting in a *p-n* junction, or diode.

As charge injection is a distinguishing feature of diode lasers as compared to all other lasers, diode lasers are traditionally and more formally called "injection lasers." When an electron and a hole are present in the same region, they may recombine or "annihilate" with the result being spontaneous emission, i.e., the electron may re-occupy the energy state of the hole, emitting a photon with energy equal to the difference between the electron and hole states involved. (In a conventional semiconductor junction diode, the energy released from the recombination of electrons and holes is carried away as phonons, i.e., lattice vibrations, rather than as photons.) Spontaneous emission gives the laser diode below lasing thereshold properties similar to an LED. Spontaneous emission is necessary to initiate laser oscillation, but it is one among several sources of inefficiency once the laser is oscillating.

The difference between the photon-emitting semiconductor laser (or LED) and conventional phonon-emitting (non-light-emitting) semiconductor junction diode lies in the use of a different type of semiconductor, one whose physical and atomic structure confers the possibility for photon emission. These photon-emitting semiconductors are the so-called "direct bandgap" semiconductors. The properties of silicon and germanium, which are single-element semiconductors, have bandgaps that do not align in the way needed to allow photon emission and are not considered "direct". Other materials, the so-called compound semiconductors, have virtually identical crystalline structures as silicon or germanium but use alternating arrangements of two different atomic species in a checkerboard like pattern to break the symmetry. The transition between the materials in the alternating pattern creates the critical "direct bandgap" property. Gallium arsenide, indium phosphide, gallium antimonide, and gallium nitride are all examples of compound semiconductor materials that can be used to create junction diodes that emit light. A simple laser diode is shown in Figure 2.27.

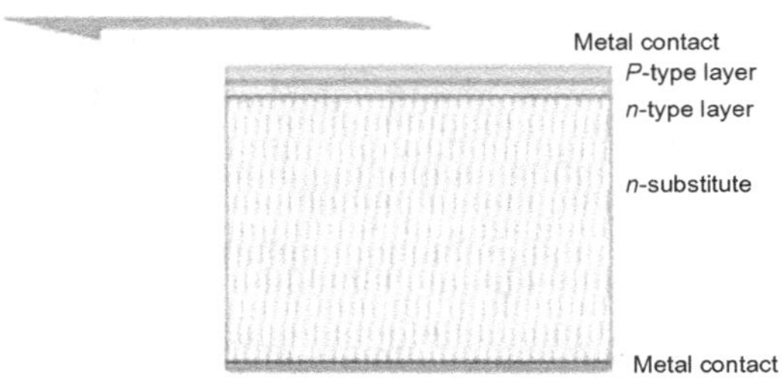

Figure 2.27 A simple laser diode

The spontaneous and stimulated emission processes are vastly more efficient in direct bandgap semiconductors than in indirect bandgap semiconductors and therefore silicon is not a common material for laser diodes.

As in other lasers, the gain region is surrounded with an optical cavity to form a laser. In the simplest form of laser diode, an optical waveguide is made on that crystal surface, such that the light is confined to a relatively narrow line. The two ends of the crystal are cleaved to form perfectly smooth, parallel edges, forming a Fabry–Perot resonator. Photons emitted into a mode of the waveguide travel along the waveguide and are reflected several times from each end face before they are emitted. As a light wave passes through the cavity, it is amplified by stimulated emission, but light is also lost due to absorption and by incomplete reflection from the end facets. Finally, if there is more amplification than loss, the diode begins to "lase".

Some important properties of laser diodes are determined by the geometry of the optical cavity. Generally, in the vertical direction, the light is contained in a very thin layer, and the structure supports only a single optical mode in the direction perpendicular to the layers. In the lateral direction, if the waveguide is wide compared to the wavelength of light, then the waveguide can support multiple lateral optical modes, and the laser is known as "multi-mode". These laterally multi-mode lasers are adequate in cases where one needs a very large amount of power, but not a small diffraction-limited beam. It is used in printing, activating chemicals, or pumping other types of lasers.

In applications where a small focused beam is needed, the waveguide must be made narrow, on the order of the optical wavelength. This way, only a single lateral mode is supported and one ends up with a diffraction-limited beam. Such single spatial mode devices are used for optical storage, laser pointers, and fibre optics. Note that these lasers may still support multiple longitudinal modes, and thus can lase at multiple wavelengths simultaneously.

The wavelength emitted is a function of the band-gap of the semiconductor and the modes of the optical cavity. In general, the maximum gain occurs for photons with energy slightly above the band-gap energy and the modes nearest the gain peak lase most strongly. If the diode is driven strongly enough, additional side modes may also lase. Some laser diodes such as most visible lasers, operate at a single wavelength, but that wavelength is unstable and changes due to fluctuations in current or temperature.

Due to diffraction, the beam diverges rapidly after leaving the chip, typically at 30 degrees vertically by 10 degrees laterally. A lens must be used in order to form a collimated beam like that produced by a laser pointer. If a circular beam is required, cylindrical lenses and other optics are used. For single spatial-mode lasers using symmetrical lenses, the collimated beam ends up being elliptical in shape, due to the difference in the vertical and lateral divergences. This is easily observable with a red laser pointer.

The simple diode described above is extremely inefficient and has been heavily modified in recent years to accommodate modern technology, resulting in a variety of types of laser diodes, as described below.

1. *Double Heterostructure Lasers (DH Lasers)*

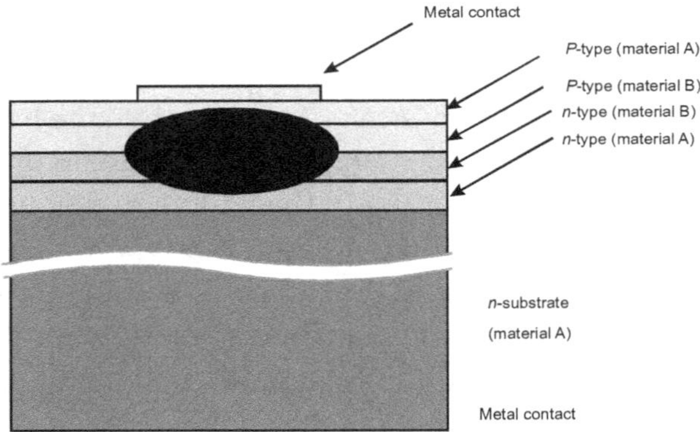

Figure 2.28 Front view of a double heterostructure laser diode

The front view of a double heterostructure laser diode is shown in Figure 2.28. In these devices, a layer of low bandgap material is sandwiched between two high band-gap layers. One commonly used pair of materials is gallium arsenide (GaAs) with aluminium gallium arsenide ($Al_xGa(1-x)As$). Each of the junctions between different bandgap materials is called a heterostructure, hence the name "double heterostructure laser" or DH laser.

The advantage of a DH laser is that the region where free electrons and holes exist simultaneously (the active region) is confined to the thin middle layer. This means that many more of the electron-hole pairs can contribute to amplification—not so many are left out in the poorly amplifying periphery. In addition, light is reflected from the heterojunction and hence,light is confined to the region where the amplification takes place.

2. *Vertical-cavity Surface-Emitting Lasers (VCSEL)* A simple VCSEL structure is shown in Figure 2.29. Vertical-cavity surface-emitting lasers (VCSELs) have the optical cavity axis along the direction of current flow rather than perpendicular to the current flow as in conventional laser diodes. The active region length is very short compared with the lateral dimensions so that the radiation emerges from the surface of the cavity rather than from its edge as shown in the figure. The reflectors at the ends of the cavity are dielectric mirrors made from alternating high and low refractive index quarter-wave thick multilayer.

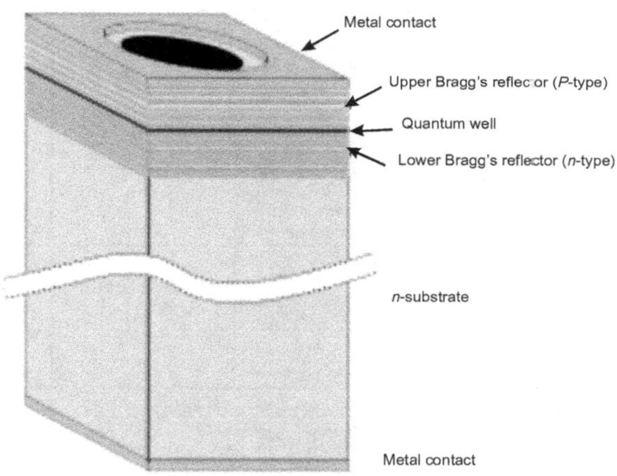

Figure 2.29 A simple VCSEL structure

Such dielectric mirrors provide a high degree of wavelength-selective reflectance at the required free surface wavelength λ if the thicknesses of alternating layers d_1 and d_2 with refractive indices n_1 and n_2 are such that $n_1 d_1 + n_2 d_2 = 1/2\ \lambda$ which then leads to the constructive interference of all partially reflected waves at the interfaces. But there is a disadvantage: because of the high mirror reflectivities, VCSELs have lower output powers when compared to edge-emitting lasers.

There are several advantages to producing VCSELs when compared with the production process of edge-emitting lasers. Edge-emitters cannot be tested until the end of the production process. If the edge-emitter does not work, whether due to bad contacts or poor material growth quality, the production time and the processing materials have been wasted. Additionally, because VCSELs emit the beam perpendicular to the active region of the laser as opposed to parallel as with an edge emitter, tens of thousands of VCSELs can be processed simultaneously on a three-inch gallium arsenide wafer. Furthermore, even though the VCSEL production process is more labour- and material-intensive, th yield can be controlled to a more predictable outcome.

Table 2.13   Different structures of diode lasers

Laser type	Laser structure	Radiation confinement
Homojunction	p-GaAs / n-GaAs — Active region ←p-GaAs	A little confinement in paper plane
Single heterojunction	Heterojunction→ p-GaAlAs / n-GaAs — Active region ← p-GaAs	Good confinement in one side in perpendicular plane (paper)
Double heterojunction	Heterojunction→ p-GaAlAs / n-GaAlAs / n-GaAs — Active region ←GaAs	Good Confinement in both sides in perpendicular plane (paper)
Gain-guided stripe	High electrical resistance material — Heterojunction, n-GaAlAs, n-GaAs, n →p-GaAs, p-GaAlAs, n or p-GaAs, Active region — Wrrent	Good. Confinement between the top and bottom horizontal planes of the active region.
Buried heterojunction (Index-guided stripe geometry)	Oxide, n-GaAs Active region, n-GaAlAs, n-GaAs →p-GaAlAs, n-GaAlAs	Good radiation confinement in both horizontal and perpendicular planes

Table 2.14 Applications of semiconductor lasers

Laser gain medium and type	Operation wavelength (s)	Pump source	Applications
Semiconductor laser diode	Wavelength depends on device material: 0.4 mm (GaN) or 0.63 mm – 1.55 mm (AlGaAs) or 3 –20 mm (lead salt)	Electrical current	Telecommunications, holography, laser pointers, printing, pump sources for other lasers. The 780 nm AlGaAs laser diode, used in compact disc players, is the most common type of laser in the world.

Review Questions

1. What are DPSSL? Explain their importance.

2. Why non-linear crystals are important? Mention the most promising non-linear crystals.

3. What is second harmonic generation? How can it be produced?

4. Mention the techniques to achieve gain in solid state lasers.

5. List the advantages and disadvantages of glass lasers.

6. Mention a few advantages of crystalline laser hosts over the glass.

7. Whar are garnets? Explain their properties.

8. Describe the construction and working of a ruby laser with energy level diagram.

9. Discuss Nd doped lasers. Explain the working of Nd:YAG laser with its energy level diagram.

10. Explain a typical Nd doped glass laser.

11. Write a note on Ti:sapphire laser.

12.   Describe the various types of pumping cavities used in laser.

13.   Explain the semiconductor laser pumping technique.

14.   Describe the construction and working of a CO_2 laser with energy level diagram.

15.   Describe the He-Ne laser and its working.

16.   What are excimer lasers? Explain.

17.   Describe the construction and working of a typical metal vapour laser.

18.   Draw a schematic diagram of a argon ion laser. Explain its working and uses.

19.   Explain the importance of a dye laser and list its applications.

20.   Write notes on (i) double heterostructure laser (ii) vertical cavity surface emitting laser.

Chapter 3

Laser Light–Tissue Interaction

INTRODUCTION

Understanding lasers begins with understanding the acronym LASER—light amplification by the stimulated emission of radiation. All states of matter—solids, liquids and gases—contain potential energy and can be stimulated to emit it in packets of light called photons. When a stimulated atom absorbs a photon, energy states of electrons change causing the emission of a series of identical photons. Argon gas, CO_2 gas, ruby crystals, Nd:YAG crystals, liquid dyes and other mediums are capable of absorbing the emitting photons of various wavelengths. Long-wavelength photons with low levels of energy and short-wavelength photons with high intensity have different biological effects in tissue. The difference in tissue effects on lasers depend on their degree of absorption in target tissue and energy delivery scheme. Ultimately thermal effects of the laser play an important role in precise surgical effects.

Laser wavelengths are found not only in the visible range but also in the infrared and ultraviolet region of the electromagnetic spectrum, and they are non-ionizing radiation. That is, laser light does not accumulate in cells and cannot cause cellular change or damage as X-rays and gamma radiation. Although laser radiation passes through the tissue, it is safe for pregnant women patients and staff. This is also the reason why no monitoring badges or shielding devices are necessary for laser radiations.

Laser light is different from ambient light because it is coherent, collimated and monochromatic. These unique properties make lasers to work as surgical tools. The coherent property of laser light uniformly absorbs, with minimal loss of energy. Coherence helps to focus a beam sharply using an optical system. Precise collimation reduces the diffusion of energy and allows delivery as an intense beam through mirrors or fibre optics. This concentrated energy does not disperse in space and produces a beam that holds its intensity until it is bent, absorbed or changed mechanically. Laser light is monochromatic — all in one colour or wavelength. It is this property that enables us to use the light to surgically alter tissue.

The effects of the laser beam on the biological tissues are as follows:

1. Thermal effects are produced by most continuous wave lasers such as CO_2, YAG and argon. The laser energy is absorbed by the biological tissue, raising the local temperature, so the tissue can be ablated, vaporized, coagulated or cut.

2. Mechanical effects arise especially when short pulses of high-power laser are used to create a "blast" by heating a small region of tissue to high temperature in a very short time. The blast creates a shock wave that disrupts the tissue nearby. This effect is used in eye treatment for disrupting posterior capsule in secondary cataract.

3. Chemical effects are used in photo-dynamic therapy (PDT). Excimer lasers are employed in reshaping the cornea.

4. Optical Processes—The parameter that summarizes the effects of laser radiation on biological tissue is fluence.

$$\text{Fluence} = (\text{Watt} \times \text{time})/\text{Spot size}$$

When a laser beam falls on matter, four processes can take place. They are 1) reflection, 2) scattering, 3) transmission and 4) absorption. Only absorption can transfer energy to the material so that there is a rise in temperature or chemical reaction.

The interaction between electromagnetic radiation and biological tissue depends on

1. The wavelength of light which determines the energy of each photon of light.

2. The intensity of radiation.

3. The shape of irradiation (continuous or pulsed).

For power levels up to few watts, the interaction is divided into three regions of wavelengths.

1.   Short UV region—the photons interact with the proteins, RNA and DNA and usually kill the biological cells.

2.   Near-UV and short visible range—cause photochemical reactions such as photosynthesis, especially with the Excimer laser.

3.   Visible and near-infrared region—thermal effects due to absorption of the radiation. When using lasers for medical treatments, a good understanding of the interaction between specific laser radiation with specific biological tissue is required.

Each wavelength interacts differently with body tissue and each brings about different surgical or medical effects. Hence, many types of medical lasers such as carbon dioxide, Nd:YAG, Ho:YAG, argon, KTP, dye, alexandrite, ruby and diode are available and no one system can perform all types of procedures. Further the type of emission whether it is continuous or pulsed is also an important factor as medical applications are concerned. The duration of the emission can vary according to the excitation duration from milliseconds to nanoseconds. The energy and the power densities are usually important. The small focal spot in which the beam is concentrated by a proper laser can reach up to hundreds of J/cm to MW/cm.

Laser light has four main characteristics that determine how each wavelength can be used in tissues. The tissue–radiation interactions are transmission, absorption, scattering, and reflection. Each of these properties affect the laser cutting, coagulation or vaporization of tissues. A thorough understanding of these four characteristics of light with tissues is necessary before the physician selects the correct laser system for a particular application.

Absorption is the way a laser interacts with biological material in tissue. The main substance that absorbs light are water, protein, melanin, and haemoglobin. Carbon dioxide laser is a multipurpose laser because it is absorbed by water. Since most body cells are composed of more than 85% water, light is easily absorbed. Light radiations develop heat when absorbed by the tissues and hence the intracellular water begins to boil. They swell continuously until they disrupt by emitting water vapour, carbon, and cellular particulates. Vaporization of cells allows for precise, rapid removal of tissue, as well as excellent excision, incision, and dissection. CO_2 laser does not coagulate well due to its affinity for water and will seal only the smallest vessels of diameter less than 0.5 mm.

Nd:YAG (neodymium, yttrium,ytterbium and garnet crystal) laser, not only passes through water but is also absorbed in tissue protein, coagulating up to

6 mm. It is the most haemostatic of all surgical lasers with the ability to seal a bleeding vessel of up to 1.5 mm. Since CO_2 laser travels so deeply into tissue, it does not cut or vaporize and can damage peripheral tissues if not carefully controlled. The CO_2 (10,600 nm) and the Nd:YAG (1064 nm) are invisible and hence they require an auxiliary low-power, visible, aiming laser beam. Most lasers use a helium–neon (630 nm) laser of very low intensity as an aiming beam. Interestingly, this aiming beam has no independent effect on tissue.

Depending on the temperature, many kinds of changes can occur in the biological system. As tissue begins to heat above 60°C, it begins to desiccate, blanch white and shrink, as proteins denature and flash boil at 100°C. Different lasers cause absorptive heating as follows:

Temp °C	Visual change	Biological change
100+	Smoke plume	Vaporization, carbonization
90–100	Pluckering	Drying, elimination of fluids
65–90	White/grey	Protein denaturation
60–65	Blanching	Coagulation
37–60	None	Warming, welding

Visible wavelengths (Argon, KTP, dyes) are absorbed by chromophores in tissues of opposite colour. The blue-green Argon (488, 514 nm) is highly absorbed in red-brown structures that contain melanin and/or haemoglobin. Argon transmits through water and is shallow in its penetration (2–3 nm) so that it can be used to coagulate superficial vessels with precision and safety.

KTP works by changing the frequency of Nd:YAG (1064 nm) by passing it through a crystal of potassium titanyl phosphate (KTP) which doubles the frequency and results in a visible green beam (532 nm). KTP works very much like Argon in absorption mechanism and tissue effects. It can be delivered through fibres and transmits easily through water and is an effective endoscopic tool.

Other visible wavelengths, such as dye lasers (575–850 nm), are more useful on light brown and pink lesions. Visible light lasers are the most effective for ophthalmic surgery and for both vascular and pigmented dermatologic lesions. A large number of these lasers are available in the market with both Q-switching and pulsed mechanisms and delivery by both articulated arms or fibre optics.

In order to work as a surgical tool, laser light must be transmitted into the tissue. Lasers are very different from electrical energy in their effects on tissue. Electrical energy travels along the path of least resistance, causing uncontrollable areas of injury. Its depth of penetration and lateral zone of destruction cannot be predetermined. It cannot produce the precise effects of laser energy which is absorbed by tissue components such as water, protein and pigment.

In summary, laser action can be obtained in almost every material within the proper operating condition. The active medium can be solid, liquid or gaseous phase. The transition can be rotational, vibrational, electronic, atomic or molecular for the different laser wavelengths. All of them possesses the fundamental property such as monochromaticity, directionality, and spatial and temporal coherence.

ForCWlasersthepoweroftheradiationdefinescompletelytheenergycontent. For pulsed lasers, a pulse duration is usually defined at full width half maximum (FWHM). The repetition rate of the pulses determines the average power as the product of the single pulse energy and the repetition rate.

The relevance of the various laser parameters in medical applications is given in the following Table 3.1.

Table 3.1 Relevance of laser parameters in medical applications

Parameter	Relevance	Effects
Brightness	Very high	Intense local heating, non-contact interaction
Spatial coherence	Moderate	Extreme focusabiligy, optical fibre coupling
Pulsed power	Moderate	Continued thermal effects nonlinear processes
Tunability	Moderate	Selective absorption, (chromophores, sensitizers)
Monochromaticity	Low	Extreme focus ability

The effects of laser on tissues can be listed as

1.   Tissue heating: a) Skin rejuvenation, b) tissue welding

2.   Coagulation :   a) Haemostasis, b)Protein with attendant necrosis

3.   Vaporization :   a) Cutting (ablating along a fine line with traction), b) Debulking (ablating volumes of tissues)

4.   Non-linear effects: a)Cold cutting–ophthalmic Nd:YAG, b) Photoacoustical "Lithotripsy" c) Fragmentation of tattoo pigment via, Q-switched lasers (Here the shock waves that rip and tear the tissues. In ophthalmic case, it creates tiny sparks in thin air which tear apart the clouded membrane behind the lens.)

5.   Photochemistry: a) Photodynamic therapy (PDT)

6.   Photodisso ciation: a) Non thermal ablation of the cornea in ophthalmology (This is vision correction laser. The laser wavelength of 193 nm removes tissue without heat generation)

In general, laser is actually vaporizing the cells when they cut or debulk tissues. Further, the way the energy is delivered in terms of its peak power, pulse duration and spot size are more important than the wavelength in the clinical choice of the laser system. Tissue reaction with lasers is shown in Figure 3.1.

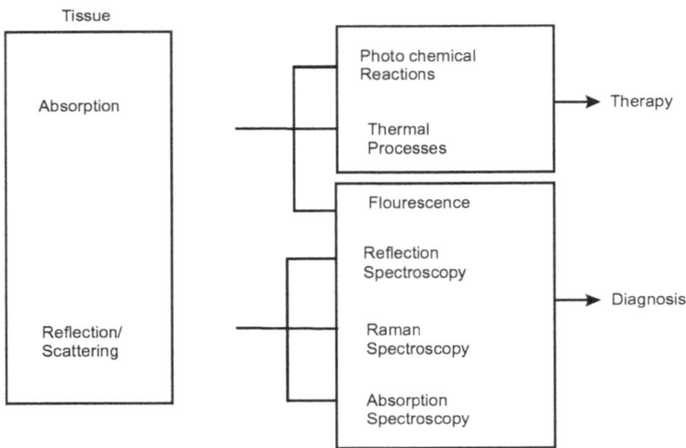

Figure 3.1 Tissue reaction with laser

3.2   PHOTOPHYSICAL PROCESS IN LASER–TISSUE INTERACTION

A good amount of research has been done on the photobiological interaction between non-ionizing radiation and living tissues in the submillimeter part of electromagnetic spectrum and in the optical region. In the specific case of laser radiation, the unique characteristic of monochromaticity of the incident field and the spatial and temporal coherence of the emission, find increasing use in medical applications, in both diagnosis and therapy. The primary interaction of laser light with tissue is shown in Figure 3.2.

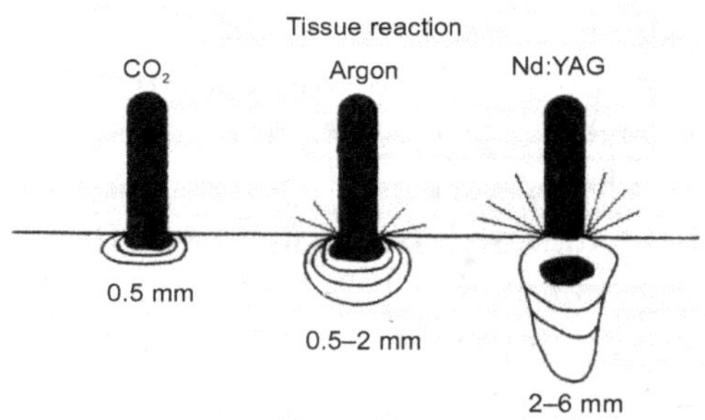

Figure 3.2   LASER –Tissue Interaction

The biological response of the irradiated tissue is due to the various process-es of conversion of the incident electromagnetic energy within biomolecules. Figure 3.3 shows a plot of power density and interaction time for different effects.

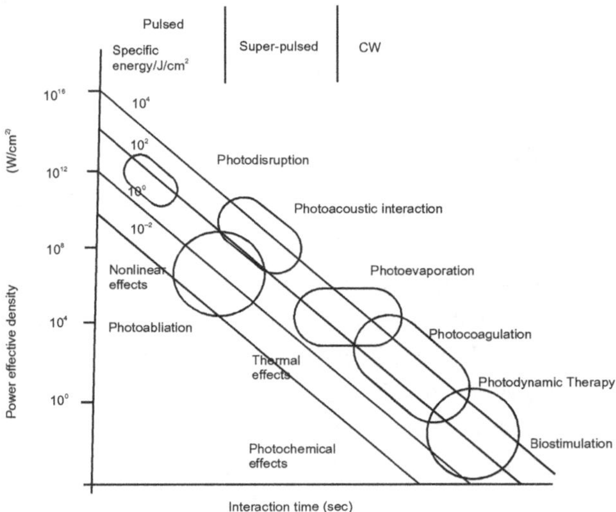

Figure 3.3   Laser–Tissue Interactions as a Funciton of Interaction

Time and Power Density

The specific modes of interaction of laser radiation with tissue characterizes the various applications in diagnosis and therapy. The effect of laser radiation on body tissue depends on the 1) absorption characteristics of the tissue, 2) the characteristics of the laser radiation and 3) biological effects consequent to the interaction. A detailed understanding has not yet been developed, although the details about interactions are well-known. The most dominant mechanism is a thermal process following absorption of the laser radiation. The mid-infrared 1.06 μm beam of the CO_2 laser is strongly absorbed by the high water content in cellular tissue. The water is heated, and vaporized tissue disrupts. This is characterized by an interaction distance of less than 1 mm for the CO_2 laser and typically 6 mm for the tunable dye (0.340–1.1μm) Nd:YAG 1.06 μm and Argon (0.485 – 0.515 μm). The intermediate absorption distance of laser radiation by tissues causes volume interaction with scattering and weak absorption. But the strong absorption distance causes surface interaction with low scattering of radiation. The wavelength, nature of absorption and nature of interaction of four commonly used lasers are given below.

Laser	Tunable dye	Nd:YAG	CO_2	Argon
Wavelength	0.340 – 1.1 mm	1.06 mm	1.06 mm	0.485–0.515 mm
Nature of absorption	Intermediate absorption	Weak absorption	Strong absorption	Scattering
Nature of interaction	Volume interaction	Volume interaction	Surface interaction	Low scattering

The absorption by water at the Nd:YAG laser wavelength is low and the beam is mainly absorbed by haemoglobin and pigmented tissue. Hence, it has an intermediate characteristic absorption distance. With absorption of the laser radiation, the tissue cells are destroyed and it is often important to minimize damage to surrounding normal tissue. When this is well-vascularized, such as in the gastrointestinal tract or in the liver, damage to adjacent tissue is limited to about 0.1 mm for the CO_2 laser, about 1 mm for the argon laser and approximately 6 mm for the Nd:YAG laser. It is seen that the effect of the CO_2 laser is highly localized and this leads to the use of the laser for surgical cutting. The interaction volume with argon laser is greater and with the Nd:YAG, it is still great. Scattering in the inhomogeneous tissue with the Nd:YAG laser leads to a volume of interaction several times larger than the laser spot size.

The thermal contraction which occurs initially causes sealing of small blood vessels and coagulation, with a reduction in haemorrhage. Coagulation with CO_2 laser is mainly by conduction from the laser beam and the largest size of blood vessel which can be sealed is limited to about 1 mm. The larger interaction volume of the Nd:YAG laser enables larger vessels to be sealed. The advantages of both good excision and coagulation with the Nd:YAG laser can be best achieved by incorporating both CO_2 and Nd:YAG lasers in a new laser arrangement.

When power levels are insufficient to produce substantial heating, biophysical effects may occur by biostimulation or through the use of tissue-sensitizing agents. Although the biostimulation mechanism is uncertain, one possible mechanism for low levels of laser radiation is to stimulate cell division so that the rate of biological process is increased (For example, in the rate of healing of skin ulcers.) This area is presently being further explored with argon and He–Ne lasers.

By various mechanisms, high-power pulsed laser interacts with tissues. The output of pulsed laser can be of duration 10^{-3} , 10^{-6} or 10^{-8} seconds or even shorter. The instantaneous high power of the laser beam when focused on the tissue produces sufficiently high electrical fields for electrical breakdown and sufficiently high temperature to form a plasma, causing disruption of the surface. Excimer lasers produce ultraviolet radiation in the range 193–315 nm, which is strongly absorbed by biological tissues and with a 10^{-7} second laser pulse, the surface can be photoablated. Since the focal spot size of the excimer laser is a few microns, a very small and well-defined region can be selectively destroyed. There are five basic types of laser–tissue interaction. They are

1. *Photothermal*   Laser light (above intensity threshold) falling on tissue produces heat and hence there is a rise in temperature. The radiations are absorbed by water, tissue pigments and proteins. Such absorption is wavelength-dependent.

2. *Photodisruptive*   The pulsed laser energy associated with acoustic energy (Photoacoustic high-pressure acoustic wave) causes mechanical interaction

with the tissue. This type of photomechanical interaction is dependent on peak power and not on wavelength.

3a. *Photochemical*   Laser radiations (low intensity and wave-length-selective) are used for photo-excitation and hence the chemical energy breaks the chemical bonds or excite the molecules to reactive state. The short wavelengths are used for photochemical interactions.

3b. *Photodynamic*   (Photochemical and photoablation—Photodynamic interaction activate singlet oxygen from specific molecules. The specific wavelengths are employed for photo- ablation.

4. *Bio-stimulation*   Low-power laser radiation is used for healing skin ulcers. Research is on the way in this area and the laser-healing mechanism will be clear in future.

5. *Photomechanical*   This term usually defines mechanical interaction of the target with the acoustic wave associated with the transient absorption of a pulsed radiation. It is used in laser lithotripsy.

Photothermal Interaction

All laser surgical applications, whether in the cutting or haemostatic mode, rely upon the conversion of electromagnetic energy to thermal energy. This is achieved by focusing a beam onto spot sizes, a few micrometres or millimetres wide. Such collimation is possible because of the spatial coherence of lasers which can supply high-energy densities. The spatially confined heating of target tissue helps in tissue removal, control of bleeding and in thermal injury. The choice of wavelength determines the depth of penetration and thus influences the interplay between tissue removal and haemostasis.

In fact, the vast majority of therapeutic application of lasers takes advantage of their capability for some spatial control over the degree and extent of tissue injury. The characterization of the photothermal biological response following laser irradiation depends, however, on the structural level that is targeted.

At the microscopic level, the photothermal process originates from the bulk absorption occurring in molecular vibration–rotation bands or in the vibrational manifold of the lowest electronic excited state, instantaneously followed by subsequent rapid thermalization through nonradiative decay. Since tissue structures may be considered as a complex condensed-phase media, rotation is hindered and vibrational amplitudes are more or less damped. Hence, energy levels are not sharp but broadened. The reaction with a target molecule A proceeds in two nearly simultaneous steps.

1.   The absorption of a photon of energy hv, promoting A to a vibronic state A*.

2.   An inelastic scattering occurring at 1–100 psec time-scale with a collisional partner M belonging to the surrounding medium.

3.   On colliding with A*, M instantaneously increases its kinetic energy to M′ by carrying away the internal energy released by A*. The microscopic origin of the temperature rise results from the amount of energy released to M. This two-step reaction can be represented as follows

Absorption: $A + hv \rightarrow A^*$ (vibronic)

Deactivation: $A^* + M(E) \rightarrow A + M(E+DE)$ (thermal)

For completeness, it should be mentioned that in standard thermodynamic conditions the kinetic energy per molecule, kT, is about 0.025 eV whereas the so-called thermal lasers such as CO_2 , Nd:YAG, and argon, have corresponding photon energies 5 to 100 times larger (**CO_2:** $\lambda = 10.6$ μm, $e = 0.12$ eV; **Nd: YAG:** $\lambda = 1.064$ μm, $e = 1.17$ eV; **Ar** : $\lambda = 514$ nm, $e = 2.4$ eV)

The photophysical parameter of interest is α (cm^{-1}) the absorption coefficient which also measures the characteristic absorption length $1/\alpha$ This wavelength or frequency-dependent coefficient $\alpha(v)$ is the product of the molecular absorption cross-section σ (cm^2) and the number density n (number of homogeneously distributed absorbing molecules per unit volume measured in cm^3).

$$\alpha(v) = \sigma n$$

The quantity is the absorbance. A more commonly used form of this law is $I = I_0 10^{\varepsilon(v)cl}$ where $\varepsilon(v)$ measured in L.Mol^{-1}.cm^{-1} is the molar (decadic) extinction coefficient characteristic of each molecular species in a given solvent and c (mol/L) is the concentration of the absorbing substance.

The absorption of tissue in the UV varies drastically depending on the concentration of DNA and aromatic residues of proteins but in general most organic molecules absorb very strongly in this range. The water absorption coefficient which typically reaches 106 cm^{-1} in the vacuum UV at 100 nm, exhibits a dramatic cut-off around 190 nm and has no significant absorption throughout the entire UV range. For physiological saline, absorption starts below about 200 nm, reaching $\varepsilon \sim 300$ 1/mol-cm at 193 nm, the wavelength of the ArF excimer laser. This absorption is, however, due to chlorine ions. Nucleic acids which constitute about 10 –15% of a cell's dry weight, are the most widespread absorbers in 190–300 nm spectral region. Infrared radiation, on the other hand, is absorbed mainly by water with increasingly stronger bands toward longer wavelengths (300 cm–1 at 3μm) with typical absorption depths as small as 10 μm in the far-IR. Between 600 nm and 1,200 nm, radiation penetrates into tissue with low losses due to weaker scattering and absorption and hence reaches deep targets.

The first mechanism by which tissue is thermally affected is molecular denaturation (e.g., proteins, collagen, lipids and haemoglobin). Table 3.2 summarizes the temperature ranges of successive transformations.

Table 3.2 Histological changes in photothermal processes (Conversion of electromagnetic radiation into heat elevation of tissue temperature)

Temperature	Effects
43 – 45°C	Conformational changes, retraction, hyperthermia (cell mortality)
50°C	Reduction of enzyme activity
60°C	Protein denaturation, coagulation
80°C	Collagen denaturation, membrane permeabilization, carbonization
100°C	Vaporization and ablation

In the neighbourhood of $T \sim 45°C$ (hyperthermic range), one observes a tissue retraction related to macromolecular conformational changes, bond destructions and membrane alterations. The range of protein denaturation is between 50°C and 60°C. As the molecule reaches its "melting temperature", the densely packed polynucleotide chain unfolds and a process called "chain melting" occurs, which is associated with a marked increase in light absorption around 260 nm.

Above the protein denaturation temperature, coagulation, necrosis and vacuolation are produced. The temperature limit at which tissues become carbonized is about 80°C. Vaporization occurs beyond 100°C, predominantly from heated free water. The high vaporization heat of water (2,530 J/g) is advantageous, since the steam generated carries away excess heat, thereby preventing further temperature increase of adjacent tissue. Vaporization, together with carbonization, yields decomposition of tissue constituents.

The major problem with material removal is to adjust the duration of laser exposure in order to minimize tissue injury and thermal damage to adjacent zones so as to obtain little necrosis. The scaling parameter for this time-dependent problem is the so-called thermal relaxation time τ associated with a characteristic diffusion length L. From heat diffusion theory, this latter quantity can be shown to be proportional to the square root of time together with a lumped physical parameter, the tissue diffusivity K(cm^2/sec), characterizing the material thermal response (thermal conductivity, specific heat and density). The relaxation time is then related to L through a relationship of the form $L^2 = 4\,KT$

For example, since the thermal diffusirity of water is $K = 1.43 \times 10^{-3}$ cm^2/ sec, heat diffuses approximately to 0.8 mm in 1 sec in aqueous media. Similarly, typical thermal relaxation times associated with 10 μm vessels are of the order of 2×10^{-4} sec, whereas for microvasculature of 100 μm size, it is approximately 1.8×10^{-2} sec. The relationship serves as the theoretical basis of a scheme, called selective photothermolysis, making use of pulsed irradiation to confine thermally mediated radiation damage to choose pigmented targets at the ultrastructural, cellular or tissue structural level. In the clinical procedure, coagulation and/or vaporization of the tissue must be obtained with minimum thermal damage to the nonirradiated healthy tissue. This requires a precise control of the temperature rise in the irradiated volume and in the surrounding zones. The temperature in the irradiated volume must reach the coagulation or vaporization limit, while it must remain below the irreversible damage limit in the untreated tissue. By adjusting the duration of the exposure to the light beam, its energy content and the repetition rate, the temperature rise in the irradiated volume and in the adjacent zones can be controlled in a sufficiently precise way.

If the pulse duration is much shorter than the characteristic time τ then the heat to diffuse along a length is nearlyequal to the penetration depth $1/\alpha$ of the optical radiation. Hence, the optical energy of the pulse is trapped in a volume

s/a (s–beam cross section) where it produces a high temperature increase. The expression of τ is given by

$$\tau = 1/4\,k\alpha^2$$

For example, for water $k = 1.4 \times 10^{-3}$ cm^2/s (approximately heat diffuses 0.8 cm in 1sec), heat of vaporization is 2530J/g at $\lambda = 10.6$ µm (CO$_2$ laser), for $\alpha = 103$ cm^{-1}; $1/\alpha = 10$ µm and thus $\tau = 179$ µs

Consequently, by pulsing the laser with pulse shorter than 179 µs it is possible to vaporize tissue directly.

Typical pulse of 10 mJ/50 µs from a CO$_2$ laser operating at 50 Hz would vaporize spots and would cut with a velocity larger than 10 mm/s.

The laser interaction with tissue under photothermal conditions are summarized in Table 3.3.

Table 3.3   Laser Radiation Interaction with Tissue Under Photothermal Conditon (Above threshold intensity)

Photothermal interaction	Effects
Laser hyperthermia	Condition of elevated tissue temperature below coagulation threshold (40–50^0 C) Enzyme activation Cancer therapy Laser thermal keratoplasty Uniform heating to 70–80°C avoiding shrinkage
Tissue weldings/Anastomoses	Irreversible damage induced by prolonged temperature rise in tissues (50 – 100°C) Permanent denaturation of proteins Tissue whitening and shrinkage Body response : dead tissue removal (not under control)
Coagulation	Coagulation of blood vessels up to effective sealing Deliberate coagulation and death of target tissue

Photothermal interaction	Effects
Haemostasis	Tissue removal through conversion into gaseous vapour
Necrosis	(T > 100° C) cutting
	Endoscopy optical fibre + suction tube
	Reduces bleeding due to haemostasis
	Heat conduction thermal time constant τ
	Surgical precision and control trades off with haemostasis
	(λ-dependent)
Vaporization	Fast water heating, explosive phase transition and mechanical disruption.
Spallation	
Selective photothermolysis	Selection of wavelength and pulsed duration to limit heating to specific structure (dermatological removal of tattoos or pigmented lesions)

Photochemical Interaction

Light may act as a reactant in a photochemical reaction. In this case, the photon energy excites a particular chromophore in a complex biological process, the final outcome of which has a therapeutical relevance. The two processes under photochemical reactions are

1. Reactions in which molecules are involved as energy carriers or as catalytic regulators after experiencing a photoexcitation. In this case the chromophore receptors are said to be photoactivated. One of the most attractive applications of this type is laser spectral sensitization in which photodynamic therapy (PDT) of malignant tumours appears to be a highly promising technique.

2. Reactions in which the chromophore molecules are modified and converted into photoproducts. An example of general importance is the photoinactivation caused by short-wavelength ultraviolet light used in the recently introduced technique of photoablative microsurgery.

A chromophore compound capable of causing light-induced reactions in molecules that do not absorb light in the same wavelength range is known as a photosensitizer. Following resonant excitation by a monochromatic source, the photosensitizer undergoes a series of simultaneous or sequential decays which result in intramolecular transfer reactions. The decays may ultimately culminate in the release of highly reactive cytotoxic species that cause irreversible oxidation of some essential cellular component and destroy affected host tissues. The essence of this photochemical interaction is photosensitized oxidation, due to the exogenous chromophore receptor which basically acts as a photocatalyst. It is first activated by resonant absorption, thereby storing energy in one of its excited states. When it deactivates, a chain reaction takes place with a reactant that is not the photosensitizer. Typical photosensitizers are haematoporphyrin derivative (HpD). The wavelength choice is red radiation 600–700 nm which penetrate deeply in the tissue.

The photochemical interaction involves low-intnsity and wavelength-selective lasers.

Wavelength	Photochemical interaction
200–315 nm	Cells and tissues absorb strongly. Unspecific excitation of many subsystems.
315–400 nm	Limited absorption by biomolecules. Some specific absorptions.
400–1000 nm	Little absorption by biomolecules. Human cells and tissue are transparent except for red blood cells. Act as optical window between 600–1000 nm.
>1000 nm	All biomolecules have specific and strong vibrational absorption bands.

The possible sequence of events following exposure of skin to non-ionizing radiation leads to beneficial and/or adverse effects as follows:

Chromophore → photochemistry → Photoproucts → altered cellfunction → mediators → biologic responses → beeficial effects and/or adverse effects

Photomechanical (Photodisruptive) Interactions

It is the mechanical interaction of the target with the acoustic wave associated to the transient absorption of pulsed radiation. This type of effect becomes significant even at 1–10 J/cm causing a characteristic vacuolization and rupture of the tissue structure. The physical principles lying behind laser-induced breakdown are 1) short laser pulse focussed at target, 2) high power density, 3) high electric field, 4) dielectric breakdown (multiphoton process), 5) plasma formation (free electron), 6) spherical shock wave propagating at low velocity and 7) localized mechanical rupture for small radius.

Basically laser pulse determines a plasma formation via a laser-induced breakdown. This sudden plasma formation couples a substantial energy to a spherical shock wave propagating into surrounding media. If the irradiation site is submerged into water, the shock wave cannot expand freely and a strong recoil force is transmitted through the tissue bulk. If this force overcomes the strength linking together different portions of a composite structure such as a urinary calculus, it becomes possible to obtain a fragmentation in smaller pieces. This is known as lithotripsy and is entirely neglecting on the excitation of a photomechanical interaction process. In photomechanical interaction, a high-power pulsed laser is used to generate a fast high-pressure sound wave which causes a mechanical impulse to the tissue. Its special features are the following:

1.   high laser power densities

2.   short pulse duration ($d\tau = 10^{-6}$ to 10^{-9} s)

3.   light concentration to small spot(focusing or fibre guiding)

4.   disruptive effect limited to surroundings of target point

The conversion mechanism is as follows: When ($d\tau > 1\mu s$) a short absorption in target tissue is required or an absorbin mechanical transducer is provided. When $d\tau < 10$ ns, laser- initiated optical breakdown occurs. This causes plasma formation and inverse bremsstrahlung absorption occurs. This leads to expansion of tissue and causes cavitation. Finally tissue disrupts. The photodisruptive interactions can be used in membranectomy, lithotripsy, calcified tissue ablation and tumour disruption.

Photoablative Interaction

As already stated, UV radiations are very strongly absorbed by most biomolecules specifically in a band extending from 200 nm to 320 nm. Table 3.4 presents the sequence of effects induced by UV radiation and leading to photodissociation and the release of molecular-scale fragments called ablation. Because of the high quantum energy of UV radiation (6.2 to 4 eV), it can modify and even convert chromophores into photoproducts by photodissociation of functionally important compounds such as proteins, nucleic acids, enzymes and pigments.

This feature has recently been exploited experimentally to produce a well-defined, non-necrotic, photoablative cuts of very small width 50 μm by exposure to excimer lasers at several UV wavelengths (ArF : 193 nm, 6.4 eV; KrF : 248 nm, 5 eV; XeCl : 308 nm, 4.3 eV), with short pulses (15 ns) focused on various tissues (cornea, skin, plaques). Similar sharp cuts with minimal thermal damage are also obtained with the third harmonic of the Nd:YAG laser at 266 nm (4.7 eV), with excellent cutting aspect owing to the high spatial quality of the beam. Control of thermal damage is clinically important since it generally produces undesirable biological effects.

Ablative photodecomposition is a new technique to make a controlled depth and shape in defined areas of specific tissue or body structure and to remove any amount of tissue by ablating that tissue to a predetermined depth. True ablative photodecomposition needs the employment of lasers emitting high peak power UV radiation. In this spectral region, laser ablation produces a trench with sharp and clearly defined boundaries by light microscopy. Among the various ophthalmological applications, the application for refractive keratoplasty is of great interest as the cornea can be reshaped to correct the most moderate degrees of hyperopia, myopia and astigmatic defects.

Table 3.5 gives the different threshold observed to ablate a typical tissue with the available excimer laser lines. It is interesting to notice that UV photoablation is inherently a pulsed process of 100 ns atmost if a requirement of minimal thermal conduction from the irradiated zone to the bulk has to be fulfilled.

In general, photoablation is a process which removes biological material with specific issues such as,

1. great depth control because each pulse etches only a few tens of microns

2. a very limited part of the incoming energy is channelled into heat so that a limited rise of temperature takes place at the border and

3. very clean and sharp edges, cuts or holes can be obtained in almost all types of tissues with ultraviolet lasers.

Table 3.4   Physical principles of laser photoablation

Nature	Effect
Short UV laser pulse (10 ns) focused on tissue	1–10 W/cm
Strong absorption in the UV (6 eV)	Absorption (proteins :amides: peptides), depth penetration to repulsive
Photodissociation	Excited state

Table 3.5   Threshold to ablate a typical tissue with excimer and other lasers

Laser ablation threshold (J/cm)	Wavelength (nm)	Penetration depth (μm)	Limiting repetition (Hz)
ArF (0.05)	193	1	37,000
KrF (0.4)	248	15	156
XeCl (1.3)	308	50	15
Dye	465, 384	8.3	10
Nd:YAG	1.064, 1.400	83	37
Er:YAG (0.05)	2.940	2	9.260
CO_2 (0.5)	10.600	20	93

Biostimulation

The low-power laser irradiation can speed up regenerative process in tissues such as wound healing or it can be an effective therapy in the management of arthritis. The biochemical and physiological mechanisms are not understood in pain relief involving biostimulation. The experimental variables in this phenomenon are not clear. Further, controlled studies to understand biostimulation are different and controversial, and end results tend to be subjective.

Until today no rigorous and firm conclusions are drawn about the claims of biostimulation.

BIOLOGICAL MOLECULES AND TISSUES

1. *Water*   It offers an excellent transmission in the region 400 to 800 nm. It gives high absorption peak in the mid-infrared region (1450, 1930, 2940 nm). Water is present in all soft and hard tissues, example, skin—70%, cartilage—75%, arteries—80%, bone—10–30%, deutin — 13% and enamel—3%.

2. *Haemoglobin*   It has wide diffusion in all tissues except cartilage and dental tissues. It strongly absorbs blue and green haemoglobin absorbs red radiation.

3. *Blood*   It is composed of water and haemoglobin. Blood absorbs the optical radiation three times higher at 1064 nm wavelength than 1320 nm wavelength.

4. *Melanin*   The biological pigment of skin and other soft tissues contain melanin which absorbs from 1000 to 400 nm.

5. *Xanthophyll*   Xanthophylls are the pigments localized in neural fibre layers (for example macula). It strongly absorbs blue radiation at 460 nm.

6. *Carbon*   While heating tissue in the presence of oxygen, charring develops carbon. This is due to inflammatory response which is undesired. Carbon strongly absorbs radiation at all wavelengths. It can alter surgical precision. Carbon formation can be minimized with suitable CW lasers.

7. *Collagen*   Collagen is the structural component of most tissue. Under mild heating, fibrils unravel and become sticky (welding and anastomoses) and expend to coagulation (haemostasis). It strongly absorbs infrared radiation at 3030 nm.

8. *Blood vessels*   They are hollow soft tissues which are effectively cooled by blood flow. Haemostasis coagulation of proteins in blood increases viscosity and denaturation of collagen. Haemostasis improves with high power density and longer pulse duration of laser and deeper penetrating wavelengths.

9. *Cartilage*   It consists of water and collagen.

10. *Bone*   Bone is a composite material consisting of collagen matrix, calcium phosphate and hydroxyapatite.

11. *Dental tissue*   It consists of enamel dentin, cementum, dental plaque, caries, water, collagen and hydroxyapatite.

12. *Atherosclerotic plaque*   It is a soft plaque deposit (yellowish colour) composed of fibrous plaque fatty deposit, collagen-calcified plaque fatty deposit, and calcium phosphate. It shows low absorption in the visible-near-infrared region.

13. *Calculus*   It is strong like deposit of inorganic salts and organic materials accumulated in organs, glands and ducts. There are great varieties in pigmentation and hence they have wide mechanical properties. Calcium oxalate is very hard while uric acid is hard but not brittle. Struvite is soft and crumbly.

RADIATION DELIVERY SYSTEMS

For every laser source proposed for a biomedical application, it is of outstanding importance to rely on a suitable beam delivery system. The system should be convenient to utilize the laser energy at the site of the irradiation by preserving all the necessary characteristics of the beam. In other words, the main requirements for a delivery system are:

1. good transmission efficiency,

2. good beam focusability and

3. ease in manipulation. In this respect both free or guided propagation can provide adequate solutions.

Optical Fibres

In practice optical fibres constitute an almost ideal solution in terms of transmission efficiency, compactness, flexibility, low cost and so on. The only limitation is due to the typical transmission window for each material constituting the core of the fibre. In silica fibres, reasonable transmission is obtained in the range $0.25 - 2$ μm. A good research has been done to develop IR fibres for transmission in the range ZrF and other fluoride glasses are proposed near 3μm. Thallium and silver halides have been proposed for 10 μm even if the former is highly toxic. The fibres should deliver maximum power and energy delivery when coupled with laser without causing a permanent and catastrophic damage. CW lasers in this respect do not suffer this damage limitations because very high CW power can be easily transmitted through suitable fibres. This is the case for Nd:YAG lasers which can easily transmit 100 W and more through a 600 μm fibre. Similar situation for Ar ion lasers, especially for medical applications where much lower power is needed.

Problems have been observed for pulsed lasers. In fact the very high peak power exerted by Q-switch operation can rise the instantaneous power density at the entrance face of the fibre up to 4 W/cm. This leads to a surface breakdown due to a severe acoustic and thermal damage and ultimately breaks the fibre. Sometimes, high-quality beams impinging on a fibre with a power density lower than the damage can cause problems inside the bulk of the fibre because of internal reflections. Another class of effects which can cause permanent damage to the fibres is due to the powerful shock wave excited on the target in a liquid environment (opaque or transmitting).

Articulated Arms

Articulated arm measurement systems use calibrated angle encoders and arm segments to determine the location of the end tip of the arm's probe. The articulated arms were used in medical tracking applications. The obstacles of manouvring these arms limited the user's motions and as a result, articulated arms are no longer the preferred choice of tracking in medical applications. Optical and electromagnetic tracking solutions offer similar benefits to articulated arms but overcome the limitations of movement.

For laser emitting out of the range 0.25 – 2 μm it is possible to use an articulated arm to provide both high transmission efficiency and a reasonable ease to manipulate the beam. A typical articulated arm has 6 arms and rotating joints. This type of articulated arm is typical of surgical CO laser. Figures 3.4 (a) and (b) presents two typical articulated arm.

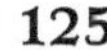

Figure 3.4   (a) and (b) Two typical articulated arm

The advantages and disadvantages of using articulated arm technology are discussed below.

Advantages

1. State good single-point repeatability

2. Available in large variety of sizes/measurement volumes

3. Independent of keyboard (mouse functions)

Disadvantages

1.   Awkward to manoeuvre.

2.   Large arms can be cumbersome.

3.   Mechanical linkages can produce unreliable results depending on joint orientation.

4.   No dynamic referencing possible—must be attached to object if movement suspected.

Review questions

1.   What are the effects of laser on biological tissues?

2.   On what factors does the interaction between electromagnetic and biological tissues depend on?

3.   What is fluence? Explain

4.   What are the four effects of light on tissues? Discuss their characteristics also.

5.   What is meant by vapourization of cells?

6.   List the visual and biological changes on tissue due to the variation in temperatues.

7.   What is the relevance of laser parameters in medical applications?

8.   Discuss photophysical process in laser-tissue interaction.

9.   What are the five basic types laser-tissue interactions?

10.   Write notes on a) photothermal interactions b) photochemical interactions c) photodisruptive interactions d) photoablative interactions, and e) biostimulation

11.   What are the special features of photomechanical interactions?

12.   Discuss in detail on the radiation delivery systems.

13.   Discuss the advantages and disadvantages of using articulated arms techniques.

14.   What are the beneficial and adverse effects of non-ionising radiation of skin?

Chapter 4

Biomedical Applications

SECTION A – MEDICAL PHOTONICS

INTRODUCTION

Following the invention of laser in 1962, laser technology began to be used in the field of medicine. Laser has opened up new prospects for both biological record and medical use. Laser therapy is a coherent therapy using low laser output. The healing process can be effectively supported through the irradiation of the appropriate point on the skin and mucosa. Laser therapy is often sufficient in itself to improve the state of the illness. Laser therapy distinguishes itself by its effectiveness, and by its ability to treat disease without causing any harmful side effects of a scientific or economic nature. In acupuncture therapy, metal needles are replaced with laser beam. The successfully applied laser therapy procedures are

1. Symptomatic laser therapy which is mainly used to relieve pain at particular points.
2. Irradiation on the skin to combat chronic and acute complaints.
3. Edge point therapy.
4. Auricular therapy.
5. Irradiation on reflex zones.

The important advantages of laser therapy are

1. No danger of infection as there is no physical contact with skin.

2. Through direct contact, the laser beam can be applied with precision to any part of the body.

3. Individual organs or organ functions can be treated precisely.

4. Short periods of therapy.

5. Controlled therapy.

6. Complete lack of pain. This is very much advantageous to children, and to nervous and very sensitive patients.

7. Minimal bleeding (bloodless operations are possible in certain cases).

8. Less postoperative swelling.

9. No decay in wound healing (grafts are well-taken).

10. Primary closure is done even in infected lesion.

Laser treatment is safe for youngest infants to adults. The laser is proving to be a powerful new tool in ophthalmology, dermatology, cardiology, dentistry and otolaryngology and wider medical uses are continuously being found. In addition to its great power, the laser has the advantage of haemostasis, precision, selective adsorption by pigments and lack of trauma to healthy tissues. Laser therapy results in reduced post-operative pain and edema. The important advantage of laser is that the laser beam applied to tissues at the focal point cuts and vapourises them without injury to the surrounding cells. Laser light can easily penetrate upto 5 cm into tissue depositing photon energy into cells without any thermal effect.

LASERS USED IN MEDICINE

Laser medicine is a rapidly growing field both in research as well as applications. The first clinical discipline that the laser entered was ophthalmology. This new technique has not only proved its success but also has showed a turning point in the field of ophthalmology. Subsequently it was introduced to dentistry. Dental laser research is progressing although it has not shown much success. Today a considerable amount of laser research is focused towards tumour treatments such as photodynamic therapy (PDT) and laser-induced interstitial thermotherapy (LIT). Due to intensive research work, laser has entered other medical disciplines like gynaecology, urology and neurosurgery. Laser's role in minimal invasive surgery (using miniature catheters and endoscopes) is significant. Laser applications in dermatology and orthopaedics are very interesting. Recently successful laser treatments have been reported in gastroenterology, otorhinolaryngology and pulmology. It is expected that lasers will spread its wings to additional clinical applications. As new lasers and technologies are emerging at a rapid rate, stagnation in laser applications is not anticipated in the near future.

Medical applications based on CO_2, excimer and solid-state lasers are assuming importance. In most cases the heat effect of light is utilised and the appropriate laser for a definite task is chosen. Recent researches reveal that Er^{2+}-doped solid-state lasers may replace CO_2 laser in many applications, since the penetration depth at this wavelength is even smaller than that of the CO_2 laser radiation due to the high-resonance absorption at this wavelength. If deep penetration is needed, Nd-lasers can be used for the purpose. In the case of pulsed lasers, depending on the energy density and power density, other interaction mechanisms may also become significant. Medical solid-state lasers are available for working in all the regions.

A big advantage of solid-state lasers in contrast to the CO_2 lasers is that the light can be guided by flexible optical fibres without any significant loss. Therefore, operation within the body can be performed without open surgery. If the quartz fibre ends up in a sapphire tip, extremely high power densities can be obtained. The tip has to be in contact with the tissues, otherwise it may melt. This technique may broaden the applications of Nd:YAG lasers into fields where almost CO_2 lasers dominated. Solid-state lasers (continuous wave and periodically pulsed Q-switched) are used in almost all fields of medical therapy.

The most widely used solid-state light source is the Nd:YAG laser. Earlier it was mainly used for coagulation–necrotization. The advantages of using lasers in medicine as compared to the classical methods are sterility, high precision, faster healing with less pain and almost bloodless operation. Table 4.1 shows a list of surgical lasers.

Table 4.1 Surgical Lasers

Laser	Region	Wavelength	Applications
CO_2	Far infrared	10600 nm	Best laser for cervical/vulvar/vaginal use in colposcopy, neurolsurgery; best for microlaryngoscopy in ENT, ultra pulse mode for skin resurfacing, vaporising bulk soft tissues
Er:YAG	Mid-infrared	2940 nm	Bone cutting, drilling—dental hard tissue—skin resurfacing, finer effects than the CO_2
Hydrogen Fluoride	Mid-infrared	2940 nm	Bone cutting and drilling, ophthalmology
Ho:YAG	Mid-infrared	2100 nm	Primary use in orthopaedic surgery, lithotripsy, ophthalmology, dentistry
Nd:YAG (harmonic)	Mid-infrared	1318 nm	Tissue welding
Nd:YAG	Near-infrared	1064 nm	General laparoscopic use with contact tips, hysteroscopy, flexible endoscopies, Q- switched types used in dermatology and ophthalmology.
Diode lasers	Variable with system	(800–900) nm	Low power version used for biostimulation and photodynamic therapy; High powers in dermatology for hair removal and general endoscopic use in urology.
Alexandrite laser	Near IR	755 nm	Both Q-switched and long-pulsed used in dermatology, primarily for hair removal.
Ruby	Deep red	694 nm	In dermatology for tattoo removal and hair removal (q-switched and long-pulsed mode)

Laser	Region	Wavelength	Applications
Krypton ion laser	Red Yellow Green	647 nm 568 nm 531 nm	In ophthalmology and dermatology
He–Ne	Red	632 nm	Used as a guide light in most IR surgical lasers and biostimulation
Gold Vapour	Red	632 nm	Used in PDT
Tunable Dye laser (variable with dyes)	Red Yellow Green	632 nm 577 nm 504 nm	PDT Pulsed dye lasers are used in dermatology for vascular lesions and surgery for lithotripsy
Copper vapour	Yellow Green	577 nm 510 nm	Used in dermatology for fine capillary lesions and pigmented lesions. A pulsed laser system; to trace individual capillaries, green used for pigmented lesions.
KTP	Green	532 nm	Used in general laparoscopy, ENT, dermatology and used to pump dye lasers for PDT
Argon	Blue green	488 nm 514 nm	Ophthalmology and used to pump dye lasers for PDT
Excimers	Ultraviolet ArF KrCl KrF XeCl XeF	 193 nm 222 nm 248 nm 308 nm 351 nm	Used in ophthalmology in corneal reshaping, cardiovascular for laser angioplasty, treating psoriasis, dentistry. They are fast pulsed lasers.

4.2 CO$_2$ LASER FOR MEDICINE

The infra-red (IR) wavelength of the CO$_2$ laser (10.6 μm), is highly absorbed by water. Since biological tissue contains 75 – 90% water, the CO$_2$ laser beam is absorbed in a very thin layer of the tissue. If the time of interaction is short, no more than 0.1 – 0.2 millimeter of tissue is influenced by the laser beam. When a focused CO$_2$ laser beam is used for cutting, the cut has very little effects on surrounding tissue. When an unfocused CO$_2$ laser beam is used for surface vaporization, it ablates thin layers, one after the other, with no damage to underlying structures. One of the main disadvantages of CO$_2$ laser for medical surgery is the unavailability of good optical fibres that can transmit high-power beam at wavelength of about 10 μm to organs inside the human body.

4.2.1 Nd:YAG Laser for Medicine

Most applications of continuous wave Nd:YAG laser in medicine were to heat a big volume of tissue to high temperature so that the haemorrhage is stopped by sealing blood vessels. One of the main advantages of Nd:YAG laser for medicine is the possibility to transmit high power of its radiation (at about 1 μm wavelength) through quartz optical fibres. This enables performing procedures inside the human body without the need to open it first. The fibre can be inserted through the body openings (such as mouth or rectum) or through a small incision and guided using medical endoscope. With the invention of synthetic sapphire tips at the end of optical fibres, a new area of contact surgery using Nd:YAG laser was opened to medical doctors. The idea is to conduct the Nd:YAG laser radiation through an optical fibre which ends with a sapphire tip of specific shape.

For each application, a different type of sapphire tip end is used.

1. A scalpel-shaped tip enables cutting and immediate coagulating with the Nd:YAG laser radiation coming out of the tip directly into the cut area.

2. Rounded or flat-surfaced tips distribute the Nd:YAG laser radiation on a large area.

3. Special frosted tips are used to cut and coagulate at the same time.

4.2.2 Importance of Erbium:YAG Laser System

1. The output of CO_2 laser (10.6 micron) heats the surrounding tissues which is a disadvantage in surgery. On the other hand, Er:YAG output (2.94 microns) absorbs water by ten times higher than that of CO_2. Er:YAG laser output wavelength is on the peak of water absorption. Hence, the surrounding tissues are not heated.

2. As collagen contains less water than normal skin cells, it has an even lower absorption coefficient than normal tissue. The barrier presented by collagen raises the risk of scarring. Er:YAG's role in skin resurfacing is due to its unmatched water absorption characteristics with pulse duration of 250 microseconds. This is shorter than thermal relaxation time of skin (estimated to be 1 millisecond). The lack of thermal scattering by Er:YAG laser is good for faster healing process and bleeding is minimal.

3. The Er:YAG can be used to perform a light peel of the epidermis without destroying basal layer. Hence, repeat treatments on a more frequency basis can be achieved with Er:YAG laser.

4. Er:YAG's small penetration depth combined with high power of the short light pulse enables erbium laser to ablate and cut soft tissue with surgical precision. The penetration depth is limited to a thin upper layer of tissue.

5. Treatments of all epidermal disorders are performed without any anaesthesia. Only in the case of tattoo removal, a 1% xylocain injection is used subcutaneously.

6. No previous therapy is required for Er:YAG laser exposure.

4.3 LASERS IN GENERAL SURGERY

In general surgery, snoring is successfully treated with lasers. Almost in every medical surgery the removal of tissue is done or a cut needs to be made. This is done with a laser. In general, the results using lasers are better than the results using a surgical knife. When a bleeding need to be stopped, a Nd:YAG laser can be used. Its radiation enters deep into the tissue and heats and coagulates a large area. When a clean cut needs to be done, an excimer laser is used. In general the common cutting tool is the CO_2 laser.

4.3.1 Advantages of laser Surgery

The advantages of laser surgery are:

1. Dry field of surgery because laser energy seals small blood vessels.

2. Operating time as well as healing time is shorter.

3. Laser surgery does less cutting and minimal damage to healthy tissues.

4. Less postoperative pain because of the sealing of nerve ends.

5. No contact with mechanical instruments, so sterilization is built-in.

6. Clear field of view because no mechanical instrument blocks it.

7. Possible wavelength-specific reaction of specific colours of biological tissue.

8. Possibility to perform microsurgery under a microscope. The laser beam passes through the same microscope.

9. Possibility to perform surgical procedures inside the body without opening it, using optical fibres to transmit the laser beam.

10. The laser can be used as a precise cutting tool. Lasers are more precise and exact than scalpels.

11. It can be controlled by a computer, and operated with a very small area of effect under a microscope.

12. No touch technique.

13. Reduced blood loss. Laser heat seals blood vessels, thereby causing less bleeding, swelling, pain, or scarring.

14. Limited fibrosis and stenosis.

15. Fibre optic delivery.

16. Potential reduction in spread of metastasis.

17. Sterilisation of impact site. The heat produced by laser is used to cut the tissues as well as to sterilize the nearby tissues. This prevents infection.

18. Reduced edema.

19. Precision.

20. Unique capabilities.

4.3.2 Disadvantages of Laser Surgery

1. Laser scientists or engineers are needed as laser safety officers. Doctors and nurses should be trained to use lasers.

2. High cost of laser equipments. Recent advances in technology may reduce their cost and size.

3. Safety precautions are the top priority in laser operation theaters.

4.4 LASERS IN OPHTHALMOLOGY

In 1961, ruby laser was used for the first time by eye doctors. It is natural that the eye was chosen to be the first organ for performing medical experiments, since the eye is transparent to the electromagnetic spectrum in the visible range. Another natural device that helps is the lens in the eye, which focuses the electromagnetic radiation onto the retina, thus, increasing the power density by orders of magnitude.

As a result of mechanical shock, the retina inside the eye can be torn, and detached from the tissue. The first application of laser for medical applications was for experiments in soldering detached retina in animals. The electromagnetic radiation from the laser heats the detached retina, and as a result the damaged blood vessels around the retina are closed and soldered to place. In 1964, the first experiments were done on human subjects, and today it is a standard treatment. Because of the focusing effect of the eye, small amount of laser power is needed to solder the detached retina. Actually electromagnetic radiation was used for this purpose for many years, starting with the middle ages where the doctors used radiation from the sun for this purpose.

The ArF excimer laser (193 nm) operates in the ultra-violet spectrum region. Since this wavelength is highly absorbed by water, and the cornea (like any other biological tissue) contains mostly water, the laser beam ablates sub-micron layers of the cornea without affecting surrounding tissue. Under computer control, it is possible to sculpture the cornea by grafting concentric circles from the cornea.

Most of the change of direction (refraction) of light rays entering the eye is performed by the cornea, since the light goes from air (index of refraction about 1) to the tissue (index of refraction is about 1.3). Thus, a small change in the radius of curvature of the cornea causes a big change in the focusing of light in the eye.

The possibility of using laser light as a useful tool in eye surgery was proposed to substitute xenon lamps for retinal pathologies. Ophthalmology is one of the successful areas for the use of solid-state lasers. They are used today for either diagnosis or therapeutic purposes. A typical application is the removal of the clouded film behind the eye lens formed usually after the insertion of a plastic lens after cataract surgery. This is done with a Q-switched Nd:YAG laser at very high power density ($\sim 10^2$ W/cm^2). At this power, laser plasma is formed which destroys the film without damaging the lens. The retina is also safe, since the laser beam is focused on the fibre and therefore the power density at the bottom of the eye is small.

Several other laser procedures have also been introduced for diseases of the anterior chamber of the eye. The use of the lasers can be divided into three categories:

1)   Retinal photo-coagulations

2)   Cataract surgery

3)   Corneal reshaping

For photo-coagulation of hemorrhagic site or point welding of detached retina, proper laser wavelengths are chosen so that they are highly absorbed by the blood vessels or by pigmented tissue. The CW argon ion laser in the blue-green region serves for this purpose. This provides just small-sized burns needed for such applications. On contrary, pulsed lasers may cause mechanical damage. Argon laser coupled to slit lamp have been used for retinal photo-coagulation and retinal surgery from 1968 onwards. For macular lesions, krypton ion laser in the red region was employed to limit the risk of unintentional photocoagulations. For the same purpose, the laser diodes of wavelengths of 900 nm were employed recently.

Cataract surgery needs a pulsed laser which is transmitted through the cornea. In order to obtain the desired vision, the lens interior must be extracted by mechanical dissipation. Q-switched Nd:YAG lasers having energies between 8 and 16 millijoules in pulse of 12 nanoseconds are successfully employed for the purpose.

Corneal reshaping is a valuable experimental technique to correct myopia. They are based essentially on very fine and precise incisions by excimer laser ablation of the cornea. Radial keratectomy provides several cuts on the cornea out of the iris to release the internal focus and to decrease the curvature and the optical power. Subsequently, a more proper corneal reshaping has been proposed in which the correction is achieved readily by removing just a few tens of microns by a centered ablation in the shape of a step negative diopter.

One important laser diagnostic tool is confocal laser microscopy which allows the detection of early steps of retinal alterations such as retinal detachment and glaucoma. The major fields of laser research in the eye surgery are detachment of the retina, treatment of glaucoma, cataract and more recently refractive corneal surgery.

The eye is the most sensitive organ of the human body. Therapeutic laser treatment of the eye can be broadly classified into front (cornea, sclera, trabeculum and iris) and rear (lens, vitreous body and retina) segments. The schematic diagram of the eye is shown in Figure 4.1.

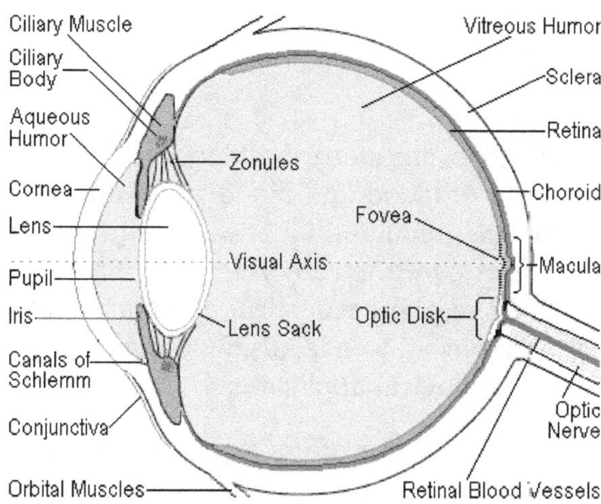

Figure 4.1 Schematic view of a human eye

The visible ophthalmological laser passes through the lens of the eye and falls on the retina when the photo-coagulation occurs, that is, heating the retina to coagulate.

As early as 1949, Meyer-Schwickerath proposed a control of neovascularisation in the retinal blood vessels with some light and subsequently with xenon photo-coagulator. This has several disadvantages when compared to the laser treatments.

i) The retinal spot size is much larger than that formed with a laser beam.

ii) The total amount of energy deposited in the eye is 20 to 50 times greater than that deposited during an equivalent laser treatment.

iii) It requires a longer exposure which causes more pain and hence local anaesthesia is required.

iv) It requires very clear optical media to be functional; mild cataracts and vitreous opacities will preclude its use.

v) It causes retinal burns of full thickness.

Campbeur and Zweng were the first to use pulsed ruby laser to weld the detached segments of retina to the choroidea during 1963/64. Ruby laser has many desirable optical properties compared to the broad spectral range and non-coherence xenon arc. The red portion of the laser beam passes through the ocular media and is absorbed by the pigment epithelium where it is converted into heat.

As the ruby laser could not close the blood vessels, argon ion laser was preferred for coagulation of blood and blood vessels because haemoglobin of blood strongly absorbs the green and blue wavelength of argon laser. The advantage of argon ion laser over the ruby laser was that it worked in a continuous wave and avoided the photoacoustical effect associated with the use of very short pulses of high power. Hence, argon ion laser is the most useful and popular laser in ophthalmological applications.

The high-power Nd:YAG laser offers a promising tool for eye surgery. It lases in the near-infrared at 1.06 μm. The advantages are that it has greater depth of penetration from 3 to 7 mm, depending on the type of tissues and can rupture any targeted tissues in the eye due to nonlinear absorption.

A typical data for argon laser used in retinal coagulation is as follows:

Exposure time	0.1s to a few seconds
Laser power	0.16 to 1 W
Spot diameter	200–1000 micrometer

The blue-green light emitted by argon ion laser are readily absorbed by the red blood vessels with minimum light scattering. Hence, the photocoagulation of the blood can be carried out without using unnecessary high-power density lasers. However, the deepest layer of the retina namely the pigment epithelium and choroid are not red and therefore absorbs more readily the red beam of the ruby or krypton laser than the blue-green beam of the argon laser.

The amount of laser energy needed for the photocoagulation depends on the spot size used. In general, the correct dose is determined visually by the ophthologist from exposure at the time of the treatment. The minimum amount of energy that causes an observable damage to the retina is known as minimal reactive dose (MRD), that is, the minimum clinical energy necessary for the protection of the human clinical photocoagulation lesions. The basic procedure for conducting laser coagulation is as follows.

Doctors always attempt laser coagulation through a slit lamp and a contact glass. The laser power is increased from a low threshold until the focused spot becomes greyish. On no account should the macula be coagulated as it will affect vision. The temperature should not exceed 80°C, in order to avoid vapourisation and carbonisation. However, to achieve good results, the surgeon can select the required energy dose for good localisation of blood vessels.

As early as 1970, krypton laser entered into ophthalmic applications. Its red wavelength (647 nm) was absorbed by choroidea while the yellow wavelength (568 nm) was strongly absorbed by pigment epithelium and xanthophyll in the macula.

The burns produced by krypton laser in the retina are different from those produced by the argon laser. Specifically, the burns from the krypton laser do not involve the inner retina. Also, krypton laser spares the nerve fibre layer near the macula. In contrast, nerve fibre layer burns are common with the argon laser. When eyes are affected with some vitreous haemorrhage, nuclear sclerosis, cataract or other media opacities, krypton laser is the best choice since it penetrates better.

The red wavelength of krypton laser penetrates through haemorrhage in a better way. Further longer wavelength (659 nm) can be focussed deeper in the choroids. The red wavelength is suitable for the treatment of ocular melanoma and retinopathy of prematurity.

The yellow wavelength of krypton laser has better penetration through nuclear sclerotic cataracts while excellent penetration through fluid and pigmentary disturbances. Minimal absorption in macular xanthophylls, accurate closure of microaneurysms, less dispersive energy in the neurosensory retina, less discomfort to the patient and greater margin of safety are the advantages of yellow wavelength krypton laser. The yellow/green wavelength is already in clinical use.

McHugh in 1988 suggested that 800 nm semiconductor diode lasers (IR radiation) can perform the same job without creating discomfort to the patient's eye. The laser treatment of retina consists of:

1) Retinal holes

2) Retinal detachment

3) Diabetic retinopathy

4) Central vein occlusion

5) Senile macular degeneration and

6) Retinal tumours.

The laser has been used in the treatment of retinal holes and tears to prevent the development of retinal detachment. When the retina is completely detached, the laser is of no help. Due to the lasers small spot size (~50 micrometer), it is possible to use the laser even in the small region where the detailed vision takes place. The laser energy produces a chorioretinal scar which causes an adhesion to form between the retina and the underlying choroid. This attachment is so strong that it prevents the subsequent retinal detachment. If necessary, this procedure can be repeated several times without much complications.

Retinal detachment occurs among myopic patients as a consequence of undetected retinal holes or tears. A reasonable detachment can be treated similar to retinal holes. If the tear is severe, the treatment aims at saving the fovea or at least a small segment of the macula which is known as panretinal coagulation. During this treatment, new membranes in the vitreous body, in the retina and beneath the retina occur which is known as proliferative retinopathy.

A laser has already been accepted as a tool for clearing the secondary opaque membrane that develops years after an extra-capsular cataract extraction is done. Prior to this, this membrane had to be surgically incised or excised to improve the vision.

Diabetic retinopathy is a complication of chronic diabetic mellitus. Eventually, nearly all patients with diabetes develop some degree of retinopathy.

During diabetic retinopathy, the oxygen concentration in the blood is considerably decreased, due to the formation of new blood vessels. This phenomenon is known as neovascularisation. Haemorrhages inside the vitreous body might lead to severe losses in vision. To prevent complete blindness, the entire retina is coagulated except fovea (panretinal coagulation). In diabetic retinopathy, neodymium frequency doubled (KTP) laser is used for resection of capillary around the macula lutea. The elderly patients get central vein occlusion as it is confined to one eye only. As a result retinal veins become dilated and severe oedema is formed in the region of the macula, leading to multiple haemorrhages with a strong decrease in vision. In 1977, Laatikainen reported that this can be treated by performing panretinal coagulation.

The primary purpose of evaluating and managing diabetic retinopathy is to prevent, retard or to reverse the effects. The diabetic retinopathy study (DRS) and the early treatment diabetic retinopathy study (ETDRS) provide the strongest support for the therapeutic benefit of photocoagulation surgery. Laser photocoagulation surgery in DRS and ETDRS was beneficial in reducing the risk of further visual loss but generally not beneficial in reversing already diminished acuity. The use of krypton laser with multiwavelengths such as red, yellow, yellow-green and green in diabetic retinopathy was already demonstrated. Certainly krypton laser is advantageous over argon laser.

Senile macular degeneration which is caused due to the formation of neovascular membranes in the choroidea is also seen among the elderly patients. This can be prevented by coagulation with the green wavelength of argon ion laser or the red wavelength of krypton laser.

Usually mechanical excisions or radioactive material implantations were used in the treatment of malignant tumours. Recently, laser treatment of retinal tumours (retinal blastome) is reported. The tumours were destroyed by using the laser radiation.

Cataract which is nothing but opaqueness of lens generally arises due to age, disease, UV radiation, food deficiencies or trauma. It is believed that the cataract occurs due to the decrease in amount of potassium and soluble lens proteins which are associated with the increased concentration of calcium and insoluble lens proteins. In ophthalmic applications of laser, cataract surgery is another important area. In order to achieve acceptable vision the lens interior must be extracted. In posterior capsulotmy, neodymium lasers are used for drilling a hole in the posterior membrane of the crystalline lens after the surgical removal of the opaque tissue. In the posterior capsulotomy, a helium – neon (He:Ne) laser is used as a reference beam.

The surgeon first focuses the reference helium – neon laser on the posterior capsule (lens interior enclosed by homogeneous elastic membrane) and then adds the cutting Nd:YAG laser. The Nd:YAG laser parameters are as follows:

a)   Pulse duration 30 ns,

b)   Pulse energies 5 mJ,

c)   Focus diameters 50 –100 μm, and

d)   Power densities exceeding 1010 W/cm^2.

After having placed several cuts, the posterior membrane opens like a zipper. The entire procedure is controlled through the slit lamp. During the surgery, the surgeon's eye is protected by a specially coated beam splitter or a filter.

Earlier, the fragmentation of human lens was carried out using ultrasonic techniques. At present picosecond Nd:YAF laser with lower threshold energy for the occurrence of optical breakdown is used for the fragmentation of the interior of the lens. In this process, the surgeon steadily moves the focus of the laser beam having the pulse energy well above the threshold without injuring the capsule.

Closed angle glaucoma increases the inner eye pressure well above 20 mm of Hg causing severe headaches, edema, degeneration of retinal nerve fibres and a sudden loss in vision. To relieve the inner eye pressure, laser iridotomy can be applied. Laser iridotomy is a general procedure which perforates the iris. The iris should be medically narrowed prior to laser exposure. This can be performed with extra argon ion lasers or pulsed neodymium lasers. The laser parameters for laser iridotomy are given in the following table:

Exposure duration	0.1–0.2 seconds
Laser powers	700–1500 mN
Spot diameter	50 mm
Argon lasers for	Dark and strongly pigmented iris
Nd:lasers for	Light iris
Pulse duration	Ns or ps pulse

The reader can refer to the book by Steinert and Puliafits (1985) for a detailed procedure. Laser iridotomy is a minor surgery with rare complication such as haemorrhage or infection.

Due to the malfunction of the trabecular meshwork, open angle glaucoma occurs. This can be treated by the technique known as laser trabeculotomy in which trabeculum is carefully perforated. Wise and Witter in 1975 reported another technique called trabeculoplasty to cure open-angle glaucoma. At present this method is widely used and finds success in primary chronic glaucoma with eye pressure below 35 mm of Hg. In this method around 100 pulses from argon ion laser with focus diameter 50 – 100 μm are applied to the surface of the trabeculum using a special type of contact glass. In continuation of open- angle glaucoma treatment, laser treatment of the sclera (internal and external scelerostomies) are also realised. Beakman in 1971 used first laser sclerostomies in glaucomatous eyes with a thermally acting CO_2 laser. Recently, pulsed Nd:YAG laser has been used to improve filtration with the method of internal sclerostomy. The laser parameters for the complete perforation of the sclera is

    a)   Number of pulses 250 – 500

    b)   Pulse duration   12 ns each

    c)   Pulse energy   16553 mJ

Here, holmium lasers can also be used for small hole drilling (sclerotomy).

The cornea and lens together account for the total refraction of the eye. However, since the anterior surface of the cornea is exposed to air with refractive index close to unity, refraction at the anterior surface of the cornea represents the major part. Corneal surgeries can be classified under two categories.

1)   Surgery pertaining to removal of any pathologic conditions, viz., treatment of irregularly shaped corneas. (For example, keratoconus, externally induced corneal injuries and corneal transplantations). Mechanical scalping is necessary before the laser exposure. ArF excimer laser makes this surgery painless and non-invasive. Very clean corneal excisions are also reported using short-pulsed neodymium lasers.

2)   Refractive corneal surgery is performed to alter refractive power. Holmium lasers are commonly used for refractive surgery (Hypermyotropy). Fjodorov and Durner reported the first corneal surgery using a diamond knife in 1979. The entire operation is known as radial keratotomy. Here radial incisions are made into the peripheral cornea so that the tensile forces are rearranged to lead to flattening of the central anterior surface.

The first medical treatments for changing the curvature of the cornea were done by cutting tiny surgical incisions along the radius of the cornea. Using a diamond-bladed knife, few cuts were made under local anesthesia. The procedure was called radial keratotomy.

In the early 80s, a new surgical technique was developed using ophthalmic laser ArF. This technique performs excisions rather than incisions. This technique was used by several groups to correct myopia and astigmatism. At present perforation is avoided due to improved application system and a more accurate pre-operative measurement of corneal parameters.

Utilising the special quality such as ablation characteristics of excimer lasers, especially ArF laser, another new technique known as keratomileusis (photorefractive keratectomy) were developed to change the optical power by carving the cornea. Since the outer layer of the cornea serves as a protective layer, a new method for PRK is by removing the outer layer as a whole piece, reshaping the inner layer, and recovering the outer layer back. This method is simpler to radial keratectomy in the sense that it achieves a direct optical correction. Further, using this method, astigmatism can also be corrected. Another new procedure is developed, using Holmium YAG laser at 2.1 μm wavelength. Using excimer laser under computer control, a change in the shape of the cornea can be precisely made, by removing sub-micron layers from the cornea. The operation is called PRK (photo-refractive keratotomy) and most of the problems with focusing the image on the retina can be repaired. This operation, which can make eyeglasses obsolete, is very popular among people who care a lot about their appearance, such as actors, politicians, etc.

Typically a single laser pulse about $0.1 - 1$ μm on corneal tissue corresponds to $0.01 - 0.1$ diopters. That is, correction of 1 dioptre is achieved with approximately 10 pulses, which takes about one second at a repetition rate of 10 Hz.

Rare earth lasers, viz., erbium, holmium and neodymium infrared lasers have been proposed for refractive corneal surgery. Erbium and holmium lasers focused on corneal tissue produce a shrinkage of the involved collagen fibres. Thus a tensile stress is induced inside the cornea evoking a change in refractive power. These lasers are widely called cosmetic lasers which are used for resurfacing skin to make one look younger. Recently an interesting technique called intrastromal ablation was proposed for refractive corneal surgery using Q-switched Nd:YAG laser. Subsequently picosecond pulse laser from a two-stage Nd:YLF laser system was also used for intrastromal ablations.

Currently extensive research was conducted in the technique of intrastromal ablations by a method called laser *in situ* keratomileusis (LASIK). LASIK utilises ArF laser and provides high performance. 100% success was achieved in treating shortsight, long sight and glaucoma with various types of emerging lasers. Hence, laser is considered the best tool in ophthalmic photonics.

4.4.1. Role of Krypton Laser on Diabetic Retinopathy

In the world of ophthalmology, the krypton laser is red or yellow light and is good for causing the regression of pre-existing neovascularisation of the disc (NVD) in diabetic retinopathy. The burns produced by the krypton laser in retina are different from those produced by argon laser. Specifically, the burns from the krypton laser do not involve the inner retina. The krypton laser also spares the nerve fibre layer near the macula. In contrast, burns of the nerve fibre layer are common with the argon laser. In eyes with some vitreous haemorrhage, nuclear sclerosis, cataract or other media opacities where krypton seems to penetrate better may be the treatment of choice. The fundus of normal human eye is shown in Figure 4.2.

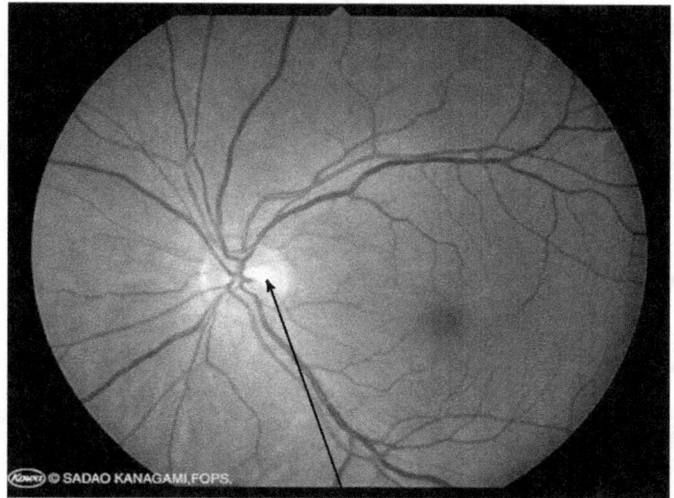

Optic disc where blood vessels converge

Figure 4.2 Fundus of normal human eye

The inner retina include the nerve fibre layer to the rods and cones layer which is clear with yellow pigments and the red blood vessels and allow laser or light of the same wavelengths to pass through them. Yellow pigments allow yellow laser light and red blood allow red light to pass through them respectively. Red wavelength has better penetration through haemorrhage and it can be focussed deeper in the choroid. It is also useful to treat ocular melanoma and retinopathy of prematurity. The yellow wavelength also penetrates better through nuclear sclerotic cataracts. It has excellent penetration through fluid and pigmentary disturbances. Further advantages of yellow light are (a) minimum absorption in macular xanthophylls producing an optimally controlled treatment, (b) accurate closure of microaneurysms, (c) less dispersion of energy in the neurosensory retina, (d) less discomfort to the patients, and (e) greater margin safety.

The diabetic status of retina is as follows:

1)   Nonproliferative diabetic retinopathy,

2)   Nonproliferative diabetic retinopathy with clinically significant macular exudates (CSME),

3)   Severe nonproliferative diabetic retinopathy,

4)   Proliferative diabetic retinopathy, and

5)   Proliferative diabetic retinopathy not amenable.

The fundus of human eye affected by diabetic retinopathy is shown in Figure 4.3 (a) and (b).

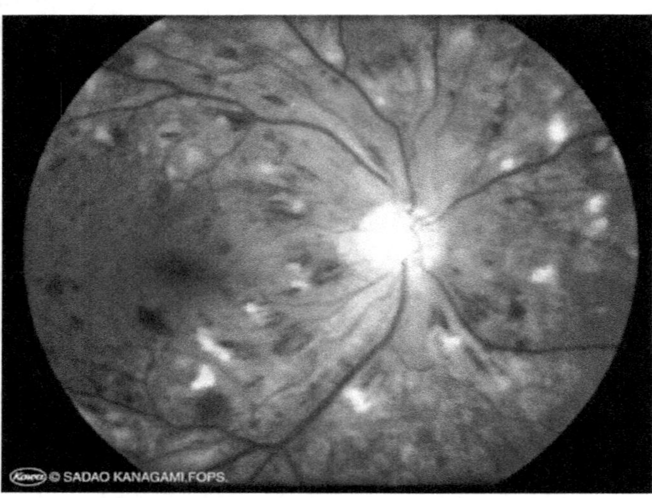

(a)

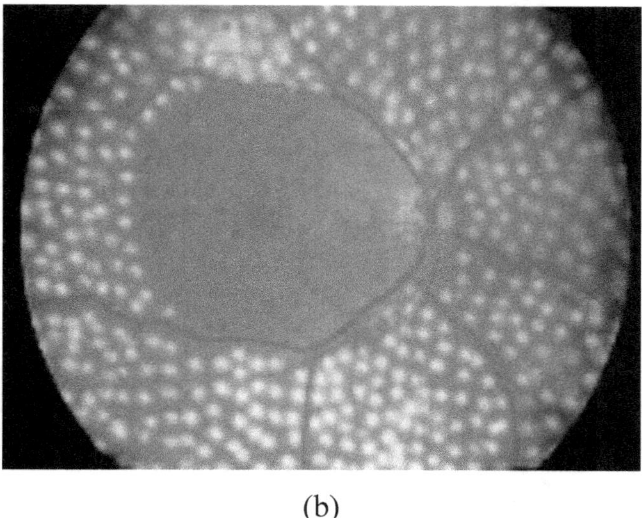

(b)

Figure 4.3 Fundus of human eye affected by diabetic retinopathy

4.5 LASERS IN DENTISTRY

The common problem in human tooth is decay or caries. Usually dentists remove the infected materials and refill a gap with gold, ceramic, alloys, or composites. Previously, the mercury amalgam was a popular alloy which was toxic. In general, the infected material is removed by mechanical drills. This causes sensitiveness to tooth nerves and there is a rise in temperature during drilling. Hence local anaesthesia is administered in caries therapy. Dental laser applications are divided between the soft tissue and the hard tissue (the teeth). Dental soft tissue treatment applications are similar to those of other soft tissue in the body and are common for many years.

In recent years this is overcome by using lasers without any physical contact between lasers and tooth. Hence vibrations are tremendously avoided. Compared to the mechanical "conventional" dental drill, the laser operates without the noise and the mechanical pressure. However, all types of lasers are not suitable for this purpose. Added to this, CW lasers and long-pulsed lasers cause thermal damage in the pulp. This can be minimised when we use ultrashort pulses.

Another important use of laser therapy is the conditioning of dental substance. This delays the occurrence of carries to certain extent. Multiwavelength argon dental laser system and CO_2 dental lasers are popular in dentistry. A non-laser light takes considerable time to cure the composites with unsatisfactory results. But an argon laser hardens the composite in seconds and cures it completely.

Lasers are used to remove decay within a tooth and prepare the surrounding enamel for receipt of the filling. Lasers are also used to "cure" or harden a filling. Lasers are used to reshape gums and remove bacteria during root canal procedures. In case of gum surgery with the laser, most of the patients suffer less postoperative pain. Further, in this surgery no stitches are required and there is almost no bleeding. Lasers can be used to remove a small piece of tissue (called a biopsy) so that it can be examined for cancer. Lasers are also used to remove lesions in the mouth and relieve the pain of canker sores.

Solid-state lasers have an assured place in medicine as an important tool. In dentistry, erbium lasers are commonly used for prevention and treatment of caries. Neodymium lasers are also used for removal of intracanal micro-organism and the final debris of dental caries by melting and vitrification of enamel tissues. In endodonty, erbium and holmium lasers are employed for endodontic surgery access, cavity preparation, etching of dental enamel and treatment of caries. Neodymium lasers are also used for gingival plastic surgery, cauterization and frenectomy in perodonty. In labial corner, neodymium lasers are used for cauterization.

Mechanical drills are commonly employed in caries therapy. Nienbe in 1993 and Piochl in 1994 showed that the ultrashot pulses can be employed in place of mechanical drills. However, research in this area is progressing to achieve better results. The other successful areas in dentistry are laser treatment of soft tissues and laser welding of dental bridges and dentures.

Compared to the traditional dental drill, lasers have advantages as well as disadvantages.

4.5.1 Advantages

1. It causes less pain and hence no need for anaesthesia.

2. It reduces anxiety in patients as the use of the dental drill is avoided.

3. It minimizes bleeding and swelling during soft tissue treatments.

4. It preserves the more healthy tooth during cavity removal.

4.5.2 *Disadvantages*

1. Lasers cannot be used on teeth with fillings already in place.

2. Lasers cannot be used in many commonly performed dental procedures. For example, lasers cannot be used to fill cavities located between teeth, around old fillings, and large cavities that need to be prepared for a crown. In addition, lasers cannot be used to remove defective crowns or silver fillings, or prepare teeth for bridges.

3. Even now traditional drills are needed to shape the filling, adjust the bite, and polish the filling (even when a laser is used).

4. Lasers do not fully eliminate the need for anaesthesia.

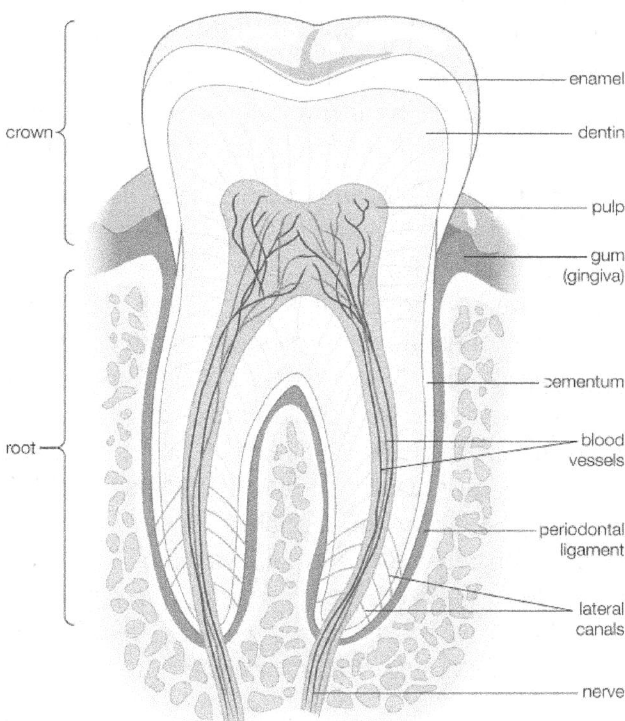

Figure 4.4 Schematic diagram of cross section of human tooth

Figure 4.4 shows the schematic diagram of cross section of human tooth. Thermally active lasers such as pulsed ruby laser and carbon dioxide lasers are employed as surgical tools for teeth. Unfortunately they produced irreversible injury of nerve fibres and tooth. Ho:YLF laser emitting 2.067 μm is very close to the water absorption peak. The stronger absorption of water at 2 μm superficially damages zones. This makes holmium laser an excellent choice for precision surgeries on cartilage and similar hard tissue. Holmium laser will be very useful to dentistry for the following reasons.

1. Holmium (Ho) laser radiation can be passed through commercial silica fibres.

2. Morphological changes in enamel and denture surfaces are observed after Ho:YLF irradiation. They are very different from those of CO_2 and Nd:YAG laser radiation.

3. Refraction data obtained with Ho:YLF laser depends on the applied energy, enamel thickness and the presence of carious tissue. No crack zones or carbonization have occurred due to Ho:YLP exposure.

4. Desired depth can be controlled by irradiation condition (750 mJ maximum) without thermal damage to the pulp. Measurements of temperature inside the pulp chamber increased not more than 2.5°C.

5. Inside the cavities, melted and recrystalised materials can seal open tubules. Denaiseu and Zeaelletel (*J. Cln. Laser Med. and Surgery*, 13, 283, 1995) concluded from their experiments that irradiating tissues by holmium laser can be useful. It causes the vaporization of organic substances, enamel etching and promotes better sealant bonding. Perforations of approximately 4 mm depth with homogeneous and smooth wall surfaces is achieved and no carbonization is obtained with holmium laser. That is, holmium laser may be useful for endodontic access and cavity preparation. During 1989, Er:YAG laser with 2.94 μm wavelength was suggested for dental application by Keller and Hibst (1989) as it matches with resonance frequency of the vibrational oscillation of water molecule in the teeth. There is a lot of scope for research in this area. At this juncture, it may be noticed that Ho:YAG and Er:YAG lasers produce severe side effects such as tooth fissures.

As a next step, ArF excimers were used in dentistry by Frentzen (1989) and Liesenhoff (1989) due to its low thermal effect caused by short pulse duration (15 ns). But the rate of ablation achieved by ArF laser was very low for clinical applications. Further, the UV radiation emitted by excimer lasers caused a great concern in its use in dentistry. During 1993, the frequency-doubled Alexandrite UV laser offered a better selectivity for carious dentine than the Er:YAG laser. Recently picosecond pulses were used for caries therapy successfully with negligible mechanical impact. Several reports are available in the literature regarding the use of CO_2 lasers in the treatment of soft dental tissue. The pulsed or CW CO_2 lasers with low power can be successfully employed due to its high absorption in the moist environment of the mouth in the management of oral malignant tissues. In the treatment, the dental surgeon is left with two choices such as excision or vaporization. The excision is advised as it provides evidence for complete removal. On the other hand, if the lesion is vaporised, doctors have to obtain the adjacent tissue to verify the complete removal. No suture to the wound is required in this treatment as the capillary blood vessels are coagulated due to laser radiation. The wound edge is also smoothened. The patient gets a complete cure within 4 – 6 weeks although it is uncomfortable for 2 – 3 weeks.

It is very difficult to treat leukoplakis in the mouth, tongue and lips using conventional surgery. A 15 – 20 watt CO_2 laser with a defocused beam treats leukoplakis very well.

High-power (20 – 30 W) CO_2 lasers are suggested for the treatment of malignant lesions. The recurrence of local tumor is reduced when CO_2 laser is used instead of scalpel. A thorough research is required to ascertain these reports. It was also suggested that Nd:YAG laser can be used for oral cancer treatment but it has not gained clinical importance so far.

In dentistry, previous filling has to be removed when a secondary decay is located beneath the filling. Infrared lasers are not advisable for removal of filling as it causes high reflection. Further the amalgam exposed to Nd:YLF laser or Er:YAG laser, melts and releases mercury vapour which is very toxic for dentist as well as to patient.

Another interesting area in dentistry is laser welding of dental bridges and dentures using high power density Nd:YAG and CO_2 lasers. The advantages of laser welding are high resistance against corrosion, ability to weld different metals, ability to weld coated alloys, reproducibility and lower heat load. It is also suggested to coat highly absorbing layer prior to laser exposure.

Recently Frederich Parkins applied Nd:YAG laser for treating apthous ulcers generally referred to as cancer sores. According to him 63% of patients treated with the laser reported immediate relief from pain and 50% reported faster healing.

Mike Wibon developed a new laser dental therapy to kill a broad range of harmful bacteria in caries and in periodontal disease using helium – neon laser (632.8 nm) and a semiconductor laser diode (630 – 680 mm) with a peak power of 7 mW and 11 mW, respectively. The principle involved in this research is as follows:

Bacterial cells are coated with chemicals which are inactive until illuminated by low power lasers. The recommended chemicals are porphyrin and phthalocyanine-based dyes that have different colours in variable states. Since blue compounds absorb strongly in the red region of visible spectrum, Wibon selected red laser light. This absorption produced single oxygen and toxic-free radicals which are believed to damage bacterial cell membranes. They have been effective at killing a dozen species of bacteria including *Staphylococcus aureus*, an antibiotic-resistant bacterium that are found in hospitals. Wibon believed that his light-sensitive compounds could easily be applied to teeth and to diseased gums by injecting the compounds near a decayed tooth. This research is at preliminary stage and these techniques may prove effective for treating wounds even in non-dental situations.

4.5.3 CAVITY PREPARATION

The Er:YAG laser was tested for preparing dental hard tissues for the first time in 1988. It was successfully used to prepare holes in enamel and dentine with low 'fluences' [energy (mJ)/unit area (cm^2)]. Even without water-cooling (Burkes et al., 1992), the prepared cavities showed no cracks and low or no charring while the mean temperature rise of the pulp cavity was about 4.3°C (Rechmann et al., 1998). In 1989, it was demonstrated that the Er:YAG laser produced cavities in enamel and dentine without major adverse side-effects. The ablation efficiency was about one order of magnitude lower than for soft tissue. It was then concluded that dentine and enamel removal was very effective with no risk to the pulp (Armengol, 2000; Cavalcanti, 2003) and the ablation rates in enamel were stated to be in the range of 20☐50 μm/pulse, and in dentine they were reported to be as high at lower fluences. Clinically, cavity preparation in enamel results in ablation craters with a white chalky appearance on the surface of the crater (Tokonabe et al., 1999). In dentine, cavity margins are sharp and dentinal tubules remain open without a smear layer. In a clinical study conducted to evaluate the efficiency and safety of the Er:YAG laser for caries removal and cavity preparation in dentine and enamel (Cozean et al, 1997), Class I, II, III, IV and V cavities were prepared for amalgam and composite restorations. It was found that the Er:YAG laser was equivalent to the air rotor in its ability to make cavity preparations in enamel and dentine and remove caries. However, the floor of the preparation was not as smooth as that achieved with the high-speed drill.

4.5.4 CARIES REMOVAL

Carious material contains a higher water content compared with surrounding healthy dental hard tissues. Consequently, the ablation efficiency of caries is greater than for healthy tissues. There is a possible selectivity in the removal of carious material using the Er:YAG laser because of the different energy requirement to ablate carious and sound tissues leaving those healthy tissues minimally affected. However, Rechmann et al. (1998) found that selective ablation of carious dentine is difficult with the Er:YAG laser. The ablation thresholds of healthy dentine and carious dentine are different. The ablation threshold of healthy dentine is two times higher than the corresponding threshold of carious dentine. Therefore, very small fluences of the Er:YAG laser energy are required to selectively ablate carious dentine. This low fluence will result in low efficiency of the ablation process (Shigetani, 2002). In another *in vitro* study investigating the effectiveness of caries removal by Er:YAG laser, it was found that the Er:YAG laser ablated carious dentine effectively with minimal thermal damage to the surrounding intact dentine (Aoki and Ishikawa et al., 1998). The laser removed infected and softened carious dentine to the same degree as the bur treatment. In addition, a lower degree of vibration was noted with the Er:YAG laser treatment. However, the study did not address the issue of selective removal of carious tissue and further studies of caries removal using lasers are indicated.

4.5.5 RESTORATION REMOVAL

The Er:YAG laser is capable of removing cement, composite resin and glass ionomer (Dostalova et al., 1998; Gimbel, 2000). The efficiency of ablation is comparable to that of enamel and dentine. Lasers should not be used to ablate amalgam restorations however, because of potential release of mercury vapour. The Er:YAG laser is incapable of removing gold crowns, cast restorations and ceramic materials because of the low absorption of these materials and reflection of the laser light (Keller et al., 1998). These limitations highlight the need for adequate operator training in the use of lasers.

4.5.6 ETCHING

Laser etching has been evaluated as an alternative to acid etching of enamel and dentine. The Er:YAG laser produces micro-explosions during hard tissue ablation that result in microscopic and macroscopic irregularities. These micro-irregularities make the enamel surface microretentive and may offer a mechanism of adhesion without acid etching. However, it has been shown that adhesion to dental hard tissues after Er:YAG laser etching is inferior to that obtained after conventional acid etching (Martinez – Insua et al., 2000). These authors attributed the weaker bond strength of the composite to laser-etched enamel and dentine to the presence of subsurface fissuring after laser radiation. This fissuring is not seen in conventional etched surfaces. The subsurface fissuring contributed to the high prevalence of cohesive tooth fractures in bonding of both laser-etched enamel and dentine.

A similar conclusion was drawn from a study that compared shear bond strength (SBS) of composite resin to dentine surfaces following different treatments (Ceballos et al., 2001). These authors reported that acid-etched specimens achieved the highest SBS values, while laser treatment showed the lowest SBS results. These findings suggest that extensive fissuring caused by laser treatment and the consequent poor bonding strength may outweigh the putative advantages of laser etching.

4.5.7 TREATMENT OF DENTINAL HYPERSENSITIVITY

Dentinal hypersensitivity is one of the most common complaints in dental clinical practice. Various treatment modalities such as the application of concentrated fluoride to seal the exposed dentinal tubules have been tested to treat the condition. However, the success rate can be greatly improved by the ongoing evaluation of lasers in hard tissue applications. A comparison of the desensitising effects of an Er:YAG laser with those of a conventional desensitising system on cervically exposed hypersensitive dentine (Schwarz et al., 2002) showed that desensitising of hypersensitive dentine with an Er:YAG laser is effective, and the maintenance of a positive result is more prolonged than with other agents.

4.5.8 CARIES PREVENTION

Several studies examined the possibility of using laser to prevent caries (Hossain et al., 2000; Apel et al., 2003). It is believed that laser irradiation of dental hard tissues modifies the calcium to phosphate ratio, reduces the carbonate to phosphorous ratio, and leads to the formation of more stable and less acid-soluble compounds, reducing susceptibility to acid attack and caries.

Laboratory studies have indicated that enamel surfaces exposed to laser irradiation are more acid-resistant than non-laser treated surfaces (Watanabe et al., 2001; Arimoto et al., 2001). The degree of protection against caries progression provided by the one-time initial laser treatment was reported to be comparable to daily fluoride treatment by a fluoride dentifrice (Featherstone, 2000). The threshold pH for enamel dissolution was reportedly lowered from 5.5 to 4.8 and the hard tooth structure was four times more resistance to acid dissolution. However, the actual mechanism of acid resistance by laser irradiation is still unclear and studies, particularly *in vivo*, to test those claims are required.

4.5.9 TEETH WHITENING OR BLEACHING

Lasers are used to speed up in-office teeth whitening procedures. A peroxide bleaching solution applied to the tooth surface, is "activated" by laser energy which speeds up the whitening process. The objective of laser bleaching is to achieve an effective power bleaching process using the most efficient energy source while avoiding any adverse effects (Sun, 2000). Power bleaching has its origin in the use of high-intensity light to raise the temperature of hydrogen peroxide, accelerating the chemical process of bleaching. The FDA approved standards for tooth whitening has cleared three dental laser wavelengths, viz., argon, CO_2 and the 980 nm GaAIAs diode. There are no reports at present about the use of the Er:YAG laser in bleaching techniques. The wavelength of the Er:YAG laser may be unsuitable for the procedures and one can take up research in this area. Table 4.2 shows dental lasers.

Table 4.2 Dental Lasers

Laser	Wavelength/Region	Applications
Argon	488 to 514 nm (Vis)	Soft tissue management and periodontal therapies.
Diode	655 to 980 nm (IR)	The many applications of diode lasers include crown lengthening procedures in cosmetic dentistry and for periodontal management by having a bactericidal effect on periodontal pockets. Oral surgeons use this laser in surgery because of its accurate and bloodless incisions for biopsies, gingivectomies, and frenectomies. It has been used for desensitizing teeth and in teeth whitening procedures in the general dentists' office as well.
Nd:YAG	1064 nm (IR)	This laser can penetrate deeper than a carbon dioxide laser and can remove soft tissue just as well. It is safe and does rapid ablation of sulcular epithelium in an infected periodontal pocket. Used for the removal of diseased or inflamed soft tissue in the periodontal pocket.
Er:YAG	2,940 nm (IR)	This laser is used for the removal of dental decay. Selectively ablate decay while preserving healthy tooth structure. Vaporizes decayed tooth structures (instead of "old" high-speed hand piece) and gives comfort to patient.
CO_2	10,600 nm (IR)	It cuts very quickly and deeply. Used by periodontists and oral surgeons for soft tissue surgeries such as frenectomies, gingivectomies, and biopsies. It is good at cutting soft tissues without causing bleeding and leaves a residue of carbon which can serve as a biological dressing for maintaining sterility of surgical sites.
Ho:YAG	10,900 nm (IR)	Vaporize, ablate and coagulate soft tissues. Its depth penetration is 0.4mm or less. Used to remove damaged discs separating the condyle of the mandibular bone from the base of the skull.

To conclude, the Er:YAG laser has been found to have applications in areas such as cavity preparation, removal of caries and restorations and etching of enamel. However, the advantages as well as limitations of the Er:YAG laser treatments have not yet been fully understood. However, there is a bright future in the coming years for the Er:YAG laser in various dental applications. Lasers may revolutionise cavity design and preparation based on development in adhesive dentistry.

4.6 LASERS IN GYNAECOLOGY

Gynaecology is one of the successful disciplines for laser applications. Cervical intraepthelial neoplasia (CIN—uncommon growths of new cervical tissue) is successfully treated with the CO_2 laser. CIN is the frecuent alteration of the cervics and should be treated immediately to avoid cervical cancers. The CO_2 laser is the standard laser source for gynaecological applications. In addition to CIN, the CO_2 laser is widely applied in vulvar intraepithelial neoplasia (VIN) and vaginal intraepithelial neoplasia (VAIN). In the literature, use of CO_2 laser for the treatment of the following are reported.

1. Vulvar intraepithelial neoplasia (VIN),
2. Vaginal intrapithelial neoplasia (VAIN),
3. Cervical intraepthelial neoplasia (CIN),
4. Endometriosis,
5. Obstruction of the uterine tube,
6. Uterine fibroids,
7. Condyloma accuminata,
6. Sterilisation, and
7. Twin–twin transfusion syndrome.

Gynaecology has the highest potential for CO_2 laser and it is used in colposcopy, operative laparoscopy and laporotomy for infertility work. It is the best laser that can be used for treating lower tract gynaecological organs like the cervix and vulva.

For gynaecological treatment, CO_2 lasers are operated in three different modes, viz., CW, chopped pulse and super pulse. Desirable surgical results are achieved by choosing the appropriate mode of CO_2 lasers. In addition to this,

CO_2 lasers are used in defocused, particle focused or highly focused mode depending upon the requirement. The tightly focused mode produce deep excision while the partially focused mode produce less deep excision but surface layer is vapourised.

In VIN, proliferated tissue is vaporised with a CW CO_2 laser in a partially focused mode. Baggish Dorsey (1981) suggested a power density of 1000 W/cm^2, for a vaporisation depth of about 3 – 4 mm. Laser should be switched off to defocused mode if there is bleeding. Similarly, to treat VAIN, a low power density radiation is suggested with a proper surgical microscope as the vaginal tissues are thinner and more sensitive.

Based on the histology, three grades of CIN (I, II or III) and cervical carcinoma are identified. If CIN II or III is diagnosed, parts of cervix must be removed to reduce the possibility of recurrence. Laser surgery is an excellent technique for treating CIN in comparision to the cryotherapy.

The cyclic growth of uterine-like mucous outside the uterus is called endometriosis which can be coagulated, vaporized or excised. The argon ion laser, CO_2 laser and Nd:YAG laser are commonly used in clinical applications. But Nd:YAG laser has the risk of injuring deeper structures due to low absorption coefficient. However, it is applied in cases of endometriosis which is associated with infertility with reasonable success. The Nd:YAG laser is used for safe sterilization by coagulating both tubes on a length of about 1 cm. Further, using CO_2 or Nd:YAG laser radiation, adhesions caused in uterine tube is vaporized to get a free tube. Tubule pregnancies can usually be managed by either salpingostomy or salpingectomy (removal of one tube). The laser treatment of tubule pregnancies was successfully demonstrated during 1989.

The optical fibres are extremely useful not only in optical communication but also in medical field, using lasers and thin optical fibres. Laser-induced interstitial thermotherapy (LITT) is used to coagulate malformations inside the uterus. Lasers with optical fibres become the most important gynecological tool especially for pregnancies.

The patients with epithelial dysplasia of cervix were treated with CO_2 lasers. The laser was irradiated to the patients who were unsuccessfully treated by electrocoagulation. The irradiation technique is as follows:

The eroded areas of epithelium and healthy tissues surrounding them up to a distance of 1 – 2 mm were exposed to an unfocussed beam with a power of 26 W. The time of irradiation depended on the size of lesion and usually was equal to 2 – 7 min. During irradiation, the lesion surface turned whitish and was covered with a thin film of coagulated tissues. New procedure is painless and does not require anesthesia and is not accompanied by bleeding either during or after operation. Epithelisation took place in all the patients after three to five weeks. In cancer patients, the laser radiation is intended to reduce the x-ray dose.

The use of argon, KTP and Nd:YAG is also useful to cut, vaporise or coagulate tissue. The bare fibre systems of the argon and KTP are among the nicest for laparoscopy using non-contact techniques. In laparoscopy, the laser provides a significant advantage in providing a method to treat mild to moderate endometriosis at the time of diagnostic look. It is good for freeing up stuck tubes and ovaries and can totally eliminate abdominal bleeding. The fibre optic argon and KTP laser systems are better for general laparoscopy while the Nd:YAG with contact probes makes a slightly better incision for ectopic pregnancies. Abdominal cysts, uterine myomas and tumours may also be excised or vaporised with these lasers. Radical procedures such as radical vulvectomies and excision of large vascular tumours are performed with laser for better haemostasis. Uterine septae may be cut with contact probes on the Nd:YAG or bare fibres with argon or KTP lasers. The use of Nd:YAG in hysteroscopy began with endometrial ablation as a treatment for chronic menorrhagia.

4.6.1 *Laser Therapy in Gynaecology (Martin DC 1990)*

Laser therapy in gynecology deals with diagnosis of female reproductive cancers, infertility, fibroids and endometriosis. The use of laser technology in gynecology has become widespread since the CO_2 laser was initially used by Kaplan. Laser is successful for a wide range of gynecological applications from the simple removal of lesions to bloodless high-precision cutting. Laser is used for the removal of HPV lesions from the cervix, condyloma treatments, balanitis treatments and other surgeries. Recent lasers are used with minimally invasive gynecological treatments for incontinence and vaginal relaxation syndrome.

4.6.1.1 *Benefits of lasers in Gynecology*

1. Minimally invasive treatments

2. Controlled coagulation

3. Greater patient comfort, less downtime and quicker healing

4. A haemostatic effect with simultaneous disinfection

5. Many treatments do not require anaesthesia

6. High precision, tissue selective treatments

7. Easy access to difficult to reach areas

In 1973, CO_2 laser was used for the treatment of cervical erosions, cervical intraepithelial neoplasia (CIN) and for microsurgery of the fallopian tube. In gynecological laser surgery, the CO_2 and thulium sources are successfully used for the treatment of many female genital tract diseases with applications in colposcopy, laparoscopy and hysteroscopy over many traditional techniques or open surgery. These procedures reduce surgical invasiveness and duration, morbidity, damage to surrounding tissue and ensure more rapid healing of patients with lower incidence of complications.

According to E. Dreher, A. Carasso and M. Meandzija, carbon dioxide laser is the most commonly used in gynaecology treatments (disease of the uterine cervix, vagina, vulva or perineum). When used in conjunction with the microscope or laparoscope during reconstructive operations on the adnexa, laser speeds up the surgical procedure and brings out the inherent advantages of this technique, namely, precise separation or destruction of tissue, absence of postoperative oedema, uncomplicated wound healing, minimal mechanical trauma, decreased postoperative pain and good haemostasis. In the treatment of premalignant epithelial cancers of the female lower genital tract, the CO_2 laser beam is used with precision through a surgical microscope for tissue ablation and excision. Intra-abdominal vaporization of abnormal tissues can be performed endoscopically through fibre optics. Surgical lasers provide thermal scalpels for haemostatic excision of malignant lesions. Photodynamic therapy is applied in the treatment of isolated malignancies persistent after conservative treatment. The advantages of gynaecological CO_2 laser microsurgery are

1. Simplicity.

2. Speed.

3. Mini-invasiveness.

4. Versatility (excisional and ablative techniques).

5. Exceedingly high average of therapeutic successes.

6. Excellent healing process.

7. Possibility of treating large lesions without abnormal scarring.

8. Almost entirely free of complications.

9. Possibility of carrying out treatments in outpatients and day surgeries (cutting health costs).

10. Possibility of operating without anaesthesia, or just with local anaesthetic (cutting costs and risks).

11. Possibility of avoiding the use of vasoconstrictors in the pre-operative phase.

12. Possibility of also operating on pregnant women and/or elderly or debilitated patients and/or patients with pacemakers.

13. Results are in accordance with standards or even better than those of other methods.

Surgical laser systems play a vital part in the treatment of gynaecologic malignancies. The use of KTP, argon, and Nd:YAG lasers became popular in the early 1980s. For precision surgery through the colposcope, the carbon dioxide laser beam appears to be useful in the control of neoplastic lesions of the vaginal mucosa and possibly of the cervix uteri. Tumor volume reduction through laser vaporization, especially when a recurrent tumor is attached to the bony pelvis, is an outstanding advantage. Adhesiolysis during myomectomy and reconstructive surgery of the fallopian tubes might be facilitated by the laser beam. Laser surgery on the vulva, both colposcopically directed and grossly with the CO_2 laser scalpel, might prove to be important for the treatment of various lesions (H.F. Schellhas, *Surg. Clin. North Am.*, 58, 151–66, 1978).

Er:YAG wavelength lasers enables a greater degree of precision as well as controlled bleeding and coagulation effects in gynecology. Nd:YAG laser wavelength penetrates deeper into tissues to create a tightening effect. Combining both wavelengths is successful in providing less invasive and more effective clinical and aesthetic gynecology treatments.

The CO_2 laser can be easily coupled to an operating laparoscope. Here the laser is aligned to the middle of the viewing lens for focusing sharply. A second or third puncture is necessary only to manipulate pelvic structures, to clear the field of plume production. It is also possible to use the CO_2 laser for second punctures by using wave guides. Research is under progress in developing a truly flexible fibre to deliver CO_2 laser energy. This is really a great challenge to fibre optics scientists although GeO_2 fibre is emerging as an alternative to silica fibres. It is still not suitable for communication due to poor mechanical strength. At present, fibre systems used in intra-abdominal laparoscopic surgery include primarily KTP, Nd:YAG and argon lasers.

An advantage of the lasers using flexible delivery systems is that they allow tactile contact with the tissue. Since every laser has a different wavelength and different absorption properties, it is necessary to understand their tissue interaction effects before they are selected for surgery.

The KTP and argon lasers share very similar wavelengths (532 nm versus 458–515 nm) and thus produce similar tissue effects. The energy produced is selectively absorbed by tissue containing haemoglobin or which is heavily pigmented. By moving the fibres closer or farther away from the tissue, one can achieve cutting, vaporization, or coagulation effects on the tissue. The main drawback of these lasers is the required use of goggles for eye protection which distorts colour discrimination.

Although the Nd:YAG laser was originally used in gynecology (hysteroscopic application), it is now used intra-abdominally with contact sapphire probes or specially made sculptured tips. These probes provide a tactile feel of the tissue and by selecting a variety of probes, one can incise, excise, vaporise, or coagulate tissue.

The gynaecological lasers have been shown to be effective in the treatment of various gynaecologic conditions such as:

1. Endometriosis,
2. Laser uterosacral nerve ablation,
3. Adhesiolysis,
4. Neosalpingostomy,
5. Fimbrioplasty,
6. Ectopic pregnancy, and
7. Uterine fibroids.

4.6.2 CERVIX—CERVICAL INTRAEPITHELIAL NEOPLASIA

Although treatment of cervical intraepithelial neoplasia (CIN) is now more commonly performed by the large-loop excisional technique, the laser was the ideal method of treatment during 1980s and still offers better option. Treatment of CIN can be performed by vaporization or by excisional conization using CO_2 laser. The major advantages of the CO_2 laser for the treatment of CIN are:

1. High degree of clinical efficacy,
2. Bloodless field,
3. Microscopic precision,
4. Sparing of normal tissue,
5. Rapid healing with minimal scar formation,
6. Small number of complications, and
7. Outpatient methodology.

The main disadvantage of the CO_2 laser is the absence of a histologic sample when vaporisation is performed.

The desired power density range for adequate ablation or excision of cervical lesions with minimal thermal damage to adjacent areas is 750–2000 W/cm^2 with an effective beam diameter of 1.5–2 mm. Super-pulse settings can be used to reduce thermal damage as well as to coagulate an area being ablated or excised. The power density delivered for coagulation may be reduced by enlarging the dot size or by reducing the power of the laser. The laser power of 10 W is sufficient to minimise scarring and lateral thermal damage for vaginal treatment or at vulva/perianal area.

In gynaecology, laser surgery is recommended for the treatment of warts (condylomata acuminata) in the anogenital area and dysplasia of the vulva, vagina and cervix (colposcopy) or for intra-uterine and endometrial pathologies (treated with hysteroscopy or laparoscopy, depending on the lesion). CO_2 laser microsurgery for gynaecology offers the best performance in the operating room.

Lasers are widely used in vaporisation, incision, and excision (e.g., conisation) of the soft tissues for the treatment of:

1. Condyloma acuminata of the cervix, vagina, anal vulvas,
2. Cysts and abscesses of Bartolin's glands,
3. Cysts of the mucosa,
4. Various degrees of CIN up to invasive or initial stage carcinomas (IA1),
5. Fornix and cupola pathologies (VAIN, vaginal endometriosis, condylomatosis),

6. VIN,

7. Bowen's disease, Queyrat's erythroplasia, Bowenoid papulosis,

8. Leukoplakia (vulvar dystrophy),

9. Polyps,

10. Perivulvar and perianal fistulas, and

11. Precancerous endoanal lesions.

Laser is successful for a wide range of gynaecological applications from the simple removal of lesions to bloodless high precision cutting. Laser is used for the removal of HPV lesions from the cervix, condyloma treatments, balanitis treatments and other surgeries. Recent lasers are used with minimally invasive gynecology treatments for incontinence and vaginal relaxation syndrome.

4.6.3 COLPOSCOPY

CO_2 laser coupled with a colposcope has become an indispensable tool for the ablation or excision of numerous lesions of the lower genital tract, especially when it is necessary to minimize tissue removal. The main applications in colposcopy are the treatment of dysplasia and warts of vulva, vagina, perineum and perianal area. In oncological gynecology, the CO_2 laser is the ideal technology for treatment of cervical intraepithelial neoplasia (CIN) by vaporisation or excisional cone biopsy (conization). The chances of complications with laser are very low. Moreover, the histological sample obtained with this method is without artefacts and therefore perfect for examination. The laser is the best choice for CIN due to:

1. Microscopic accuracy (ability to select the level of ablation with sub-millimetre precision).

2. High clinical effectiveness and clean surgery.

3. Minimal damage to healthy tissues surrounding the lesion.

4. Rapid healing with minimal scarring, even for the treatment of large lesions.

5. Reduced incidence of complications.

The most common treatments with CO_2 laser in colposcopy also include treatment of vulva intraepithelial neoplasia (VIN) and vaginal intraepithelial neoplasia (VAIN). The use of lasers in these cases is the best and excellent option in comparison to other surgical treatments. It is used in the treatment of cervical, vaginal, vulvar and anal acuminate condylomas, cysts and abscesses of Bartolin's glands, cysts of the mucosa, VIN, vulvar dystrophy, polyps, perivulvar and perianal fistulas, precancerous endoanal lesions and dysplasia of lower genital tract.

4.6.4 LAPAROSCOPY

This minimally invasive surgical procedure allows surgeon to perform surgery through small incisions. By using a laparoscope (a thin lighted telescope), gynecologic surgeon can make a small incision in the abdomen, rather than a long cut. The laparoscope is inserted through one or more small incisions into patient's abdomen. This type of surgery is not suitable for all patients.

Laser can be coupled with an operative laparoscope for intra-abdominal surgical treatments. The advantage of CO_2 laser in gynecological laparoscopy is the minimal lateral thermal damage and complete control of action depth. The CO_2 falls in the category of "WYSIWYG" (What You See Is What You Get) lasers. Interestingly, the operator can constantly monitor the penetration depth during surgery. The lasers are the best choice for laparoscopic surgery on critical areas such as those adjacent to the intestine, ureter and bladder. Optical fibres also play an important role in laparoscopic surgery. It is used in endometriosis, adhesions, myomas and uterine fibroids, ovarian fibromas and operations of salpingostomy, fimbrioplasty, fallopian tube microsurgery, oophorectomy, ovariectomy, ovarian drilling (for ovarian polycystosis), metroplasty, ablation of the uterosacral ligaments, hysterectomy, sacrocolpopexy, sacrocervicopexy, and sacrouteropexy (for genital prolapse).

Laparoscopy is also used for vaporisation, incision, excision, and photocoagulation of the soft tissues for treatment of:

1. Endometriosis,

2. Adhesions,

3. Myomas and uterine fibroids,

4. Ovarian fibromas,

5. Salpingostomy,

6. Fimbrioplasty,

7. Fallopian tube microsurgery,

8. Oophorectomy and ovariectomy,

9. Ovarian drilling (for ovarian polycystosis),

10. Metroplasty,

11. Ablation of the uterosacral ligaments,

12. Hysterectomy, and

13. Sacrocolpopexy, sacrocervicopexy, and sacrouteropexy (for genital prolapse).

The advantages of laparoscopy include minimal incisions, less pain, quicker recovery and reduced risk of infection. Laparoscopy is used in the following surgical situations:

1. Endometriosis diagnosis and treatment

2. Symptomatic ovarian cyst

3. Hysterectomy

4. Exploratory surgery for possible infertility causes

5. Ectopic pregnancy

6. Pelvic pain

7. Tubal ligation

The lasers are effective in the treatment of numerous pathological conditions including endometriosis. Endometriosis is a benign condition. Endometrial tissue (the tissue that lines the uterus) grows outside the uterine cavity and can attach itself to reproductive or abdominal organs. The patches of endometrial tissue swell with blood during menstruation as if they were still in the uterus, causing severe pain. Further, areas may bleed causing adhesions and cysts that can cause scarring and damage to nearby organs. Endometriosis is a common disorder, and most often occurs in women between the ages of 25 and 40. Symptoms vary and may worsen with time. They tend to improve during pregnancy and cease with menopause. Symptoms of endometriosis are:

1. Pain in the vagina, lower abdomen, and lower back (pain often begins just prior to monthly periods, continues during menses, and worsens just after the cessation of blood flow).

2. Abnormal or heavy menstrual bleeding.

3. Vaginal pain during sexual intercourse.

4. Infertility (endometriosis is one of the most common causes of infertility).

The treatment for endometriosis depends on the severity of symptoms, age and whether patient wants to have children, etc. Hence treatment depends on:

1. Low-dose oral contraceptive pills to suppress ovulation,

2. Hormone suppressing medication for 3–6 months to shrink endometrial tissue, and

3. Surgical removal of the tissue (laser laparoscopy, hysterectomy and oopherectomy).

The areas affected by endometriosis can be vapourised or removed by CO_2 laser which is most suitable for endometriosis treatment from phase I to IV (as per the classification of the American Fertility Society). The main reason is its high safety margin due to precise penetration depth control coupled with the minimal thermal damage to healthy tissues. These characteristics make it particularly suitable for operations in sensitive areas such as those adjacent to the ureter and intestine.

4.6.5 ADHESION

Pelvic adhesion disease can result from previous infections or after-effects of surgery. Both CO_2 and thulium diode laser systems are good choices for adhesiolysis. In particular, they are ideal tools for the lysis of vascular adhesions as they are able to perform excision and coagulation simultaneously by limiting the trauma of peripheral tissue.

4.6.6 UTERINE FIBROIDS AND OVARIAN FIBROIDS

For the removal of myomas (uterine fibroids) and ovarian fibroids, the CO_2 and thulium diode lasers are the best choices for the improved haemostasis, decreased tissue trauma and lower incidence of adhesion formation.

4.6.7 OVARIAN CYSTS

An ovarian cyst is a fluid-filled sac that forms in the ovary. They are common and generally benign (noncancerous). Ovarian cysts can be of different sizes and can occur at different sites in the ovary. The most common type develops when an egg-producing follicle does not rupture and release the egg but instead swells with fluid and forms a follicular cyst. Ovarian cysts often disappear on their own without treatment, but in some cases they may require laser surgical removal. In rare cases, a cyst that twists or ruptures can cause serious complications and emergency surgery may be necessary.

4.6.8 TUBAL DISEASE

Tubal disease is a common infertility condition. The fallopian tubes have blockages (usually adhesions) that prevent the fertilised egg from travelling into the uterus for implantation. Doctors diagnose tubal disease with a hysterosonogram, a radiological procedure that can diagnose tubal blockage. Alternatively, doctor view the obstructed tube through laparoscopy. Gynaecological surgery removes the blockages that are preventing from becoming pregnant.

4.6.9 HYSTEROSCOPY

Hysteroscopy is a procedure that allows the doctor to see the inside of uterus. Lasers equipped with a flexible fibre enter easily through the hysteroscope. Hysteroscope is used for endouterine surgical procedures, viz., removal of fibroids and polyps, resection of uterine septum, lysis of intrauterine adhesions, and endometrial ablation. The advantages of laser hysteroscopy are operation speed, limited blood loss, absence of abdominal and uterine scars, minimal morbidity and the absence of reduction in intra-uterine volume. It is used in the treatment of myomas, polyps, and uterine malformations (septate uterus, uterine synechiae and adhesions). Hysteroscopy is performed by using a hysteroscope (a thin, lighted telescope); the doctor will check the inside of the cervix and uterus. The hysteroscope is inserted through the vagina, so there are no incisions. The doctor may also collect different samples of tissue from the vagina, cervix and uterus to examine under the microscope to ascertain the evidence of irregular cells.

The reason for examining the uterus and cervix (inside) is to know the cause of irregular bleeding, for endometrial ablation and to remove fibroids and polyps. Endometrial ablation is used to burn away the lining of the uterus. It destroys most or all of the lining. The following Figures 4.5 (a), 4.5 (b) and 4.5 (c) show the treatment of endometriosis performed with CO_2 laser.

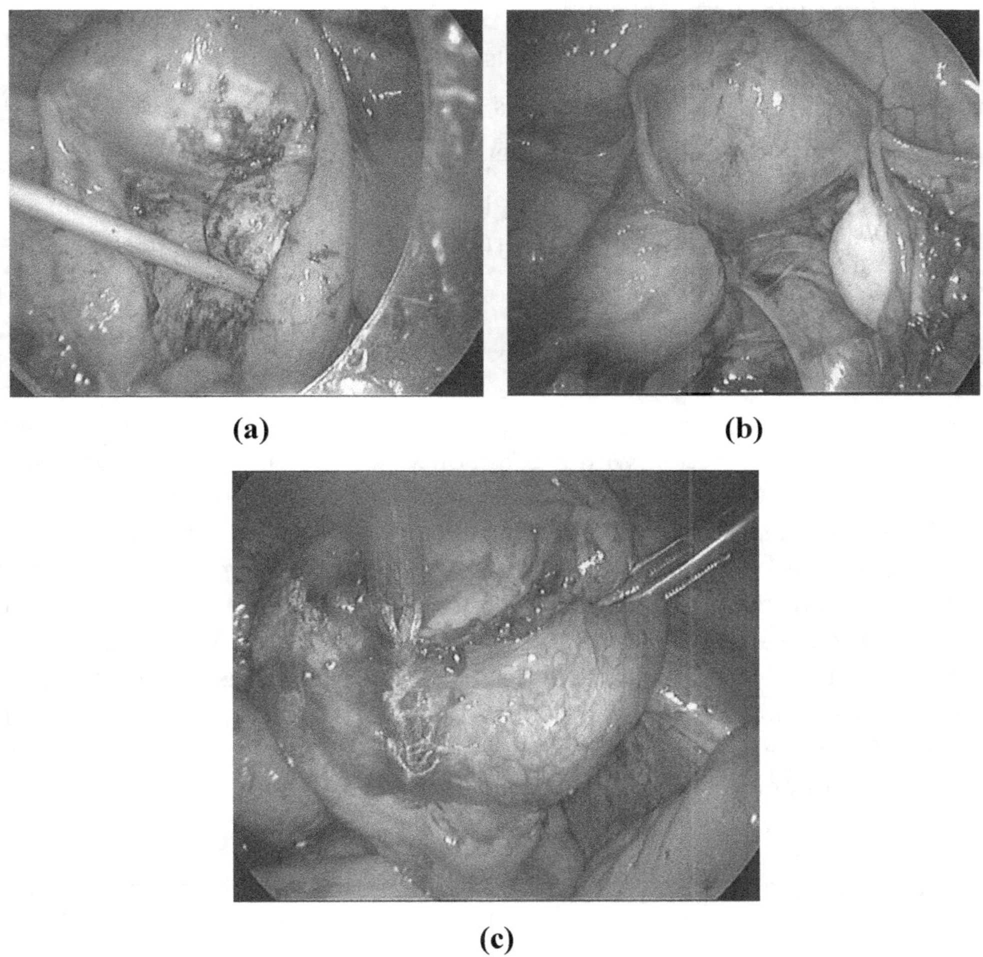

(a)

(b)

(c)

Figure 4.5 Treatment of endometriosis performed with CO_2 laser[Courtesy of M. Rosati, M.D. Director of the Operating Unit of Gynaecology and Obstetrics Spirito Santo Hospital, Pescara, Italy]

4.6.10 ECTOPIC PREGNANCY

An ectopic pregnancy occurs when a fertilized egg implants in the fallopian tubes, instead of the uterus. This is extremely dangerous, as the tube can burst, endangering a woman's life and future reproductive health. The symptoms of an ectopic pregnancy are:

1.   irregular vaginal bleeding,

2.   breast tenderness (which is also a symptom of early pregnancy),

3.   cramping or pain in the pelvis, especially on one side, and

4.   sharp pain felt in one shoulder.

To remove the ectopic pregnancy, laparoscopy or a laparotomy is carried out. If the ectopic pregnancy has not ruptured, medical treatment may be an option.

4.6.11 CERVICAL DYSPLASIA

Cervical dysplasia is the presence of precancerous cells on the cervix. A sexually transmitted infection with a common virus, the Human Papillomavirus (HPV) causes it. Cervical dysplasia can lead to cervical cancer which is the third leading cause of cancer death in women. HPV vaccine provides protection against HPV. There are usually no symptoms of cervical dysplasia. The results of a pap smear can diagnose cervical dysplasia. Mild dysplasia is often followed conservatively with no treatment. In many cases, the dysplasia will regress completely and the patient will clear the HPV virus. More severe lesions, known as high-grade squamous intraepithelial lesion (HGSIL), are often treated. There are several treatment options for woman with cervical dysplasia leading to the removal of the precancerous cells. They are:

1.   Laser—the laser can burn away the precancerous cells.

2.   LEEP (Loop Electrosurgical Excision Procedure)—this procedure uses cauterization (burning) to remove the precancerous cells.

3.   Cone biopsies—surgery removes the abnormal tissue.

4.   Cryotherapy—uses freezing to remove the precancerous cells.

4.6.12 LASER SAFETY

1.   For CO_2 laser of the external genitalia or cervix, the patient is draped in damp towels to absorb any misdirected laser beams and the patient's eyes are protected with wet gauze or protective glasses. All personnel, except the physician operating the microscope, should also wear eye protection accessories.

2.   The cervix, vagina, or vulva is bathed in a 3% solution of acetic acid, and abnormalities are noted with the microscope before the laser is fired.

3. A smoke evacuator system is used to remove the vapour plume. This is accomplished most efficiently with (a) a suction catheter attached to the speculum with a conduit toward the cervix to maximize plume removal or (b) a suction tip placed as far into the vagina as possible without interfering with the laser beam. Custom specula with smoke evacuation attachments are commercially available.

In future, HPV may be treated in a nonsurgical fashion with photosensitising drugs and a dye laser or gold vapour laser. It is known as photodynamic therapy which is widely used to diagnose and treat cancer. But it is applicable to many other areas.

4.7 LASER IN UROLOGY

In 1969, Miissiggang was the first to investigate the alterations caused by laser beams in kidney, bladder and prostate tissue using CO_2 and Nd:YAG laser. Lasers are used in the following areas in urology.

1. Bladder tumours
2. Urethral structures
3. Condyloma acuminata
4. Penile carcinoma
5. Laparoscopic procedures
6. Interstitial cystitis
7. Ureteral calculi
8. Prostatectomy
9. Vasectomy reversal (investigational)
10. Partial nephrectomy

The commonly used lasers in urology are CO_2, argon ion, Nd:YAG and dye lasers.

CO_2 lasers	Precise in cutting tissues
Nd:YAG lasers	For the coagulation of large tissue due to its deep penetration power
Q-switched Nd:YAG lasers	Standard tool in lithotripsy
Argon ion laser	Used for the coagulation of vascularies, tumours or malformations

In 1973, Nalt first demonstrated fibre optic endoscopic applications of lasers for destruction of bladder tissues. The urologic laser treatment extends from the external genital, the lower urinary tract (urethra), the bladder, the upper urinary tract (urethra) to the kidney. Lasers were successfully employed in treating benign hyperplasia of type 4 prostate.

The ultrasonic technique is conventionally used in lithotripsy of urinary calculi. In recent years urinary lithotripsy operation is based on the principle of laser-induced shock waves. The aim is to fragment urinary stones. The shock waves required to crush the stones are generated by optomechanical energy conversion. The energy from a Q-switched Nd:YAG (or Nd:GGG) laser (1.06 μm) is coupled into a thin fibre. This flexible fibre can be inserted into the patient's urinary track with the aid of small endoscopes. The energy of the short (0.025 ns) pulse at the end of the fibre produces plasma bubbles in the applied fluid (the process is in the laser-induced breakdown). The spontaneous expansion of the plasma causes the required shockwaves. During this treatment, no appreciable heating occurs even with long-duration irradiation.

In the biliany lithotripsy operation mode, the thermal effect of laser pulses is utilised. The relatively long (0.1 – 10 ms) laser pulses are applied directly to the calculus via a thin fibre under endoscopic control. The thermal, a photo-acoustic effect produces an interaction with the concrement where the pulsed laser light is absorbed and transformed into heat and stresses. First with relatively small energy (0.5 J) laser pulses, a hole is drilled into the stone until the center is reached. When the tip of the fibre reaches the center of the stone a few high energy pulses with about 2 J energy are applied. As a result of the thermally induced pressure and internal stress, the stone breaks up into several fragments. Recently Q-switched Alexandrite lasers are also used for stone breaking. They operate at wavelengths around 0.7 μm with a pulse duration varying in 30 ns – 50 μs range. Although the high repetition rate is destructive to urinary and biliary tissues, the damage to them is very minimal.

Urinary bladder carcinomas can be treated with argon ion and Nd:YAG lasers. But Nd:YAG laser is superior for applications because of its capacity to penetrate deeper, with light tissue-clearing effect. Nd:YAG laser is also used in endoscopic irradiation of bladder tumours with gas-filled or water-filled bladders. The irradiation effect is seen from a pale coloration and slight shrinkage of the tissue. The following irradiation effects can be observed during laser treatment of urinary bladder:

(i)   Nitrogen gas offers excellent view during irradiation. Charring is observed during irradiation.

(ii) Air-filled bladder can judge the alterations on the tissue surface. However, cooling effect must be considered.

(iii) The water-filled bladder charring occurs frequently and alterations in the tissue surface cannot be easily judged.

In general, one has to check the diagnosis by means of sample incisions from several areas of the tumour before the laser coagulation can be performed. From the literature it is clear that the endoscopic application of lasers is advantageous especially for destruction of small multiple tumours on the posterior wall of the bladder. The special advantages of endoscopic application of lasers compared to conventional technique is the low degree of bleeding or its absence and the deep homogeneous necrotization of the bladder wall with one perforation. The major disadvantage of the laser method is its high expenditure on apparatus. This situation is likely to change in the near future due to the new family of lasers—fibre lasers and new fibres.

Nd:YAG laser has the capacity for deep penetration and homogeneous irradiation on the tissue with development of total necrosis. A 40 watt and 600 μm focal spot size laser is suggested for the destruction of early stage penis carcinoma. Hence, the risk of performing partial amputation is avoided. But at an advanced stage, tumor is at first mechanically extricated. Subsequently, the remaining tissue surface should be additionally coagulated. The Nd:YAG laser has been used clinically to treat bladder tumours, penile carcinoma, urethral strictures and prostate cancer.

Lower urinary tract diseases are stenoses induced by inflammation and tumour growth of unknown origin. In these cases the CO_2 laser urethrotomey by endoscopic control is performed. The results from the technique are far satisfactory. The credit of using Ho:YAG laser (30 pulses within energy of 370 mJ with 1ms time) of urethral stenoses goes to Wieland (1993) and Nicolai (1995). According to them, this technique is a good alternative to mechanical urethrotomey in virgin stenoses as well as restenoses.

Tumours of the bladder are very difficult to treat, since they tend to relapse after therapy. Further, bladder tumours break bladder wall. Hence, a treatment is successfully provided to remove tumor completely without perforating the bladder wall or damaging the adjacent intestine. The CO_2, Nd:YAG, and argon lasers can be used on bladder tissues while Nd:YAG has proved to be the best laser, in coagulating bladder tumours. Even advanced tumours can also be efficiently removed with Nd:YAG lasers since the homeostatic treatment guarantees best vision. Nd:YAG laser with 30 – 40 w power and a working distance between 1 mm and 2 mm is suitable for treating bladder tumours. The tumour should be irradiated until it becomes pale. Afterwards, coagulated necrotic tissue is mechanically removed. For safety reason, the remaining tissue surface should also be coagulated. The laser treatment is extremely safe because perforations of the bladder wall are unlikely and the function of the bladder remains unaffected.

Very recently photodynamic therapy gained importance in the treatment of bladder tumours. Photodynamic therapy is considered as a useful supplement to other techniques since it enables the resection of tumours which are not visible or otherwise. The ability of simultaneous diagnosis by means of laser-induced fluorescence and the treatment of tumours are the key advantages of photodynamic therapy. It is certain that photodynamic therapy in urology will improve substantially in future with novel photosensitizers.

Recently research in urology is increasingly focused on diseases of the prostate (benign hyperplasias or carcinoma). Conventional therapies including photodynamic therapy are employed in the diseases of the prostate. However, the laser treatment is given only if the tumour cannot be completely eliminated.

Very recently the demand for minimally invasive techniques significantly increased. In the treatment of benign prostatic hyperplasia (BPH), two important procedures, viz., transurethral ultrasound-guided laser-induced prostatectomy (TULIPO) and laser-induced interstitial thermotherapy (LITT) were attempted. Out of these two, LITT is an excellent therapy for BPH.

Lasers have proved very successful in urological surgery. Cutting renal parenchyma by conventional techniques causes severe haemorrhage. Lasers have proved their particular usefulness, in performing nephronomy without harmful haemorrhage. With laser, it is possible to preserve the tissue adjacent to parenchyma tissue which ensures the smallest possible damage to the tissue.

Laser also plays an important part in the laser bladder surgery. The removal of endobladder papillon for smaller formations can be done by the vaporization of tissues using low-power laser beam (slightly out of focus on the tissue surface). The destruction was carried out gradually on subsequent thin layers. The advantages of laser technique in bladder surgery are the following:

1) Absence of sear retractions.

2) Absence of substantial reduction of bleeding.

3) Risk of squeezing the tumour avoided.

4) No physical touch with tumour.

Holography is a photographic technique that creates images which are much more realistic than the photographs produced by an ordinary camera. Holography is a three-dimensional photography. Holographic interferometry can be used not only in materials testing but also for early diagnosis of alterations in the bladder wall (such as bladder tumours) and ulcers precisely. Although there are many different approaches to holographic inspection, all use the same basic techniques. Two holograms are created from the object and these two holograms are superimposed and viewed simultaneously. Any change in the object that occurred between the two holograms shows up as interference fringes due to the alteration of internal pressure. That is, this area can be used for medical diagnostics. If endoscopic interferogram are produced by these techniques, organ systems which can be made accessible to the laser beam such as ulcers in the intestine or stomach, can be analysed.

The use of Nd:YAG laser for treatment of superficial bladder tumor is progressing. There will be no bleeding and the patient will not need a catheter. Urethral strictures have been successfully treated with both argon and Nd:YAG lasers, with the argon and KTP having worked better for the long strictures. The vapourising contact probe with the Nd:YAG laser may be an excellent approach to strictures but little experience has been acquired. Laser-assisted prostatectomy utilises the Nd:YAG laser for coagulation and/or ablation of the prostate. The laser is fired circumferentially around the prostate to close feeding vessels.

A combination of Ho:YAG/Nd:YAG laser is now being used so that coagulation/haemostasis of the prostate is achieved with the Nd:YAG and immediate recanalisation achieved with the Ho:YAG wavelength. In laser prostatectomy, VLAP (Visual Laser Ablation of the Prostate) has become more widely accepted because it is performed with mostly conventional instrumentation and the use of side firing fibres or contact probes. The prostate is directly visualised and the laser used circumferentially to photocoagulate the prostate. Additionally the obstructing prostate may be immediately ablated with contact tips or probes or the Ho:YAG laser.

A pulsed dye laser producing green light at 504 nm is used to fragment kidney stones. The laser impact develops a type of shock wave that mechanically disintegrates the stone. It works on impacted stones and those within the pelvis areas that are more difficult for extracorporeal shock wave lithotripsy (ESWL) to handle. It is also approved for use on biliary stones and sees use during endoscopic retrograde cholangiopancreatography (ERCP) for impacted common stones. More recently Ho:YAG, alexandrite and pulsed Nd:YAG laser systems have been used for lithotripsy.

4.8 LASER IN NEUROSURGERY

Although lasers were used in surgery, it took a long time for its use in neurosurgery. Heppner was the first to carry out the first successful tumour extirpation on humans in 1976 by using CO_2 laser. From that time onwards, the role of lasers has become more and more important, particularly in surgery. Neurosurgery is mainly dealing with the diseases of the central nervous systems. The main advantages of lasers in neurosurgery are due to its ability to cut, vaporize and coagulate tissue without mechanical contact. This is of great significance when dealing with very sensitive tissues. Simultaneous coagulation of blood vessels eliminates dangerous haemorrhages which are extremely life-threatening when occurring inside the brain. Further this area of operation is sterilized as lasing takes place at operation spot. The advantages and disadvantages of various lasers used in neurosurgery are listed below.

Laser type	Advantages	Disadvantages
Nd:YAG (1.319 μm)	Coagulation of blood vessels. Very precise tissue cut can be performed.	
Argon ion when combined with 200 μm fibre	Effective in coagulating blood vessels.	Strongly scattered inside brain tissue.
Er:YAG (2.94 μm)	Soft brain tissue which contains high water content is suddenly vaporised.	*Mechanical damage is pronounced* Thermal alteration on adjacent tissues

Laser type	Advantages	Disadvantages
Picosecond Nd:YLF	*Removal of tissue by plasma-induced ablation. *No thermal or mechanical damage to adjacent tissue.	
CW laser	Does not remove brain tumours but only coagulates them	Necrotic tissue remains inside the brain leading to the occurrence of severe oedema
CO_2 laser	Ideal for microscopic use, long reach into small holes and precision. Its ability to vaporise is useful in debulking tumours. Used to dissect muscle for spinal surgery.	

An interesting technique called stereotactic neurosurgery which is a well-established clinical discipline, is reported in the literature. By means of a stereotactic head ring, a laser probe is inserted into the brain. CT and NMR data are used to position the distal end of the probe inside the tumour. Stereotactic techniques are not only applied in combination with lasers but also with alternative therapies. Stereotactic surgery is certainly a favoured treatment of minimal invasive surgery (MIS).

Jain (1980) developed yet another technique of suture microvascular anastomosis using Nd:YAG laser of 18 W power, 0.3 mm focal spot size and 0.1 s single exposure. This is performed in some cases of cerebrovascular occlusive disease.

Spinal surgery is another important area of neurosurgical treatment. CO_2 laser was successfully used in treating tumours of the spinal cord. Such tumours can be coagulated without severe complications. Neurosurgery is expected to show a breakthrough with miniaturized surgical instruments in the near feature. The highly sophisticated endoscopes and appropriate lasers will create a revolution in neurosurgery in the years to come.

4.9 LASERS IN CARDIOLOGY

From laser studies, we know that patients operated with lasers need fewer blood transfusions than patients operated on with scalpel. Lasers can be used in angioplasty treatment. Angioplasty is nothing but the treatment of a narrowed or obstructed blood vessel, the latter typically being a result of atherosclerosis. The degree of obstruction is obtained in percentage by 100 x intimal area / (internal area + space available for blood flow).

Judkins (1964) performed angioplasty to femoral arterial using a special type of catheter. This technique was modified and extended to coronary arteries by Gruntzig (1979). This was considered to be a major contribution as the atherosclerotic plaques on the vessel wall are life-threatening. This technique increases the size of the vessel through cracking, splitting and disrupting plaque. Although this method is safe, there occurs some short-term and long-term complications. Apart from by-pass surgery, atherectomy and high-frequency rotational coronary angioplasty (HFRCA) are a few surgical treatments for coronary arteriosclerosis. By-pass surgery involves a complicated open heart surgery with the interruption of heartbeat. The atheroclony involves mechanical abrasion.

In the eighties, an attempt was made to use thermal lasers such as argon ion, CO_2 and Nd:YAG laser in angioplasty. Laser radiation was applied to the plaque by means of optical fibres which caused severe thermal injuries such as extensive coagulation necrosis of vascular tissue vessel wall. Subsequently, laser catheter was modified by enclosing distal and optical fibre metallic cap. This arrangement converts laser energy into thermal energy by absorption. Hence, the plaques are homogeneously removed. But subsequent research revealed the occurrence of vasospasm (thermally induced shrinkage of the vessel wall). In general, these vasospasms are not predictable and they can induce severe secondary obstructions.

The pulsed excimer laser XeCl was also employed for performing efficient plaque ablations with minimal thermal injury of adjacent tissues. Although it appeared to be successful, after three years the excimer laser angioplasty caused a severe restenosis which led to an actuate myocardial infarction. Hence medical community totally rejected excimer laser angioplasty.

In 1992 Ho:YAG laser was attempted in laser angioplasty and found that its clinical use is extremely limited. Mirohseini et al. (1992) proposed CO_2 laser systems to create additional channel for the blood supply of heart. These channels originate from the epicardium and remain open after laser treatment. Although this method proved to be successful, further researches are required regarding blood flow and recovery before a general acceptance of the method.

As on today, laser diagnosis plays an important role in angioplasty. It is widely accepted that laser endoscope is a very sensitive method when compared to X-ray ultrasonic angioplasty doppler angiography. The development of powerful miniaturised and sensitive laser endoscopes with visible laser radiation will create a new era in laser endoscope for angioplasty.

Electrophysiology technique in curing palpitation will be replaced by photophysiology using He+Ne or ruby laser in the near future.

Laser uses in cardiovascular medicine generally include:

1. Peripheral laser angioplasty
2. Transmyocardial revascularisation
3. Laser welding
4. Coronary laser angioplasty
5. Laser thrombolysis
6. Arrhythmic node ablation.

Argon lasers with hand-held fibres at 0.5 to 3 watts output is used to weld arteriotomies with good results. Pulsed Ho:YAG and excimer lasers are used for reopening of blood vessels because these can remove tissues precisely without generating excessive heat in the process.

4.10 LASERS IN DERMATOLOGY AND PLASTIC SURGERY

Modulation of the laser exposure time to the skin is very important. The prolonged exposure time beyond thermal relaxation time leads to excessive heating. The basic concept in tissue damage is

$$\text{Heat energy} \times \text{exposure time} = \text{Tissue damage}$$

The thermal property of laser radiation is successfully used in coagulation and vaporization in dermatology. Since absorption and scattering are wavelength-dependent, one can induce various types of tissue – radiation interaction with argon ion laser, dye laser, CO_2 laser, ruby laser and Nd:YAG laser. The specific use of lasers in various treatments in dermatology is illustrated below:

Lasers	Applications via absorption/scattering
Argon ion laser	Strong absorption by pigmentation and melanin (dark tissue). Penetrates the skin 0.5 to 2 mm. 1. Superficial treatment of haemangiomas and melanin vascularised lesions. 2. Removing port wine stains. 3. Removing tattoos.
Tunable dye laser 577–585 nm (yellow)	Mostly used because of the tunability of the wavelength, which can be adapted to the organ to be removed. The specific wavelength which has maximum absorbance in the defective tissue can be chosen, while at the same time it should have low absorbance in normal tissue. Most efficient and less painful treatment of port wine stain (but costly). Selective applications in vascular skin lesions.
CO_2 laser	1. Tissue removal by vaporization. 2. Treatment of external ulcers and refractory warts. 3. Removing tattoos.
Ruby laser	Removing tattoos.
Nd:YAG laser	Significantly less scattered and absorbed 1. Treatment of the deeply located haemangiomas and semi-malignant skin tumour.
Copper vapour laser (578 nm, 514 nm)	Administered as a more of a fine pinpoint to trace vessel.

Active research is on the way, regarding biosimulative effects of laser radiation. The contribution of biostimulation on wound healing is under progress. The mechanism of biostimulation is not yet understood clearly and hence one has to be careful in using the laser for biostimulation work. If very low power laser is used, its effect becomes unnoticed. It is believed that the ongoing research in this area will throw some light on biostimulation and wound healing in the coming years.

The main advantages of lasers in dermatology are (1) almost no bleeding and (2) almost no scars left after removal of defects.

Lasers can remove almost all the defects such as pigmented skin, abnormal skin growth and blemishes on the skin. Sometimes the laser is the only instrument to perform a specific procedure. With the wide variety of lasers in use, tattoos can almost completely be erased from the skin. Different wavelengths are used to remove different ink colours from the skin. The specific laser wavelength is selectively absorbed by the specific colour, without damage to surrounding cells. Usually the treatment is made in a number of sittings. What was left in the damaged skin is checked after each and every sitting. Most dermatological procedures are done in an outpatient clinic, under local anaesthesia. Use of lasers in dermatology and plastic surgery include:

1. Port wine stains
2. Hemangioma
3. Nevus ad benign skin lesion
4. Scar revisions
5. Reduction of wrinkles
6. Hair removal
7. Tattoo removal
8. Café–au–lait spots
9. Telangiectasia
10. Superficial varicosities
11. Skin resurfacing
12. Non-ablative skin rejuvenation
13. Verruca
14. Actinic cheilitis
15. Laser blepharoplasty

Pulsed dye lasers of about 510 nm are used for pigmented lesions to the 585 nm used for vascular lesions. The short pulse lasers for benign pigmented lesions are given below:

Laser	Wavelength (nm)	Indication
Short pulse dye	510	Epidermal lesions
Q-switched Nd:YAG	532, 1064	Epidermal lesions, dermal lesions
Q-switched ruby	694	Epidermal or dermal lesions
Q-switched alexandrite	755	Epidermal or dermal lesions

Epidermal pigmented lesions may also be treated satisfactorily with continuous or pseudo-continuous lasers. They are given below:

LASER	Wavelength (nm)
Argon	488, 515
Tunable dye	504 or greater
Copper vapour	511
Krypton	521, 531
KTP	532

Nd:YAG, diode, alexandrite, ruby and intense pulsed laser systems are used for hair removal. Tattoos can be removed with argon, KTP and CO_2 lasers. Pulsed Nd:YAG, pulsed Nd:YAG doubled to green light, ruby, and alexandrite laser systems are also used to provide better fragmentation of the dye granules. There are advantages and disadvantages to each system depending on the preferences of the user. These aesthetic treatments are discussed in the next section under cosmetic photonics.

4.10.1 Eczema and Dermatitis

Eczema describes skin which is red, dry, scaly, cracked, blistered or cozing and any other combination thereof. Eczema is just a skin description. Determing the cause of eczema constitutes a diagnosis and permits rational treatment. There are several common types of eczema and they are:

1)   Allergic contact eczema.

2)   Irritant contact eczema.

3)   Atopic dermatitis—This is due to the scratch that itches which causes skin inflammation. Basically, it is an immunologic disease of hyperactivity of the skin to many exogenous antigens.

4)   Dishydrotic eczema—The sudden appearance of water blisters along the fingers, palms and soles. These blisters are quite itchy at first and then flatten out and become scaly. Stress is often an exacerbating factor.

Eczema is also due to circulatory problems in the legs (stasis dermatitis), dry air, xerotic eczema and scalp disease (seborrhoea). Laser therapy that delivers a concentrated beam of ultraviolet light may help ease a hard-to-treat form of eczema. An excimer laser 308 nm is used for treating atopic dermatitis and certain other skin conditions, including psoriasis and vitiligo. It works by emitting a concentrated beam of ultraviolet B (UVB) light directly to patches of affected skin, avoiding the healthy surrounding skin. The purported advantage of the excimer laser over traditional UVB therapy is that it more precisely targets the problem areas of the skin. The patients received weekly twice laser treatments for 10 weeks.

4.10.2 Warts Removal

Warts that affect human skin are common and in most cases they are benign. Warts are of two main types. One is due to the human papovavirus and the other wart virus (pox virus) causes molluscum contagiosum.

There are 70 types of HPV and they occur anywhere on the body. They are named by their location—plantar, when it is at the bottom of the foot and genital when they are on or near the genital areas. Although warts are contagious, the virus is so ubiquitous that it is usually not reasonable or possible to pinpoint the source of infection. However, infection in the genital area is an exception.

Warts often regress spontaneously. Most warts can be destroyed by burning, freezing or by acids. For stubborn warts, several types of lasers may be used. Carbon dioxide or erbium YAG lasers vapourise the top layers of the skin. Vascular lasers may also be helpful in that they target the dilated blood vessels at the base of the wart. Laser warts removal treatment is effective and permanent on fingers, finger nails, face, feet, hands, elbows and knees.

4.10.3 Moles and Melanoma

Moles appear during the early years. Almost everyone has pigmented spots on their skin. Most adults have approximately twenty five moles—some have none and others have hundreds. Moles generally appear between childhood and the mid-twenties. Pigmented spots or moles present at birth or in the first year of life are called 'congenial'. They seem to have a higher chance of becoming malignant; however the exact percentages are in dispute. Certainly, congenital moles should be evaluated and in many cases removed. Most benign moles are small and symmetric with even borders and bland coloration. Normally they do not itch, burn or bleed. Moles which change, which become inflamed or whose border and /or colour is irregular should be evaluated. Despite advances in photography and digital imaging, the gold standard of evaluation of a mole remains biopsy with microscopic evaluation. When examined under a microscope, a mole may be 1) Benign (harmless), 2) Atypical or dysplastic (appear unusual under the microscope), and 3) Malignant melanoma (tumor). It shows features of asymmetry, border irregularity, colour variation and diameter larger than 6 mm. If diagnosed early, it can be cured.

4.10.4 PSORIASIS

Psoriasis is a genetically determined, chronic, inflammatory disease of the skin. It may be limited to small areas such as the elbows or scalp or it may be extensive and generalized. The nature of disease may change over the years. It may be made worse by stress, infection or even sunburn. Many forms of treatment are available. Therapy is tailored to the patient and the severity of the disease. In any psoriasis therapy, control—but not cure—should be expected. Untreated skin on thigh and treated skin is shown in Figure 4.6.

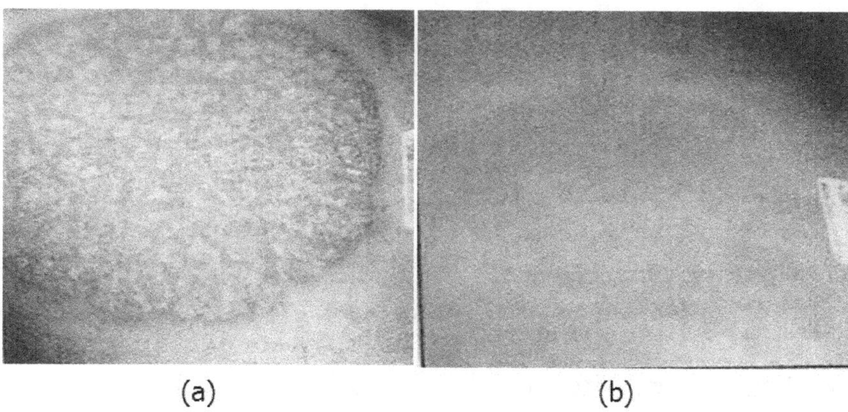

(a)   (b)

Figure 4.6 Psoriosis is treated successfully with excimer lasers (a) Untreated skin on thigh and (b) Treated skin (Courtesy: The Gange Centre, Massachusetts Hospital)

Prior to laser use, patients requested up to 25 treatments with UVB radiation (λ = 311 to 312 nm) to remove silvery over-grown skin patches characteristics of the disease. With excimer lasers, as few as four to six treatments can be effective to cure psoriasis. Using λ = 340 and 400 nm, atopic dermatitis and morphea (skin becomes thick and forms depressions) are treated.

4.10.5 Skin Cancer Treatments

The three major forms of skin cancer are a) basal cell carcinoma, b) squamous cell carcinoma, and c) malignant melanoma. The common skin cancer among these is basal cell carcinoma.

i)   Basal cell carcinoma

It usually appears on the skin exposed to the sun and looks like a flesh-coloured or pink bump or a sore that bleeds but does not heal. There is a great variability in its location and appearance. It is diagnosed by biopsy and surgically removed.

ii)   Squamous cell carcinoma

The next common carcinoma of skin is squamous cell carcinoma. It also appears on sun-exposed skin. Generally it starts as crusted patch that refuses to heal. Biopsy and surgical treatment is the common choice for this cancer.

iii) **Malignant melanoma**

The most serious type of skin cancer is malignant melanoma. Although it appears in the sun-exposed skin, it occurs anywhere in the body including the eye. If detected early, it is 100% curable. If the lesion has a) asymmetry, b) irregular borders, c) colour variation, and d) diameter larger than 6 mm, then it is malignant melanoma.

Apart from surgical cancer removal and skin immunotheraphy, photodynamic therapy of skin cancer is becoming popular.

4.10.6 *Photodynamic Treatment of Skin Cancer*

In photodynamic therapy, a photosensitizer is applied to the skin. This is absorbed preferentially by certain structures in the skin, such as hair follicles, oil glands, bacteria or rapidly growing cells; illumination with a high-intensity or laser causes a photochemical reaction in the skin, resulting in destruction of the targeted tissue. Photodynamic therapy has been effective in the treatment of actinic keratoses, some types of skin cancer, sun-damaged skin, acne and oily skin with sebaceous gland enlargement.

During PDT, the skin is washed several times and the activated substance is applied. Either of these may cause stinging. During therapy, burning may occur and local anaesthesia may be used to prevent this. Following treatment there may be some transient itching and burning. After PDT, a small amount of activated substance remains in the skin for 24 to 48 hours. Sunlight and even indoor light may affect this and cause redness and itching. Use of sunscreen and a hat may diminish the undesired effects. Most people experience mild burning and itching for about one hour after procedure, although this can last a day or two. Mild to moderate redness may be experienced for 24 to 48 hours. Routinely, gentle emollients should be applied to the skin. Areas most likely to swell are around the eyes. This will subside within several hours. Application of ice or cold packs may help. Peeling of treated skin may occur several days after the procedure and can be alleviated by gentle washing and application of a slightly thicker moisturizer.

In other technique, photosensitizing agent is injected into blood stream. It is absorbed by cells all over the body but stays in cancer cells longer than it does in normal cells. Approximately 24 to 72 hours after injection, most of the agent has left normal cells but the agent remains in cancer cells and the tumor is exposed to light. The photsensitizer in the tumor absorbs the light and produces an active form of oxygen that destroys nearby cancer cells. Apart from killing cancer cells, PDT appears to shrink or destroy tumours in two other ways. It damages the blood vessel in the tumor so that nutrients are prevented from reaching blood vessel. Second, PDT activates the immune system to attack tumor cells. The laser light is used for PDT. Laser light can also be directed through fibre optic cables to deliver light to areas inside the body. Fibre optic can be inserted through an endoscope into the lungs or oesophagus to treat cancer in these organs. LEDs can be used for treating surface tumours such as skin cancer. Porfimer sodium (Photofrin) is used to treat symptoms of esophageal and lung cancer.

PDT has its own limitations. They are:

(1) The light needed to activate most sensitizers cannot pass through more than one centimetre. Hence, PDT is used to treat tumours just under the skin or on the lining of internal organs or cavities.

(2) PDT is less effective in treating large tumours.

(3) PDT is a local treatment and generally cannot be used to treat cancer that has spread.

The side effects of PDT are as follows:

Patient must remain out of direct continued sun exposure for 5 days following treatment. Porfimer sodium makes the skin and eyes sensitive to light for approximately 6 weeks after treatment. Hence, patients are advised to avoid direct sunlight and bright indoor light for atleast 6 weeks. Although damage to healthy tissue is minimal by PDT, it causes burns, swelling, pain and scaring in nearby healthy tissues. Other temporary side effects are coughing, trouble swelling, stomach pain or painful breathing.

4.10.7 Lasers and Plastic Surgery

Histological and histochemical examinations of stained fragments cut by laser shows no evidence of tissue necrosis or any other cellular damage. The cut surface is identically same to that obtained by scalpel. Therefore a cut made by laser may be sutured and will heal normally just as any cut made by scalpel. The same is true to a skin flap prepared by laser. While cutting, laser beam automatically give rise to haemostasis, sealing blood vessels with free blood flow, up to a diameter of 1.5 mm and upto 2 mm when blood flow is stopped. This type of automatic haemostasis considerably reduces operation time and complications. Further, the laser beam seals lymphotic vessels at the same time as it seals blood vessels without touching the tissues. The patients recover from an operation with less pain and recovering time is fast. Hence, surgeons throughout the world are of the opinion that lasers can be used. Experience also shows that the use of laser leads to sterilisation of the wounds thus facilitating and shortening any subsequent treatment of infected wounds, phagedenic ulcerations and bed sores, etc. These properties are helpful to use laser in plastic surgery.

Laser has made a significant contribution in the treatment of serious burns. By using lasers, necrotic tissues can be excised without much blood loss so that patient's haematic, proteinic and electrolyte levels are balanced. Subsequently, vital surfaces are covered with dermo-epidermic grafts which save the patient from terrible pain and fast recovery. The burnt surfaces can be given grafts at a later date.

The CO_2 laser which has a wavelength of 10.6 mm in the near infrared region is best suited for plastic surgery. These lasers at 10.6 mm possess high absorption coefficient, poor penetration, no colour discrimination and delivery by mirror reflections which are the required properties for surgery. Hence, with minimal coagulation, neurosis at the edge of the cut is good enough to seal vessels up to 0.5 mm in diameter providing good haemostasis. The rapidity of evaporation limits the size and depth of the cut as well as thermal side effects. It should be remembered that the CO_2 laser is not as effective as the argon or the Nd:YAG laser systems for bleeding because of its deeper penetration (short wavelength). The latter two systems have larger thermal effects and hence there is a wide coagulation necrosis and the sealing of bigger vessels up to 1– 3 mm in diameter. These latter two systems are more adoptable for parenchymatous tissue cutting and coagulating as well as for fibre optic endoscopy.

The CO_2 laser beam in the face lift procedure is very impressive. It is very neat, smooth and precise cutting with almost no oozing. The surgeons have to control and clamp bigger vessels. The risks of haematomas and infection are minimal, particularly with proper handling of tissues. In fact the level of swelling, oedema and discomfort are very little. An abdominoplasty and lipectomy are body contouring operations where CO_2 laser with 40 W CW beam can be useful and is highly recommended. The same laser was also successfully used in eyelid plasty and mammoplasty.

4.11 LASER IN ORTHOPAEDICS

At present, bone excisions (osteotomics) are done in orthopaedics using saws, milling machines and mechanical drill. All these instruments make physical contact and cause severe mechanical vibration and haemorrhages. Since lasers possess unique property, they can be used in the place of mechanical instruments in osteotomics. The high water content (sharp absorber of IR radiation) in the bone gives a clue that CO_2, Er:YAG and Ho:YAG lasers can be used for this purpose. Ho:YAG laser (pulsed) is used for joint arthroscopy and spinal work. The research has proved that CO_2 laser was successfully employed in osteotomics. The only disadvantage is the delayed healing. It was concluded that the thermal damage of the bone rim was responsible for the delay. It is to be remembered that wavelength and pulse duration play an important role in osteotomics. The other types of lasers used in orthopaedics are:

Laser	Advantage/disadvantage	Clinical use
Ho:YAG	1. Causes higher thermal damage. 2. Radiation is efficiently transmitted through flexible fibres.	Used in ablation.
Er:YAG	Causes very low thermal damage.	Used in microsurgery in the inner ear.

The excimer lasers have also been proposed for the removal of bone material due to their high precision in removing tissues. Unfortunately the efficiency of these lasers is low for clinical applications. Further, they cause severe thermal damage and hence a considerable delay in healing due to laser-induced bone excisions.

Lasers can also be used for arthroscopic treatments. Transmission of lasers through flexible fibres is regarded as a mandatory requirement for an efficient surgical procedure. Due to this constraint, CO_2 lasers are not suitable for arthroscopic treatments. Nd:YAG laser combined with ceramic contact process was used in arthroscopic treatment of the jaw joint. Hence, optical delivery system for all IR lasers plays an important role in arthroscopic treatments.

The recent researches on arthroscopic treatment using Ho or Er lasers encourage a positive trend. The success of Ho:YAG laser for the ablation of cartilage was reported by Trauner during 1990. Er:YAG laser operating at 2.79 μm is effectively used for tissue ablation although it is strongly absorbed by water. The encouraging results of holmium and erbium lasers in minimally invasive arthroscopic surgery indicate a bright future for these lasers as valuable surgical tools.

Laser surgery in fact proves to be particularly useful in the treatment of haemophiliac patients with articular lesions. These patients develop a characteristic arthropathy mainly affecting knee, elbow and ankle joints. In these cases, the laser enables surgery with a minor blood loss which considerably reduces medical collateral therapy. Further, a marked reduction of post-operative pain and a shortening of hospital stay have been observed.

Orthopaedic lasers are used in

 (1) Joint arthroscopies (all types),

 (2) Low level laser therapy for pain,

 (3) Endoscopic carpel tunnel release, and

 (4) Laser discectomy (decompression).

An exciting prospect for reconstructive orthopaedic microsurgery is the use of laser to achieve tissue fusion. Low power density carbon dioxide lasers and argon lasers do this job.

4.12 LASERS IN OTORHINOLARYNGOLOGY AND PULMOLOGY

Otorhinolaryngology deals with the diseases of the ear, the nose and the throat. The most significant application of lasers in otorhinolaryngology is microsurgery of the larynx. Laryngeal carcinoma is the most frequent malignant tumours of the throat. The five major origins of this carcinoma are:

 1. Epiglottis

 2. Vestibulum

 3. Ventriculis laryngis

 4. Glottis (vocal cord)

 5. Infraglottis

Diagnosis and treatment of laryngeal carcinoma are performed by means of laryngoscope. It was already established that benign and malignant lesions of vocal cords can be safely removed with CO_2 lasers instead of mechanical means. But laser therapy aims at a palliative treatment for the advanced cases. When patients are treated with laser under complete anaesthesia, the inflammable gases causes complication. For a proper operation of the intubation tube, metal tubes provide highest security. Laser treatment of patients with various laryngeal lesions showed several advantages (M.S. Strong and G.J. Jako, *Ann. Otol.* 81, 791 1972).

Laser surgery in the larynx first reported using CO_2 lasers in the treatment of various lesions of the vocal cords and CO_2 lasers has the following advantages:

1. CO_2 laser energy can be applied in extremely accurate doses to exactly the right spot,

2. There is no post-operative oedema,

3. Rapid healing, and

4. Virtually there is no blood loss in this operation.

The laser can also be successfully used to enlarge the air way in the case of stenoses. The laser is also extremely useful in the treatment of laryngeal carcinoma. Further, recent researches proved that the laser is undoubtedly useful in the palliative management of patients with malignant lesions which causes obstruction of the airway. Lasers were employed in the treatment of patients for whom surgery or radiotherapy was impossible. Hence, laser can offer favourable results from primary laser therapy of small malignant neoplasm confined to a single vocal cord. If the lesion is very extensive, one can go for laser excision to remove the tumour.

Recently, it was established that CO_2 laser is superior to conventional therapy when treating laryngeal or subglottic stenoses. If the stenoses are of the order of several centimetres in size, it should be subjected to conventional surgery. The ability of laser to perform surgery and coagulation of blood vessels is utilised in laser treatment of the nose. Highly vascular tumours such as haemangiomas or pre-malignant alterations of the mucosa can be treated with argon ion or carbon dioxide lasers.

Laser was used to treat otosclerosis which is a bone disease of the inner ear. Otosclerosis affects the stapes and finally leads to hearing impairment. There are two types of treatment available, viz., stapedectomy and stapedotomy. In the former, the stapes of footplate in the inner ear are mechanically removed and replaced by an artificial implant. In the latter, a microhole is drilled into the stapes using miniature drills or with suitable lasers. Laser stapedotomy is considered as a typical method of minimally invasive surgery (MIS). Since laser technique is a non-contact method it is best suited for stapedotomy. The type of laser used in stapedotomy and their advantages are listed below:

Laser	Advantages	Disadvantages
Argon laser		Strongly absorbs only in highly pigmented tissue, efficiency in ablating cortical bone is very weak.
Frequency doubled Nd:YAG laser		Efficiency in ablating cortical bone is very weak.
CO_2 laser		It cannot be guided through optical fibres.
Er:YAG and Er:YSGG laser	Strongly absorbed in bones. Can be transmitted through ZrF_4. Edge of perforation is very precise and does not indicate mechanical damage. Efficiency is good.	

In stapedotomy, one can expect risks due to the rise in temperature of the perilymph and induced high pressure on cochlea. The technology helps us to overcome the problem of the power output of Er:YAG laser which is limited to 10 J/cm². The increase in temperature can be controlled to the order less than 5°C. Similarly erbium lasers permit a safe pressure level if their fluence is limited to 10 J/cm². In recent times, KTP laser play a vital role in all ENT treatments.

Pulmology is connected with diseases of the lung. The resection of tracheobronchial tumours is conveniently performed with a rigid bronchoscope. Severe and life threatening haemorrhage is often inevitable. Apart from this, mechanical removal, electrocoagulation and cryotherapy are also performed. In the last decade, treatment of tracheobronchial lesions was attempted with

Nd:YAG laser and a flexible fibre. Since Nd:YAG laser provides the surgeon with the ability of immediate coagulation, the occurrence of severe haemorrhage is significantly reduced.

Doctors believe that Nd:YAG laser is a valuable supplement in the therapy of tracheobronchial tumours although it is usually limited to a palliative treatment. The research on lasers and clinical studies are progressing steadily in this area for alternative lasers. Further, the advances in the development of photosensitisers such as 5-aminolaevulinic (ALA) paves the way for laser treatment in tracheobronchial tumours.

4.13. LASERS IN GASTROENTEROLOGY

Gastroenterology covers the diseases concerning ulcers and tumours of the oesophagus, stomach, liver, gall bladder, ileum, colon and rectum. Any kind of ulcer or tumour can be treated with lasers if it is accessible with endoscopic surgery. Depending on the nature and size of the tumour, laser application is restricted. For a nonresectable tumour, laser treatment is palliative so that patient experiences relief in pain. Argon, KTP and Nd:YAG lasers have been used endoscopically in the treatment of gastrointestinal disease. However, the Nd:YAG plays the primary role in the treatment.

In gastroenterology, laser is used in the following areas:

1. Esophageal obstructions
2. AV malformations
3. Fistula repair
4. Hemorrhoidectomy
5. Pilonidal cysts and sinuses
6. Hemorrhagic telangiectasia
7. Colonoscopy
8. Colorectal tumours
9. Fissure repair abscesses

The CW thermal Nd:YAG laser is used in the treatment of gastrointestinal haemorrhages and benign, malignant or non-neoplastic stenoses. At low power, it stops bleeding by coagulation and at high power it serves in recanalisation of stenoses. The other lasers such as argon laser and CO_2 lasers (not suitable as it cannot transmit through optical fibres) were also attempted in gastroenterology without significant advance. The dye laser is employed only in photodynamic therapy. Very recently electron speckle interferometry technique using low power laser was employed to diagnose the stomach ulcer successfully.

Stenoses of the oesophagus can be treated with lasers. Even if endoscope cannot pass the stenoses, it can be widened mechanically through dilatators and subsequently coagulated using Nd:YAG laser with quartz fibres. Unfortunately stenoses of oesophagus occur frequently and can be treated with radioactive source. Laser coagulation for malignant oesophagus tumours, esophagectomy or palliative treatment was suggested. After esophagectomy, an artificial tube can be installed. The Nd:YAG laser finds its application in the endoscopic treatment of bleeding from peptic ulcers.

Obstructions may be coagulated in a noncontact fashion, then debrided. Care must be taken at the anterior wall because of the deep Nd:YAG scatterer, to avoid tracheal–esophageal fistulas. Obstructions can also be opened with the use of contact vapourising probes.

Cryotherapy is the conventional technique used for the treatment of lower gastrointestinal tract. In general, the treatment is carried out under complete anaesthesia in contrast to laser treatment. But laser therapy causes an enhanced formation of oedema. However, such oedema can be treated medically.

Laser therapy for haemorrhage is widely reported in literature. Using lasers, all localised and acute haemorrhages can be coagulated. The suggested powers for such lasers are:

Rectum	50 – 70 W
Stomach	70 – 100 W

Immediately after the clearance of blood source, tissue can be coagulated. There is no time limit for this procedure. Following laser treatment, patients should be supervised for at least three days in ICU.

Sandeer in 1988 developed a technique to treat ulcers or haemorrhages using a combination of laser beam and water jet. The laser beam is guided through a water jet to the site of applications. This technique appears to be useful for other kinds of tissue coagulation.

Although Nd:YAG lasers are widely used in gastroenterology, a few reports are appearing in the literature about the complications from its use. Hence, active research is on the way to find alternative lasers to Nd:YAG lasers. In the years to come, one can expect a few more lasers for the treatment in gastroenterology.

As discussed earlier, photodynamic therapy (PDT) is successfully used in modern gastroenterologic treatment. Rhodamine dye lasers pumped with an argon ion laser is used for this purpose. This area of study is becoming very popular due to the development of novel photosensitisers which have a very high efficiency in the red and near infrared. One has to keep in mind that the success is inversely related to tumour size at the time of treatment. With an early diagnosis of tumour, nearly 75% of cases can be completely cured. The major advantage of PDT is that fewer endoscopic sessions are usually required, compared to treatments with the Nd:YAG laser. Therefore overall duration of a PDT treatment is significantly shorter and easier to tolerate. This area shows a great promise for laser as well as medical community.

4.14 LASERS IN PODIATRY (DISORDERS OF THE FOOT, ANKLE AND LOWER EXTREMITY)

The CO_2 laser is the most commonly used in podiatry, though the HO:YAG laser show much interest for ankle arthroscopy. Lasers are used in podiatry for:

1. Verrucae plantaris
2. Heel fissures
3. Matrixectomy
4. Excision of neuromas, cysts, etc.
5. Heel spurs
6. Callus, cysts, corns, etc.
7. Fungus nails
8. Subungual hematoma
9. Scar excision
10. Ankle arthroscopy

4.15   RECENT MEDICAL APPLICATIONS USING LOW POWER LASER

Laser therapy may be considered as an alternative to heart surgery in treating ischaemic heart disease because it increases the contractile power of the heart and restores blood supply to the heart, as before. It reduces viscosity of blood. As an antioxidant, it reduces the stickiness of plaque and gradually reduces high blood pressure, thereby reducing the chances of the rupture of soft plaque. It reduces cholesterol by acting on lipid metabolism and increases micro-circulation. It also reduces the amount of soft and hard plaque. Prakash Katariya, President of Indian Institute of Laser Medicine successfully demonstrated Laser Therapy on Ischaemic Heart Disease. Several doctors employ low power laser successfully in various diseases. Kazuyoshi Zenba, President of Isehara Threrapeutic Institute successfully treated Tennis Elbow and Low Back Pain by low power laser. Takao Igarashi, President of Ikarashi Pediatrics Allergy Clinic treated 'Atopic Dimentia' by using low power laser. Kazuyoshi Zenba, also the President of Isehara Clinical Research Institute treated 'Chronic Rheumatoid Arthritis' using low power laser.

Low power laser therapy is the best non-invasive and more expensive treatment for diabetic arteriopathy (DA) which was done by Cristian Zaharia, President of Laser Medical and Praxis Medical Modern Association (Romania). Analgesic effect of low power laser for chronic rheumatoid arthritis was successfully done by Jyunichi Obata, President of Japan Rheumatism Laser Research Institute. Kazushi Nishijo, President of Tukuba College of Technology successfully conducted low power laser and acupuncture. Lasers commonly employed in medicine are listed below.

Lasers commonly employed in medicine

Lasers	Wavelength in nm	Nature of laser	Use in medicine
Ruby	694	Pulsed	Holograms; tattoo coagulation
Nd:YAG	1064	Pulsed	Coagulation
Ho:YAG	2130	Pulsed	Surgery; root canal

Er:YAG	2940	Pulsed	Surgery, dental drill
KTP	532	Pulsed; continuous	Dermatology
Alexandrite	720–800	Pulsed	Bone cutting
GaAs	904	Pulsed	Biostimulation
GaAlAs	780–820–870	Continuous	Biostimulation; surgery
InGaAsP	630–685	Continuous	Biostimulation
Dye laser (tunable)		Pulsed	Kidney stones
Rhodamine	560–650	Pulsed; continuous	PDT; dermatology
He–Ne	633, 3390	Continuous	Biostimulation
Argon	350–415	Continuous	Dermatology; eye
Carbon dioxide	10600	Continuous; pulsed	Dermatology; surgery
Excimer	193, 248, 308	Pulsed	Eye; vascular surgery
Copper vapour	578	Continuous; pulsed	Dermatology

A parallel light beam with small diameter is by far the most dangerous type of beam. It can enter the pupil, in its entirety and be focused by the eye's lens to a spot with a diameter of hundredths of a millimeter. The entire light output is concentrated on this small area. With a 10 mW beam, the power density can be up to 12,000 W/cm^2. It is obvious that a powerful laser (many watts) is more hazardous to stare into than a weak laser.

The lasers average power output is of importance, especially in terms of dosage calculation. The peak pulse power value is of some relevance for the maximum penetration depth of the light. Manufacturers specify the peak pulse output in their technical specification to make it more impressive. For example, 70 watt peak pulse output means 35 mW average output. This comes from the rule of thumb, i.e., watt peak pulse power is divided by 2 to get the average output in mW. Typical lasers suited for a particular job are given below:

Laser type	Suited job
He–Ne (3–10 mW) or InGaAlP laser	Dentistry
He–Ne (0.5–1.0 J/cm^2 around the edge of the wound and approximately 0.2 J/cm^2 in the open wound).	Wound healing, skin wounds, wounds to mucous membrane, herpes simplex, herpes zoster (shingles), gingivitis, pains in the skin, mucous membrane, conjunctivitis, neuralgia
GaAs Can also be used in combination with He-Ne of InGaAlP with low dosage (under 0.1 J/cm^2).	Treatment of pain and inflammations (even deep-lying ones) and is less suited to the treatment of wounds and mucous membrane. Functional disorders in muscles, tendons and joints (e.g., epicondylitis, tendonitis and myofacial pain, gonarthrosis, etc.).

4.15.1 Laser Penetration into the Tissue

The depth of penetration of laser light depends on the light's power and wavelength (whether it is super-pulsed or not).

Laser	Penetrating Depth
HeNe laser (3.5 mW)	6–8 mm depending on the type of tissue
HeNe laser (7 mW)	8–10 mm depending on the type of tissue
GaAlAs	3.5 cm with 5.5 cm lateral spread
GaAs	20 and 30 mm (sometimes down to 40–50 mm)

Due to increased circulation there is usually an increase of 0.5–1 °C locally. The biological effects have nothing to do with heat. GaAlAs lasers in the 300–400 mW range may cause a noticeable heat sensation, particularly in hairy areas. The coherence of the laser light does not disappear when entering the tissue. The length of coherence, though, is split into very small coherent 'islands' called speckles. These speckles remain coherent and will penetrate deeply into the tissue. A laser designed for the treatment of humans is rarely suitable for treating animals with fur.

4.16 LASERS IN CANCER TREATMENT

Laser light can be used to remove cancer or precancerous growths or to relieve symptoms of cancer. It is used most often to treat cancers on the surface of the body. Laser therapy uses high intensity light to treat cancer and other illnesses. Lasers can be used to shrink or destroy tumours or precancerous growths. Lasers are most commonly used to treat superficial cancers (cancers on the surface of the body or the lining of internal organs) such as basal cell skin cancer and the very early stages of some cancers, such as cervical, penile, vaginal, vulvar, and non-small-cell lung cancer. Lasers also may be used to relieve certain symptoms of cancer, such as bleeding or obstruction. For example, lasers can be used to shrink or destroy a tumor that is blocking a patient's trachea (windpipe) or oesophagus. Lasers also can be used to remove colon polyps or tumours that are blocking the colon or stomach. Laser therapy can be used alone, but most often it is combined with other treatments, such as surgery, chemotherapy, or radiation therapy. In addition, lasers can seal nerve endings to reduce pain after surgery and seal lymph vessels to reduce swelling and limit the spread of tumor cells.

Laser therapy is often given through a flexible endoscope (a thin, lighted tube used to look at tissues inside the body). The endoscope is fitted with optical fibres (thin fibres that transmit light). It is inserted through an opening in the body, such as the mouth, nose, anus, or vagina. It treats cancer or precancerous growths inside the trachea (windpipe), oesophagus, stomach, or colon. Laser light is then precisely aimed to cut or destroy a tumor. Organ laser therapy causes less bleeding and damage to normal tissue and lower risk of infection. However, the effects of laser surgery may not be permanent, so surgery may have to be repeated.

Laser induced interstitial thermotherapy (LITT), or interstitial laser photocoagulation, also uses lasers to treat some cancers. LITT is similar to a cancer treatment called hyperthermia, which uses heat to shrink tumours by damaging or killing cancer cells. During LITT, an optical fibre is inserted into a tumor. Laser light at the tip of the fibre raises the temperature of the tumor cells and damages or destroys them. LITT is sometimes used to shrink tumours in the liver. Photodynamic therapy (PDT) is another type of cancer treatment that uses lasers. In PDT, a photosensitiser or photosensitising agent is injected into a patient and absorbed by cells all over the patient's body. After a couple of days, the agent is found mostly in cancer cells. Laser light is then used to activate the agent and destroy cancer cells. Because the photosensitiser makes the skin and eyes sensitive to light afterwards, patients are advised to avoid direct sunlight and bright indoor light during that time.

Three types of lasers, viz., carbon dioxide (CO_2) lasers, argon lasers, and neodymium:yttrium-aluminium-garnet (Nd:YAG) lasers are used to treat cancer. The laser can shrink or destroy tumours and can be used with endoscopes. CO_2 and argon lasers can cut the skin's surface without going into deeper layers. Thus, they can be used to remove superficial cancers such as skin cancer. In contrast, the Nd:YAG laser is more commonly applied through an endoscope to treat internal organs, such as the uterus, oesophagus, and colon. Nd:YAG laser light can also travel through optical fibres into specific areas of the body during LITT. Argon lasers are often used to activate the drugs used in PDT.

Lasers are more precise than scalpels and do less damage to normal tissues. As a result, patients usually have less pain, bleeding, swelling, and scarring. With laser therapy, operations are usually shorter and performed on an outpatient basis. Further, the healing is faster and the patient is less likely to get infections.

Laser therapy also has several limitations. Surgeons must have specialized training before they can do laser therapy, and strict safety precautions must be followed. Laser therapy is expensive and requires bulky equipment. In addition, the effects of laser therapy may not last long, so doctors may have to repeat the treatment for a patient to get the full benefit.

4.16.1 Treating Cancer with Lasers

Lasers can be used in two ways to treat cancer:

a)   To shrink or destroy a tumor with heat.

b)   To activate photosensitizing agent which kills only the cancer cells (photodynamic therapy or PDT). Though lasers can be used alone, they are most often used with other cancer treatments, such as chemotherapy or radiation.

4.16.2 Shrinking or Destroying Tumours Directly

The CO_2 and Nd:YAG lasers are used to shrink or destroy tumours inside the body using endoscopes. Lasers can be employed with low power microscopes and micromanipulator to cut an area as small as 200 microns in diameter very precisely. Lasers are used to treat or to remove polyps, small growths that might become cancerous. Early cancers of the oesophagus, colon, cervix, vagina and vulva as well as precancerous tissues are treated well with CO_2 lasers. Cancers of the head, neck, airways, and lungs can be treated with the help of Nd:YAG lasers. Laser-induced interstitial thermotherapy (LITT) uses heat to shrink tumours by damaging cells. In LITT, the laser light is passed through an optical fibre right into a tumor which damages or kills cancer cells. It is used to treat tumours in the liver.

4.16.3 Photodynamic Therapy

The special drug (photosensitising agent) injected into the bloodstream is absorbed by body tissues. The drug stays in cancer cells for a longer time than in normal tissue. Exposure of specific wavelength of light (e.g., argon laser is used for 1 cm penetration alone) on the cancer cells with drug kills the cancer cells. PDT has some advantages over other treatments:

1. Cancer cells can be singled out and destroyed but other normal cells are spared.

2. The damaging effect of the photosensitizing agent happens only when the drug is exposed to light.

3. It has no long-term side effects when used properly.

4. It is less invasive than surgery.

5. It usually takes only a short time and is most often done in the outpatient ward.

6. It can be targeted very precisely.

7. Unlike radiation, PDT can be repeated many times at the same site if needed.

8. There is usually little or no scarring after the site heals.

9. It often costs less than other cancer treatments.

10. The side effects are fairly mild. However, PDT as it's currently used is not without its problems. The photosensitizing agents used today can leave people very sensitive to light, causing sunburn-like reactions even after a very brief exposure to sun.

PDT is used to treat cancers as well as pre-cancers of oesophagus, and certain kinds of lung cancer. PDT is being studied for use in other cancers, such as those of the brain and prostate. Researchers also are looking at different kinds of lasers and new photosensitiser drugs that might work even better. The other disadvantages of PDT are:

1. PDT can only treat areas where light can reach. This means it's mainly used to treat problems on or just under the skin, or in the lining of organs that can be reached with a light source.

2. PDT cannot be used to treat cancers that have spread to many places.

3. The drugs used for PDT leave people very sensitive to light for some time, so special precautions must be taken after the drugs are put in or on the body.

4. PDT cannot be used in people who have certain blood diseases, such as any of the porphyrias (a rare group of diseases that affect the skin or nervous system) or people who are allergic to porphyrins.

4.16.4 Drugs used in PDT

1. Porfimer sodium (Photofrin®)—most widely used and activated by red light from a laser.

2. Aminolevulinic acid (ALA or Levulan®)—special blue light, rather than laser light, is used to activate this drug.

3. Methyl ester of ALA (Metvixia® cream)—activated with a red light.

4. Researches are being carried out for using PDT in cancers of the skin, cervix, bladder, prostate, bile duct, pancreas, stomach, brain, mouth, larynx (voice box), head and neck, vagina, and vulva (the outside part of a woman's genitals).

4.16.5 FUTURE OF PDT

Newer photosensitising drugs now being studied may have advantages over the ones available today.

1. They may be able to treat tumours that are deeper under the skin or in body tissues.

2. They may be more selective for cancer cells as opposed to normal cells.

3. They may collect in cancer cells more quickly, reducing the time needed between getting the drug and the light treatment.

4. They may be removed from the body more quickly, reducing the time people need to worry about photosensitivity reactions.

Added to this, the researchers are on the way to invent different types of lasers and other light sources. Researchers are also looking more closely at how PDT works and how the cancer cells respond to its effects. Understanding how cells respond to PDT may allow doctors to enhance those effects that promote cancer cell death and suppress or counteract those that protect the cancer cells. There may also be ways to pre-treat the tumour to make it more susceptible to certain PDT treatments.

4.17 OPTICAL FIBRES

In practice optical fibre constitute an almost ideal solution in terms of transmission efficiency, compactness, flexibility, low cost and so on. The only limitation is due to the typical transmission window for each material constituting the core of the fibre. In silica fibres, reasonable transmission is obtained in the range 0.25–2 μm. A good research has been done to develop IR fibres for transmission in the range 2–10 μm. ZrF and other fluoride glasses are proposed near 3 μm. Thallium and silver halides have been proposed for 10 μm, even if the former is highly toxic. The fibres should deliver maximum power and energy delivery when coupled with laser without causing a permanent and catastrophic damage. CW lasers in this respect do not suffer these damage limitations because very high CW power can be easily transmitted through suitable fibres. This is the case for Nd:YAG lasers which can easily transmit 100 W and more through a 600 μm fibres. Similar situation for Ar ion lasers, especially for medical applications where much lower power is needed.

Problems have been observed for pulsed lasers. In fact the very high peak power exerted by Q-switch operation can rise the instantaneous power density at the entrance face of the fibres up to 4 W/cm. This leads to a surface breakdown due to a severe acoustic and thermal damage and ultimately breaks the fibre. Sometimes, high quality beams impinging a fibre with a power density lower than the damage can cause problems inside the bulk of the fibre because of internal reflections. Another class of effects which can cause permanent damage to the fibres is due to the powerful shock wave excited on the target in a liquid environment (opaque or transmitting).

The recent invention of the flexible CO_2 laser delivery system shown in Figure 4.7 overcomes many limitations of CO_2 lasers such as general anaesthesia and reaching areas of the head and neck. The flexible system's greater control over laser angulations potentially results in decreased thermal damage to surrounding tissues. Further, the flexible fibre may decrease blood loss and offer better tissue coagulation, rapid wound healing and reduced inflammation. The gas flow from the distal tip and through the fibre hollow core minimizes the smoke plume and bleeding. Added to this, flexible CO_2 laser delivery system offers much smoother cut edges. However, with newer lasers, the benefits of this new delivery system depend on surgical techniques.

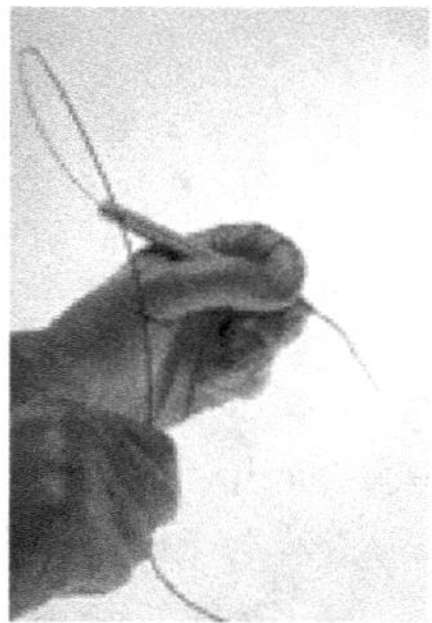

Figure 4.7 Flexible CO_2 laser delivery system (Image courtesy of Omni Guide)

4.18 REMOVAL OF TUMOURS OF VOCAL CORDS

Figure 4.8 illustrates human larynx, trachea and oesophagus. Tumours that grow on the vocal cords, irrespective of cancerous or benign are often removed with invasive surgery. Tumours can be cancerous or noncancerous. Noncancerous tumours can be caused by a virus or they may be unusual growths of body tissue that cause voice problems. Cancerous tumours are most likely to occur in smokers and people who drink too much alcohol. Cancerous tumours are life-threatening if not caught and treated early. Most cancer experts agree that vocal cord cancer starts likely as small areas of abnormal cells (dysplasia) which undergoes sequential changes and ultimately leads to the development of cancer. Pre-cancerous lesions may appear as a white or red plaque (called leukoplakia or erythroplakia) on the vocal cord and a biopsy should be done to rule out the presence of cancer. Removal of pre-cancerous lesions reduces the risk of developing cancer. The symptoms of vocal cord cancer are a sore throat, sensation of something stuck in throat, voice change, trouble in breathing, trouble in swallowing with associated weight loss, and the appearance of one or more lumps in the neck. The treatment for this tumor is either surgery or radiation therapy. Instead of surgery and radiation therapy, laser destroys tumours in less than 30 minutes. The red laser targets the blood supply and eliminates the blood supply to any tumor in the body. Hence the tumor is cured.

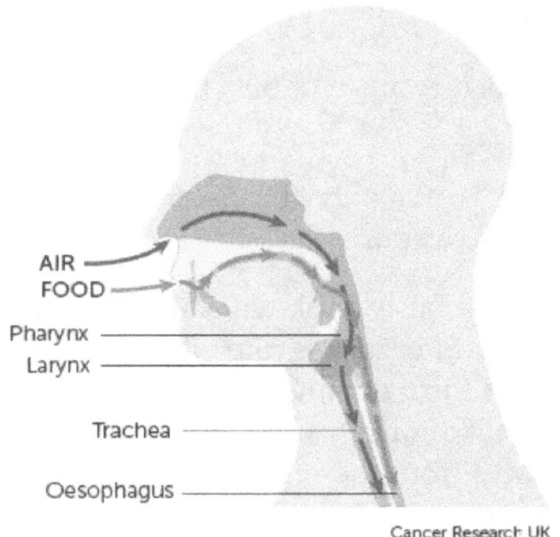

Figure 4.8   Human larynx, trachea and oesophagus

The inflamed larynx and vocal cords are shown in Figure 4.9.

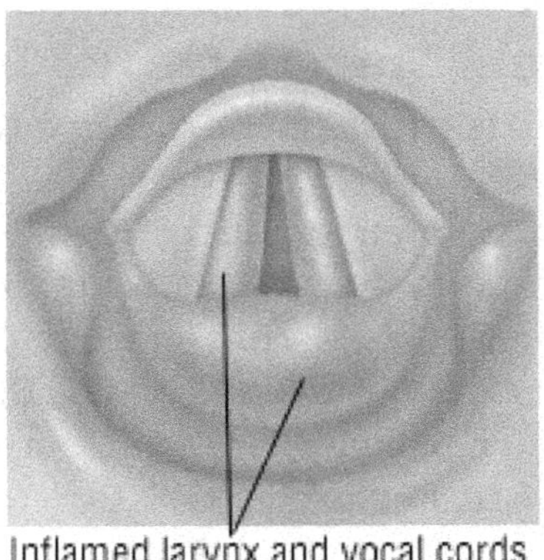

Figure 4.9   Inflamed larynx and vocal cords

Earlier there were two options such as laser surgery or radiation to treat patients diagnosed with early vocal cord cancer. Vocal cord cancer is classified according to size, location, and whether or not they spread beyond the larynx. The different types of vocal cord cancers are:

T1—very superficial, with normal mobility of the vocal fold.

T2—tumour has spread a little deeper and wider and this reduces movement of the vocal fold.

T3—the tumour replaces much of the vocal fold, and the vocal fold is fixed (immobile).

T4—the vocal fold is not only fixed, but there is evidence of cartilage framework (voice box) invasion.

T1 and T2 cancers are fairly "isolated" immunologically and hence spread to lymph nodes or to distant organs is rare with early tumours. The cell type of cancer in this location is virtually always squamous cell carcinoma. An alternate term, epidermoid carcinoma, is used interchangeably. These terms signify that the tumor originates from the mucosa, or surface layer of the vocal fold. The most common cause of this tumour is tobacco use. Another known cause is HPV (human papillomavirus) infection.

For early squamous cell carcinoma of the vocal folds, specifically T1 and T2 tumours, one uses endoscopic laser surgery accomplished through the mouth during general anaesthesia or radiation therapy.

4.18.1 CO_2 Laser Surgery for the Treatment of Vocal cord Carcinomas in early Stages (T1, T2)

According to Drs. Shvero J, Koren R, Zohar L, Hadar T, Feinmesser R, and Segal K the standard treatment for patients with early vocal cord carcinoma has been radiotherapy. In recent years, encouraging results with CO_2 laser surgery has changed treatment strategy in selective cases. During the past four years at the Rabin Medical Center, patients with carcinoma of the vocal cord during early stages (T1, T2) were treated using CO_2 laser surgery. Table 4.3 illustrates the modes of treatment for early vocal fold cancers.

Table 4.3   Modes of treatment for early vocal fold cancers

Point of Competition	Radiation	Laser Surgery
1. Cure rate with initial single-modality treatment (Failure of first treatment does not imply that the tumor will win, but only denotes that you will need a second treatment modality.)	Approximately 85% "cure." The remaining 15% needs more treatment.	Approximately 85% "cure." The remaining 15% needs more treatment.
2. Convenience	Approximately 30 visits to the radiation therapy facility.	One outpatient surgical procedure under general anaesthesia, or, uncommonly, two.
3. Early side effects	Little to none for two weeks, then skin of neck goes from pink to red to somewhat tanned; the inside of the throat becomes sore. There may be a period of radiation laryngitis lasting a month or so, as well as a sore throat when swallowing. You may lose some weight due to swallowing discomfort.	Sore throat from the laser surgery, typically for a few days following the procedure. Voice may be quite weak for a few weeks until healing is established. Approximately one in ten patients develop exuberant "proud flesh" healing response, which delays voice recovery, but does not change final result.

Point of Competition	Radiation	Laser Surgery
4. Later untoward consequences, potentially permanent	1) Persistent throat dryness. 2) A rare progressive fibrosis—what we call a "leatherization" process that makes tissues stiff, and voice progressively harder to produce, usually starting several years after radiotherapy was completed. 3) A rare stenosis where raw surfaces—either vocal folds, or upper oesophagus—stick together, causing poor voice or swallowing difficulty. However may be treated successfully. 4) A radiation-induced malignancy called sarcoma. It occurs rarely, many years after treatment is complete.	None, other than (for some, not all) persistent huskiness that is usually less than that caused by the tumour itself.
5. Cost	An estimated five times the cost of surgery	An estimated one-fifth the cost of radiation

Point of Competition	Radiation	Laser Surgery
6. Voice result	Usually quite good after recovery from radiotherapy. Most voices are a little deeper in pitch and "drier."	After healing, the typical voice result rivals that achieved with radiotherapy provided not more than one-third of the bulk of the fold is removed. In those with larger resections, an implant can be placed to improve voice.
7. Implications of treatment failure	Since radiation therapy cannot be repeated, the second treatment is necessarily some form of surgery: endoscopic laser or partial laryngectomy, or, rarely, even total laryngectomy.	All surgery options, including a second laser excision, remain. So does radiation therapy.

4.18.2   Laser Therapy—a new Option for Vocal Cord Cancers

With the emergence of the Pulsed Dye Laser (PDL) and Potassium Titanyl Phosphate (KTP) laser, new applications of lasers in laryngeal surgery are emerging rapidly. A new laser treatment for early vocal cord cancer, targets tumour blood vessels while preserving and restoring patients' voices, according to Massachusetts General Hospital researchers. They have also reported that radiotherapy or surgery can permanently damage vocal quality. According to Dr. Steven Zeitels, director of the MGH Voice Center, "We had previously adapted pulsed Potassium-Titanyl-Phosphate (KTP) laser that target blood vessels to treat precancerous vocal cord dysplasia and a variety of benign vascular lesions. We have now applied that experience to treat vocal cord cancer, which is diagnosed in several thousand American patients each year". More than 90 percent of patients with early vocal cord cancer can be cured with pulsed-KTP laser treatment. Thus, laser surgery is a versatile method of treating early and medial stage laryngeal cancer.

Zeitels et al. demonstrated that the thulium laser is also a useful tool for extensive endolaryngeal resections, offering improved haemostasis and the option of cutting tangentially. However, further studies must be done to minimize tissue damage by determining optimal power settings and cutting parameters and developing ways to decrease thermal damage.

4.19 SURGERY FOR BRAIN TUMOURS

Surgery is the primary treatment for brain tumours that can be removed without causing severe damage. Many benign (non-cancerous) tumours are treated only by surgery. Most malignant (cancerous) tumours, however, require treatment in addition to the surgery, such as radiation therapy and/or chemotherapy.

The following is a general overview of surgical treatment for brain tumours. There are different types of surgeries and techniques available for brain surgery. Types of surgeries for brain tumours are:

1.   Imaging and monitoring techniques
2.   Surgical techniques
3.   Strategies to improve treatment
4.   Laser brain surgery

4.19.1 Procedure in Brain Surgery

i)   Biopsy

A biopsy is a surgical procedure to remove a small piece of tumor in order to confirm the diagnosis. The sample is examined under the microscope by a pathologist who determines the type of the tumor. A biopsy can be performed as part of the surgery to remove the tumor or as a separate procedure.

There are two different approaches for performing a biopsy for brain tumours. An open biopsy involves exposing the tumor and then removing a small portion of it. A needle biopsy is performed by making an incision in the skin, drilling a small hole into the skull, inserting a narrow, hollow needle through the hole and into the tumor, and drawing up a small amount of tumor into the needle.

A needle biopsy may also be conducted with the assistance of computers and scanning equipment, including MRI or CT, in order to increase the precision of the procedure. This procedure is called stereotactic needle biopsy and is useful for patients with deep or multiple tumours.

ii)   Craniotomy

The most commonly performed surgery for removal of a brain tumor is called a craniotomy. "Crani" means skull, "otomy" means cutting into. In preparation for a craniotomy, a portion of the scalp is usually shaved and an incision is made through the skin. Using specialized equipment, a surgeon removes a piece of bone to expose the area of brain over the tumor. The dura mater (the outermost layer of the brain tissue) is opened, the tumor is located and then removed (resected). After the tumor is removed, the bone is usually replaced and the scalp stitched shut.

In a conventional craniotomy, surgeons guide themselves by what they see, their knowledge of anatomy, and their interpretation of the pre-operative scans. During stereotactic surgery, surgeons may rely on a computer to help direct the craniotomy.

iii)   Laser surgery

Before surgery, the location of the brain tumor in relation to other structures and blood vessels must be determined as precisely as possible. To achieve this, a variety of tests are performed. These may include:

1. Computerized tomography (CT),

2. Magnetic resonance imaging (MRI),

3. Positron emission tomography (PET), and

4. Angiography (to map blood vessels).

Using the information obtained from these tests, the surgeon can plan and even rehearse the operation in order to obtain optimal results. Evaluation of outcomes in elderly patients who had undergone surgery for brain tumours indicates that those who underwent preoperative MRI experienced better outcomes than those patients who were not evaluated with MRI before surgery.

Using a laser during brain surgery is a relatively routine practice. The aim of laser surgery is to direct the laser beams at the cancer and destroy it with heat. Because the light beams cannot penetrate bone, the laser can be used only during surgery. Lasers are used in addition to, or in place of, a scalpel. Lasers are capable of immense heat and power when focused at close range. Lasers destroy tumor cells by vaporising them. Stereotactic, or computer-assisted techniques, are frequently used to direct the laser. Lasers are chiefly used in the treatment of tumours that have invaded the skull base or are deep within the brain, with hard tumours that cannot be removed by suction, or with tumours that break apart easily.

4.19.2 Photodynamic Laser Surgery

A laser is also used in photodynamic therapy. Photodynamic therapy combines a drug that increases a tissue's sensitivity to light and laser surgery. Prior to surgery, the photosensitizing drug is injected into a vein or artery. It travels through the blood system to the tumor, accumulating in the cells of the tumor. The patient is then taken to surgery for removal of the tumor. During the operation, the treated tumor cells appear fluorescent. The physician aims a laser at the tumor cells, activating the drug. The activated drug then kills the tumor cells. Only operable tumours can be treated with this procedure. Tumor cells not seen by the surgeon or not sensitive to the drug are not affected by this treatment. This is a local form of therapy because some parts of the tumor might not be exposed to the light. Because of the danger of swelling, tumours near the brain stem cannot be treated with this technique.

4.19.3 Destroying Cancer Cells with Laser-Directed Heat

[Courtesy: Clevland Clinic, Rose Ella Bur Khardt Brain Tumor and Neuro-Oncology Center]

When tumours are in hard-to-reach brain areas or are close to areas that control vital functions, traditional surgery may be too risky. MRI scans produce detailed images of internal organs without the use of radiation. This innovation allows physicians to see and direct the progress of tumor destruction such that tumours will be completely treated. Laser interstitial thermal therapy (LITT) transmits heat to coagulate, or "cook," brain tumours from the inside out. This technology is not new in cancer treatment but early approaches posed challenges with limiting the laser energy only to tumours. With Monteris Medical Inc.'s NeuroBlate system, the surgeon can "steer" and monitor the effects of the laser beam, thus sparing surrounding healthy tissues. Unlike conventional open surgery, this therapy is minimally invasive. It takes place with the patient in an MRI machine because the laser system is guided, positioned and monitored with MRI.

The patient will be placed under general anaesthesia. With great precision, a thin, high intensity laser probe will be inserted through a small hole in skull, deep into the patient's brain. The tip of the probe emits laser energy sideways, heating and destroying brain tumour tissue in one direction while cooling to remove heat and protect normal tissue in neighbouring areas. Each burst of laser energy lasts from 30 seconds to a few minutes. The laser generates heat up to 160 degrees Fahrenheit, which is sufficient to coagulate and kill the tumor cells. On a computer screen, surgeon will monitor the tumor destruction as it occurs. An advance known as MRI thermometry measures temperature in and around the tumor, providing valuable feedback to the surgeon throughout the procedure. After surgery, the patient will remain in the hospital for one or two days, which is typically half the time the patient would have been hospitalized after conventional surgery. Any type of brain surgery poses some risk such as some temporary swelling around the treated area, which can be managed with medication.

This thermal therapy:

1. Is less invasive than even the most minimally invasive open operations.

2. Enhances patient safety.

3. Promotes quicker recovery.

4. Has the potential to help some patients whose tumours had been considered too risky to treat, whose tumours did not respond to alternate treatments or who had otherwise been deemed poor candidates for surgery.

5. Offers a therapeutic option when radiosurgery fails.

6. May allow for multiple treatments.

7. Is less costly than traditional surgery.

The integration of technologies represents a significant advance in patient safety, reduced procedure time and better outcomes. Figure 4.10 shows laser brain surgery operation theatre at Clevland Clinic.

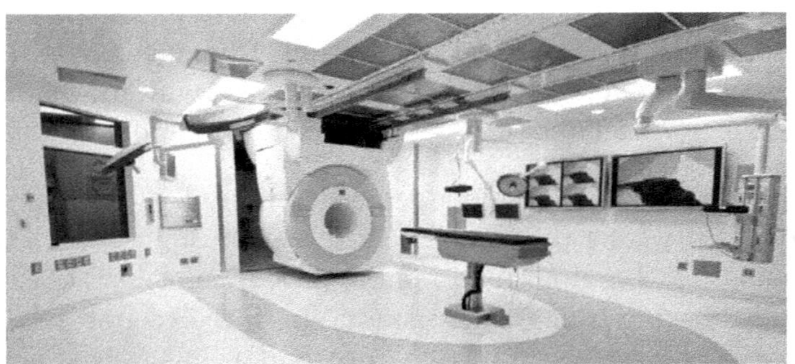

Figure 4.10 Laser brain surgery Operation Theater at Clevland Clinic, Rose Ella Bur Khardt Brain Tumor and Neuro-Oncology Center (clevelandclinic.org/neuroblate.)

4.20 IMAGE-GUIDED LASER TECHNOLOGY FOR NEURO-SURGERY

The procedure is as follows:

1. Lesion has been previously located and identified.

2. Laser probe is in the target area and patient is in MRI unit.

3. Neurosurgeon has a very accurate estimate of the length and desired temperature of the treatment.

4. Treatment begins. Neurosurgeon observes live temperature maps, minimizing damage to healthy tissue.

5. Treatment typically lasts a few minutes. When done, neurosurgeon gets to see the results immediately with MR Imaging.

4.21 LASERS IN PLASTIC SURGERY

Plastic surgery is defined as any procedure used to correct or restore either form or fraction of a body part. It deals with body modification and reconstruction surgery as well as surgery for aesthetically pleasing purpose. Body reconstruction surgery was done as early as 2000 BC by the famous Indian surgeon Sushruta. Nose and ear reconstruction were done for the first time in plastic surgery. Harold Gilles of New Zealand and Vilary Blair of USA are the fathers of modern plastic surgery. Gilles even performed the first male to female sex surgery operation in 1951.

The cosmetic photonics treats the effect of sun damage and ageing of the face, thus it reduces fine wrinkles, uneven pigmentation and rough skin. It also slightly tightens the skin. It is moderately effective in treating facial scars such as shallow acne scars. Certain early skin cancers can be treated by CO_2 laser where the aesthetic result is particularly important.

The replacement of skin during skin loss from burns, major trauma or infection is known as skin grafting. Cosmetic surgery such as nose correction, face lifts, botox, breast agumentation and tummy tucks enhance the appearance. A facelift (rhytidectomy) lifts tissue and removes surplus skin. It is particularly good for the jaw and the neckline which is inaccessible to the laser. Excess skin is removed more precisely in an eyelid reduction (blepharoplasty) and the bags or bulging fat can be removed. The CO_2 laser will reduce fine wrinkles and tighten the skin of the lower eyelids generally rather than precisely. Plastic surgery is also used in body modification, tattoo and genital modification including circumcision, etc. Skin rejuvenation is done using (1) ablative lasers CO_2 and Er:YAG and (2) non-ablative lasers for sub-surfacing.

However, commonly used lasers in plastic surgery are ruby (694 nm), Nd:YAG (1064 nm), KTP (532 nm), Er:YAG (2940 nm), diode (800 nm), alexandrite (755 nm), Cu vapour (578 nm), yellow dye (585, 595 nm), green dye (510 nm), argon (488, 514 nm), He:Ne (633 nm), CO_2 (10600 nm) and excimer (ultraviolet).

4.21.1 Ablative Lasers

They are used for:

1. Removal of pigmentations and superficial wrinkles.
2. Ablation of thin layers of epidermis.
3. Ablation by water (selective photothermolysis).
4. Vapourisation of cells and ablation of thin and exact layers of tissue.

Advantages of Er:YAG ablation laser are:

1. It emits in 2940 nm,
2. Cold ablation means no effect in subcutis,
3. Better and quicker healing of treatment area,
4. Advantage against peeling,
5. Better control in depths of ablation, and
6. No styptic effect.

Lasers that non-specifically destroy tissue can be used to remove skin lesions or layers of skin, usually with minimal blood loss because the dermal vessels are coagulated as the tissue is vaporized. CO_2 laser light is absorbed by intracellular water, which vaporizes tissue as the water turns to steam.

4.21.1.1 *Vascular Lesion Lasers* Oxyhemoglobin absorbs green and yellow light, spawning a variety of lasers appropriate for treating dermal vessels. Historically the argon (blue/green) laser was the first clinically useful laser but yellow light has become the preferred colour (oxyhemoglobin absorption peaks at 577 nm yellow light), with the pulsed yellow dye laser (intentionally adjusted to 585 nm and 595 nm for greater dermal penetration). The high energy/short duration pulse causes vascular disruption as the blood rapidly heats up and expands. The KTP laser (532 nm; green light) also targets oxyhemoglobin but the pulses are much longer in duration and tend to coagulate rather than disrupt vessels. Pigmented lesion lasers target melanin.

4.21.2 Non-Ablative Lasers

The properties of non-ablative lasers are:

1.   It emits 16,600 nm radiation.

2.   Effective in subcutis by heating of collagenous tissue.

3.   Collagen shrinking to one-third of original length.

4.   Increasing of number of collagen fibres.

5.   Activity of fibroblasts increases.

6.   Styptic effect.

4.21.3 Cosmetic Photodynamic Therapy

The use of light-activated drugs to treat acne and other skin conditions currently is best represented by levulan. The compound is metabolised by sebaceous glands into porphyrins. The acne bacteria itself also produces porphyrin, and the use of blue, green or red light stimulates the production of oxygen-free radicals that destroy the bacteria and suppress sebaceous gland activity.

4.21.4 Non-Laser Phototherapy

Intense pulsed light is not actually laser light. Xenon flash lamps generate multiwavelength noncoherent light that is partially modulated by a series of filters. Intense pulsed light is used for sun-related pigmentary changes, telangiectasias, and for hair removal

The Figures 4.11 and 4.12 show typical wrinkles and pigment change due to sun damage and the result of subsequent laser application.

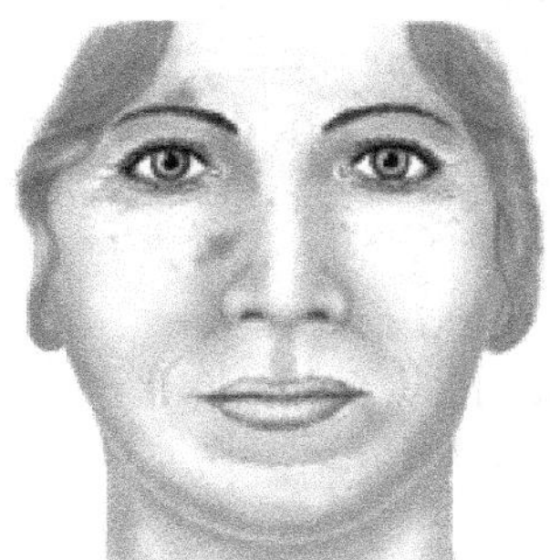

Figure 4.11 Typical wrinkles and pigment change due to sun damage

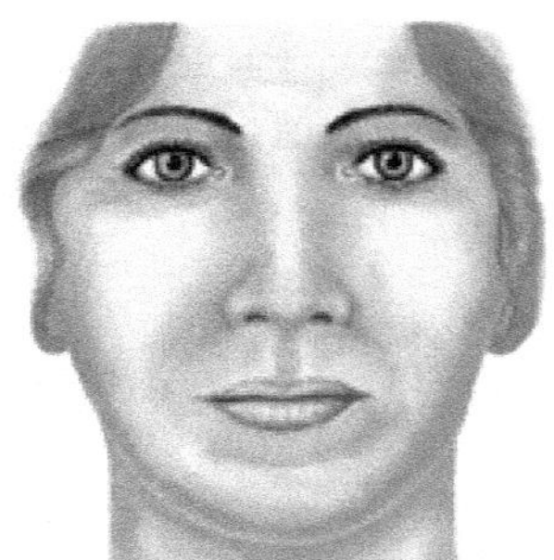

Figure 4.12 The laser can be directed to trace specific areas or more commonly the whole face excluding the neck

Laser resurfacing technology has come a long way since its first implementation in the 1980s to continue to look youthful. The recent technology of the CO_2 and Er:YAG lasers decrease side effects and increase therapeutic results to make one look beautiful.

4.22 LASERS IN ONCOLOGY

Oncology is the branch of medicine that researches, identifies, and treats tumours. The word *"onco"* means bulk, mass, or tumor while *"logy"* means study. Doctors who practice oncology are called cancer specialists or oncologists. They help in diagnosis of the cancer, help in staging the cancer and grading the aggressive nature of the cancer. The most important part of the diagnosis is the clinical history of the patient. Common symptoms that point towards cancer include fatigue, weight loss, unexplained anemia and fever of unknown origin, etc. Oncology mainly depends on diagnostic tools like biopsy or removal of bits of the tumour tissue and examining it under the microscope. Other diagnostic tools include endoscopy for the gastrointestinal tract, imaging studies like X-rays, CT scanning, MRI scanning, ultrasound and other radiological techniques, Single Photon Emission Computed Tomography, positron emission tomography and nuclear medicine techniques, etc. Common methods include blood tests for biological or tumor markers. Rise of these markers in blood may be indicative of the cancer.

Oncology has three primary clinical disciplines, viz., medical oncology, surgical oncology and radiation oncology.

1. A medical oncologist specializes in treating cancer with chemotherapy.
2. A surgical oncologist specialises in the removal of the tumor and surrounding tissue during an operation as well as biopsies.
3. A radiation oncologist specializes in treating cancer with radiation therapy.

Added to this, the American Society of Clinical Oncology (ASCO) also recognises other types of oncologists:

1. A gynecologic oncologist focuses on the care and treatment of women with gynecologic cancers, such as uterine cancer and cervical cancer.
2. A paediatric oncologist specializes in the treatment of children with cancer. (Some types of cancer occur most often in children and teenagers, such as certain brain tumours, leukaemia, osteosarcoma, and Ewing's sarcoma. However, they occasionally occur in adults. In these instances, an adult may decide to be treated by a paediatric oncologist).
3. A haematologist–oncologist specializes in the diagnosis and treatment of cancers of the blood, such as leukaemias, lymphomas, and myelomas.

There is no place for mechanical and ablative interactions in oncology. Thermal lasers have been in routine use in oncology for the last 20 years. These lasers (visible or infrared) are used to produce three basic effects such as hyperthermia, coagulation and vaporization. Other energy sources beside lasers can also be used to produce these tissue effects but lasers seem to possess certain basic advantages. In comparison with monopolar or bipolar diathermy and heater probes, lasers can deliver more power accurately and precisely at the target tissue with better control of damage and a wider range of effects. In comparison with microwave and ultrasound therapy, lasers are again more precise and can be used with more compact and accurate delivery devices. In endoscopic surgery, laser light is delivered through an optical fibre within the endoscope. Recently, the laser fibre can be placed directly within tumour tissue for interstitial thermal therapy of liver metastases, pancreatic tumours and brain tumours.

Recently Bandieramonte et al. (1978) reported laser microsurgery in oncology (lower genital tract, lesions of the larynx and oral cavity and skin lesions). According to them the use of the microscope for laser resections (CO_2 lasers) under magnification was recognised to be preferable in routine surgical oncology practice. Short- and medium-term clinical results with laser microsurgery were comparable to those with conventional surgery. Power (1992) recently reported current status of lasers in neurosurgical oncology.

During the last two decades, the photothermal and photochemical effects of several medical lasers have been studied for the clinical treatment of benign and malignant, primary and secondary central nervous system tumours. Increased precision and haemostasis during tumor excision are possible with the microsurgical carbon dioxide, argon, and frequency doubled neodymium:YAG lasers. Computerized tomography and magnetic resonance imaging aided the volumetric tumor removal precisely. Photodynamic therapy with hematoporphyrin derivative as the photosensitiser and neodymium:YAG laser hyperthermia are currently under evaluation for the treatment of residual and recurrent malignant tumours. Laser surgery in gynecologic oncology was reported by Helmut F. Schellhas (1995). In the treatment of premalignant epithelial cancers of the female lower genital tract, the CO_2 laser beam is used with precision through a surgical microscope for tissue ablation and excision. Intra-abdominal vaporization of abnormal tissues can be performed endoscopically through fibre optics. Surgical lasers can be used for hemo-static excision of malignant lesions. Photodynamic therapy is applied in the treatment of isolated malignancies persistent after conservative treatment. Surgical laser systems are important tools in the treatment of gynecologic malignancies. They were treated with laser oncology using CO_2, Nd:YAG and argon lasers. Experimental data regarding tumor cell spread through lymphatic and hematic channels and cell viability in the fumes after CO_2 laser irradiation are reported. Due to the optical properties of the laser beam, physical measurements of the delivered energy and mathematical calculation of the energy per tissue volume unit to be ablated increase the precision in microsurgery. The main applications of surgical oncology are reported in otolaryngology, gynecology, and endoscopy.

4.22.1 Head & Neck Oncology

Since 1970's, lasers have been increasingly used in oral and maxillofacial/head and neck surgery. Their effect on tissue is determined by their wavelength and the tissue-specific absorption. The commonly used lasers include carbon dioxide (CO_2), neodymium:yttrium-aluminium-garnet (Nd:YAG) and argon lasers. They are also used for the diagnosis of mucosal lesions. CO_2 laser is primarily suited for transoral resections of premalignant and early oral carcinomas. It is the most useful laser in oral and maxillofacial/head and neck surgery practice.

Due to the unique characteristics of Nd:YAG laser (its ability to coagulate and ablate but it is not as precise a cutting tool as the CO_2 laser), it has specific advantage in the treatment of large oral vascular malformations. Laser therapy is the choice for oral leukoplakia since the mid-1980s.

Laser surgery is superior for morphological and functional recovery. Pain control and non-postoperative complications were better with lasers. The use of lasers in the management of oral disorders has been implemented for several years. The advantages of this approach include minimal damage to adjacent tissues, delayed acute inflammatory reaction, and reduced myofibroblast activity, leading to reduced wound contraction and scarring. Reduction of collagen in the postoperative phase maintains soft tissue movement. The laser-treated area can be left exposed to granulate, thus obviating any need for skin grafting or wound dressing. During the laser dissection, more normal oral tissues are preserved and hence greater preservation of oral function such as swallowing and speech, etc.

When laser is used, the operating time is reduced. Patients require a shorter hospital stay. Laser can be used again even if there is a recurrence or malignant transformation. Laser can also be used with conventional surgery, chemoradiation and/or photodynamic therapy. The thermal damage from the laser on the borders of the biopsy specimens did not interfere with the pathologist's establishment of a firm diagnosis. This suggests that laser surgery is an appropriate instrument for excisional biopsies of oral soft tissue lesions.

Over the past few decades, the use of lasers among oral and maxillofacial/ head and neck surgeons has grown dramatically and new procedures find a common place in oral and maxillofacial/head and neck surgery.

4.22.2 Radiation Oncology

Radiation oncology focuses on the use of radiation to treat cancer and other diseases. Radiation treatment remains a powerful weapon against cancer in its many manifestations, resulting in increased cancer cures and lessening the suffering for patients. A radiation oncologist uses ionizing radiation (such as megavolt X–rays or radionuclides) in the treatment of cancer. Radiation therapy uses carefully targeted and regulated doses of high energy radiation to kill cancer cells. Radiation causes some cancer cells to die immediately after treatment but most die because the radiation damages the chromosomes and DNA so that the cells can no longer divide and the tumor cannot grow.

Radiation oncology is made up of three unique medical specialties namely radiation oncologists, radiation therapists and radiation physicists. These professions involve the following:

1. Radiation Oncologist—a medical doctor attends cancer patients, specifically using radiation therapy.

2. Radiation Therapist—a health professional who designs, calculates (plans) and provides the radiation dose to patients and is responsible for ongoing patient care and wellbeing of the patient over the length of treatment.

3. Radiation Oncology Medical Physicist —a scientist who creates, implements and monitors the delivery of radiation in cancer treatment.

4. New technologies in radiation oncology are due to the advances in physics and engineering sciences. A typical radiation oncology treatment room is shown in Figure 4.13

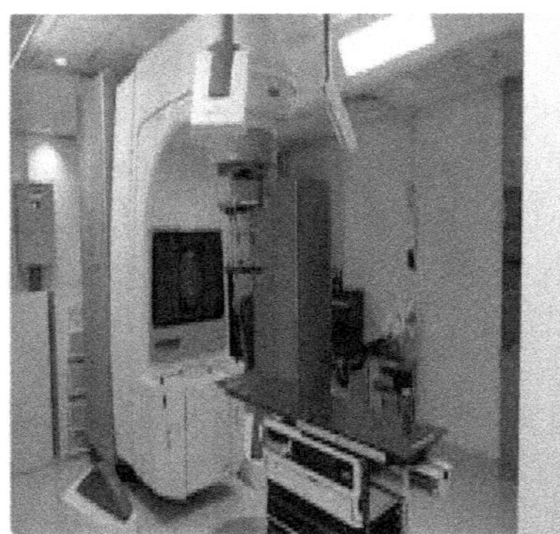

Figure 4.13 Radiation Oncology treatment room (Courtesy: park waycancer centre.com)

4.22.2.1 *Radiation Therapy* Radiation therapy is a safe, effective way to treat cancer. Radiation therapy offers clear benefits to patients. It allows organ preservation, preserves quality of life, reduces pain and improves survival. Radiation therapy can be used to treat almost all cancers, anywhere in the body. It can be used alone or with other treatments like surgery or chemotherapy. Radiation therapy cures cancers or gives symptom relief in the absence of cure. More than 50% of cancers can be cured using radiation therapy. Radiation therapy aims to kill cancer cells but avoids damage to the structure and function of nearby healthy tissues.

Cancer patients are exposed to radiation by radiation oncologist after consulting doctors from other specialities such as surgery and medical oncology. Patients having radiotherapy have multidisciplinary team care because they have complex needs. The team is made of radiation oncologists, medical physicists, radiation therapists, nurses and allied health professionals. The multidisciplinary team is focussed on quality, the patient's needs and achieving the best possible outcomes for the patient.

Recent scientific advances help radiation oncologists to view 3D images of tumours. That is they can direct radiation beams very precisely so that less normal tissue is affected. Intensity Modulated Radiation Therapy (IMRT) and Image-Guided Radiation Therapy (IGRT) allow radiation oncologists to target tumours. The radiation dose can be closely fitted to the tumour. This reduces radiation dose to important structures like the spinal cord or parts of the brain. Radiation therapy is usually given as an outpatient treatment. New technological advances in radiation therapy have made life better for cancer patients in recent years.

4.22.3 Laser Oncosurgery

Laser oncosurgery is the advanced laser treatment for lung cancer, liver cancer, bone cancer, oral cancer, breast cancer, head and neck cancer and soft tissue sarcoma. It is also the treatment of choice in cancers like basal cell carcinoma and squamous cell carcinoma of skin. There is now a separate field in MRI-guided laser ablation of brain tumours.

Liver carcinoma is being increasingly handled by laser over surgery in several specialized centres. Breast carcinoma is being handled by many centres internationally by ablation rather than open surgery. Surgeons all over the world have accepted laser as the best, precise, fast, bloodless, and convenient tool with practically no pain. Today lasers can be used in 70% of nonlaparoscopic general surgery though the expertise (laser scientists, engineers and laser safety officers) is extremely limited at present.

4.22.3.1 *Tumour in late stages*   Late stage cancer has always been an enigma to handle for oncosurgeons. Late stage is defined as any tumour in stage 3 or 4. Tumour handling in late stages is not intended for cure but for palliation, i.e., relief of symptoms. Although there are several ways to achieve this, it essentially follows the principle of cyto-reduction or ablation or debulking. Cyto-reduction is a simple concept that decreases the size of advanced tumour. Radiotherapy and chemotherapy are more effective in treatment of advanced cancer. The other methods are a) Surgery, b) Radiofrequency ablation, c) Cryosurgery, d) Laser, and e) Microwave. These procedures should also accompany chemotherapy and radiotherapy which are handled by the concerned professionals. The usage of laser technologies depends on the adaptability of the surgeons.

SECTION B – COSMETIC PHOTONICS

4.23 INTRODUCTION

The broad area "Photonics" is now divided into several branches such as material photonics, biophotonics, medical photonics, cosmetic photonics, veterinary photonics, entertainment photonics, military photonics, communication photonics, food photonics and industrial photonics. However, lasers have gained popularity in cosmetics because they enable cost-effective skin treatments which are not easily achieved with other technologies. The wider new applications reduce equipment cost and products. This enables lasers to play an even broader role in cosmetics in the future. In recent years a number of important advances, including the development of versatile solid-state materials and nonlinear crystals, offered a major impact on cosmetic and medical laser technology. This opened the door to a wide range of new instrumentation and treatment capabilities. Cosmetic lasers are used in skin resurfacing and in plastic surgery. Laser skin resurfacing, viz., 'laser peel' of the face is a popular type of plastic surgery. Dermatologists began performing laser resurfacing as an alternative to dermabrasion. Most commonly a CO_2 laser is used to vaporize the top five cell thick layer of epidermis. To speed healing, some doctors use an Er:YAG laser that does not penetrate very deeply. With CO_2 laser, the initial redness may take up to three months to fade away while with Er lasers it is generally less than two weeks.

In our modern world, huge amounts of money are spent to make skin look younger, more beautiful and healthier. Recently, a doctor from Hollywood recommended the combination of full face CO_2 laser skin resurfacing with surgical face lift to obtain younger looking skin. Thus a 60-year-old woman can now appear to be physically young using laser skin resurfacing. A few years ago, doctors used dye lasers to treat varicose veins. Now their attention has shifted to frequency-doubled Nd:YAG to perform this treatment. The common cosmetic/dermatology lasers available at present are as follows:

Laser type	Wavelength	Applications
Alexandrite	755 nm	Hair removal
CO_2	10.06 mm	Ablative skin resurfacing
Diode	800–1000 nm	Hair removal and teeth whitening
Er:YAG	2.94 mm	Ablative skin resurfacing
Flash lamp pumped dye	585–600 nm	Vascular and pigmented conditions
Nd:YAG	1.064 mm	Hair and dark skin removal
Nd:YAG/Freq. Doubled	532 nm	Vascular and pigmented conditions
Ruby	694 nm	Hair removal
CuBr & pulsed dye	Yellow/Green	Vascular lesions, for brown pigmented lesions

Lasers have also been used to remove unwanted decorative tattoos and benign pigmented skin marks and lesions. The pulsed dye lasers are widely used for this purpose. Traumatic discolouring caused by accidents, gun shots or explosives, with various materials becoming embedded in the skin, can be extremely difficult to correct. Recently Dr. Agneta Troilius, a Swedish doctor has achieved good results in the removal of such marks with Q-switched Nd:YAG laser treatment.

Hair removal is one of the largest potential markets for laser applications and treatment. This is going to be of great help not only to doctors but also to men and women who spend a vast amount of money on razor blades, electrolysis and hair removal creams. On the other hand, hair transplants are also possible with lasers. In laser-assisted hair transplantation, laser creates skin pockets that can accept hair follicle transplants.

Nowadays people are interested in having white teeth. They do not want discoloured teeth. Argon and CO_2 lasers (low intensities) are widely used by dentists for teeth whitening. Since injections cause pain and possibility of infection, there has been interest in delivering drugs without injection. Now the 694.3 nm Q-switched ruby laser delivers drugs without injection. This new approach could be useful in application for drugs such as insulin for diabetic patients. In short, lasers provide better cosmetic care at a lower cost in the years to come.

Cosmetic laser surgery has been successfully done in the following areas.

1. Laser birthmark removal
2. Skin resurfacing
3. Laser scar removal such as acne scars, surgical and traumatic scars
4. Facial blood vessel treatment
5. IPL photofacial treatments
6. Laser hair removal
7. Laser removal of Nevi (moles)
8. Laser stretch mark removal
9. Laser tattoo removal
10. Thermage thermalift

4.24 LASER BIRTHMARK REMOVAL

Discolorations in skin such as port wine stain, nevus of ota and café au lait are known as birthmarks. Five percent of population including newly born possess skin discolorations. Brown pigmented birthmarks (café au lait) and blue-black birthmark (Nevus of ota) are commonly seen at birth or develop in the first few years of life. Photonics made a major breakthrough to remove or improve port wine stains hemangiomas, café au lait lesions and nevus of ota. Congenital birth marks are composed of blood vessels (port wine stain or hemangiomas), pigmented cells called café au lait (coffee and cream) or blue-black dermal stains called nevus of ota. Port wine stains can occur anywhere on the body and may rarely be associated with underlying abnormalities of the eye and the brain. Port wine stains show diffuse collections of dilated capillaries in the dermis and hence they are called capillary haemangioma. Use of pulsed yellow, green light, diode, alexandrite and Nd:YAG lasers can improve or eliminate many of these lesions. Selection of lasers depends on size, colour and anatomic location. Pigment birth marks are divided into superficial (café au lait) or deep (nevus of ota) varieties. A typical port wine stain before laser treatment and after laser treatment are shown in Figures 4.14 and 4.15.

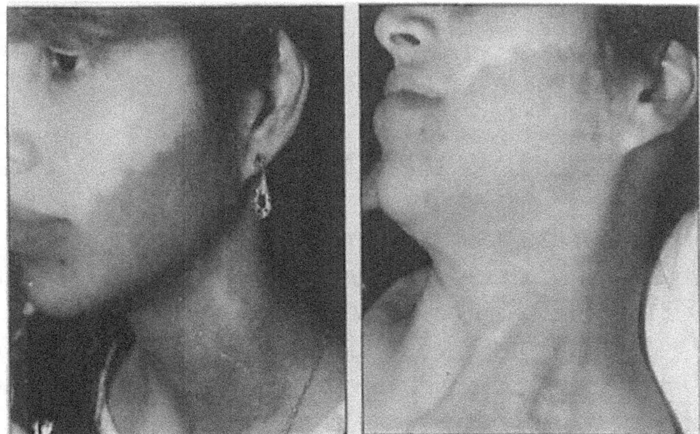

Figure 4.14 Port wine stains before and after laser treatment   (Courtesy: Biophotonics)

Multiple sittings are required to eliminate the collection of pigment cells in the deep dermis. Café au lait birth marks arise by excess melanin deposits and pulsed green lasers are suitable for treatment. Nevus of ota shows good response for ruby, alexandrite or Nd:YAG lasers.

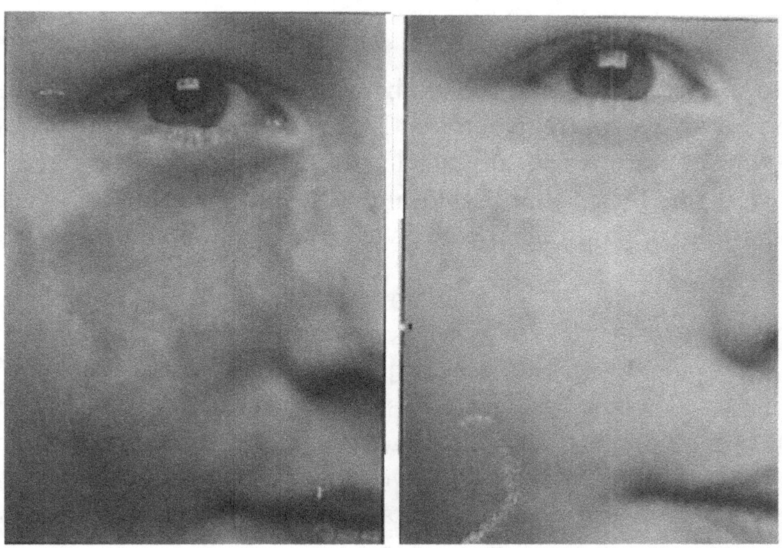

Figure 4.15 Port wine stains before and after laser treatment (Courtesy: Biophotonics)

The cutaneous surgical lasers operating at a wavelength of 585 nm is effective for the treatment of port wine stains, hemangiomas, facial spider veins, scars, warts and other vascular abnormalities.

4.25 LASER SKIN RESURFACING (FACIAL REJUVENATION)

Our skin reveals our age. Older skin is loose, shows fine and deep lines, larger pores and or blotchy pigmentation. There are intrinsic causes of aging that cannot be avoided but may be affected by general health, nutrition and exercise. Extrinsic causes of aging are predominantly sun and cigarette. We practically see the gradual descent of the face into folds around the eyes, jaws and neck. This happens due to the gradual loss of subcutaneous fat volume. The lines of facial expression are due to emotions such as anxiety, happiness, shocks, depressions and worries. They are crow's feet, brow furrows, and smile lines. With reference to time, the texture of skin suffers.

Traditional cosmetic procedures which included chemical peels and dermabrasion helped to remove the dead surface layers of skin to expose the still living dermis. Chemical peels literally burned away the top layer of the skin with little control over the chemical's penetration while dermabrasion uses abrasive compounds to clear off dead skin cells. Both techniques are often ineffective, carry risks and are very expensive.

Due to the limitations of these methods, laser skin resurfacing is becoming a popular choice for skin rejuvenation. Laser reduces the effects of sun, aging and the environment on delicate facial skin. Laser treatment reduce or eliminate wrinkles, fine lines, skin discoloration, hyperpigmnetation, hypopigmentation, facial redness and facial blood vessels as well as improve overall skin texture and appearance.

This technique has produced dramatic results. In laser resurfacing, a physician typically uses a pulsed laser to deliver hundreds of milliwatts of energy in less than the thermal relaxation time of skin which is estimated at 700 μm. This energy ablates the surface layers of skin and shrinks collagen strands embedded in skin by about one-third. The result is smoother skin with fewer fine lines, wrinkles and age spots. This technique produces consistent and predictable improvements in facial skin quality. This can also be used to remove irregular scar contours.

Skin resurfacing is done using ultrapulse CO_2 and Erbium:YAG laser system. The pulsed Er:YAG laser fulfil the basic requirements for skin rejuvenation. The laser emits a wavelength with a maximum water absorption peak. It delivers laser energy in a time duration short enough to prevent heat conduction damage and enough energy is delivered to the tissue to obtain the desired cosmetic results. Since ablation is possible without significant thermal necrosis, the incidence of complications would be quite rare. Er:YAG laser (2940 nm) produces maximum power of 20 W, pulse duration of 350 microseconds, and spot size of 2.5 –7.0 mm. These characteristics produce an output energy level of between 100 – 1700 mJ per single pulse.

The advantage of laser-induced tissue ablation over chemical peeling and dermabrasion, lies in the laser's precise well-controlled ability to remove thin skin layers. The laser heats the skin, peeling off the outermost layers and at the same time it heats the collagen in the dermis. The heated collagen shrinks and the newly synthesized collagen protein gradually replaces it. The new collagen tightens the skin and wrinkling caused by sun damage or aging is removed. Larger, deeper wrinkles like brow furrows may tend to recur to some degree.

The procedure is usually not painful but produces a red and raw look that may last up to four months. The continuing redness indicates the construction of new collagen and reflects the formation of a new blood supply to the new collagen.

A coherent CO_2 laser was used to vaporise areas of elevated skin around the scars to induce a local inflammatory reaction that causes epithelial cells to multiply and to smoothen out skin in the long term. Individual wrinkles were treated in a single pass of laser light with energies from 300 to 400 mJ per pulse. When the entire face needed resurfacing, the best results were obtained by using up to two passes of 300 mJ per pulse of light. For the thinner skin around the eyes, a single sweep of 200 mJ per pulse was used. No special skin care was applied before surgery and water compresses were used to sooth the skin after surgery. The full-face laser resurfacing with face lift surgery is another milestone in the cosmetic laser research. This approach is adopted to correct sagging skin and to improve the quality of the skin.

Recently, an 'UltraPulse" CO_2 laser which emits high infrared energy in very short pulses was used to eliminate or reduce the chances of scarring associated with the conventional CO_2 lasers. Dr. Adrian was one of the first physicians in the world to perform laser resurfacing in 1993. In his technique, laser induces new collagen formation in the dermis post-operatively over a period of 3 to 6 months enhancing the effects of the laser resurfacing procedure.

To start with, α-hydroxy acids are applied as a light chemical peel to remove dead tissue and expose new skin. Then deep moisturiser is applied. This is followed by resurfacing the skin with a coherent laser. The best results were achieved using light doses of 300 mJ per pulse delivered in a single pass for areas around the eyes. The obvious advantage in this method is the considerable decrease in healing time. Figure 4.16 illustrates the triple helical structure of collagen molecule.

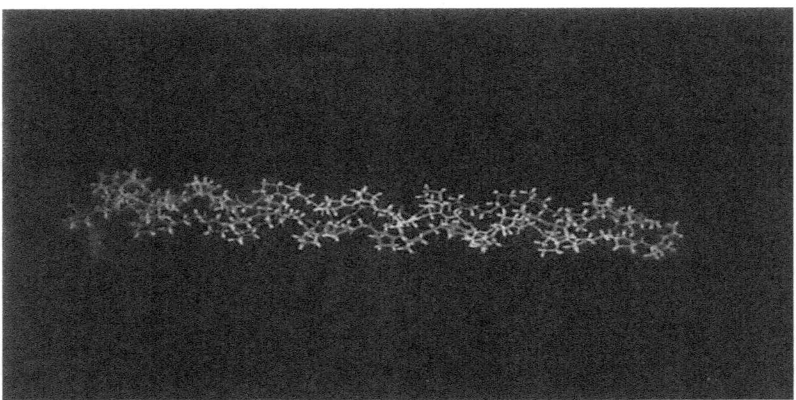

Figure 4.16 Triple helical structure of collagen molecule

The skin resurfacing done on a lady with CO_2 laser is shown in Figure 4.17.

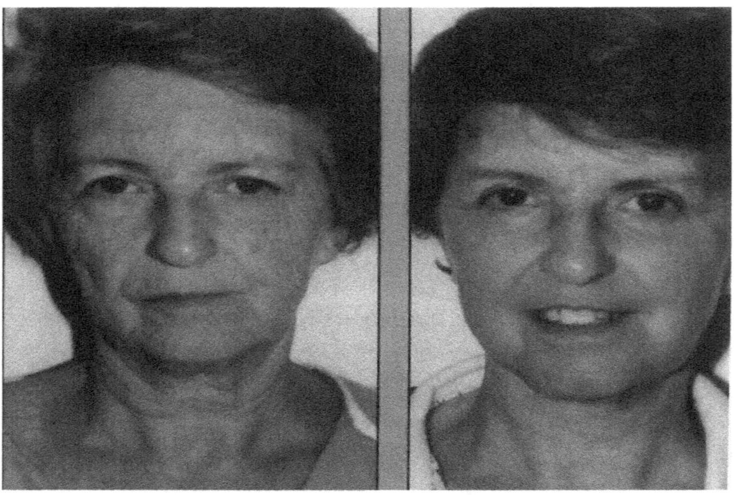

Figure 4.17 Full face skin resurfacing (Courtesy: Biophotonics)

Pulsed dye lasers operating at 577 to 585 nm have proved useful for treating patients with red to pale pink port wine stains on the face, head and neck. The port wine stains that involve small capillary tube vessels can easily be treated with dye lasers.

4.26 CO_2 LASER VANQUISHES SKIN WRINKLES

Face is the index of the mind. Dynamic wrinkles are caused by contractions of the delicate underlying facial muscles every time we smile, laugh or frown (wrinkle one's brows when worried). The more emotions we show, the deeper these wrinkles and lines are likely to be. Wrinkles are caused by a host of factors including loss of collagen and elastin, stress, sun damage, smoking, alcohol use, pollutants in air, illness and hormonal changes. Skin changes may also be part of the natural aging process but no one has the option to reduce the visible signs of aging and wrinkles.

If these lines are untreated, they become permanent. Now-a-days frown lines, crow's feet and forehead lines can be dramatically softened or eliminated. This procedure is known as cosmetic denervation.

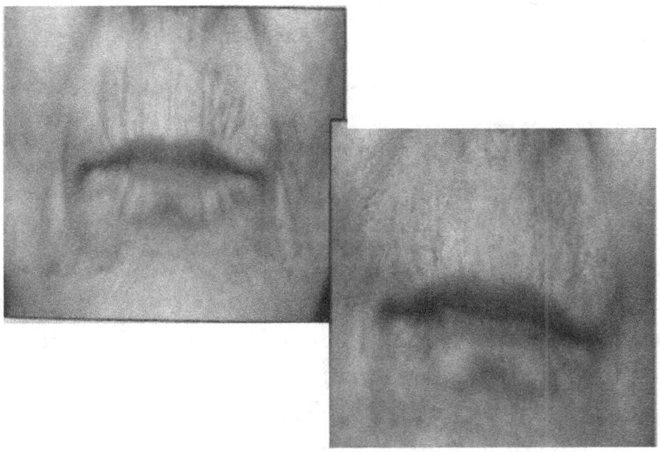

Figure 4.18 Laser resurfacing of lips removes wrinkles (left) leaving a smoother version (right) (Courtesy: Biophotonics)

The anatomy of a wrinkle is as follows. The skin dermis layer, a mere millimeter or less in thickness on the face, consists of large tough fibres of collagen protein and stretchy fibres of elastin protein. With age, particularly in a person who has spent considerable time in the sun, the epidermis dries and thins. Excessive sun exposure leads to abnormal, disoriented elastin fibres, robbing the skin of its support and elasticity. The epidermis folds and wrinkles are born. The lip lines before and after treatment is shown in Figure 4.18.

4.26.1 Role of LEDs

Light emitting diodes (LEDs) photomodulation is the interaction of light delivered to activate cells causing them to produce collagen and multiply. By building collagen, wrinkles are reduced and skin retains a more youthful, radiant appearance. LED photomodulation suppresses collagen degrading enzymes that assist in the aging process. Further, it offers a totally natural, non-ablative method for skin rejuvenation. The treatment is quick, very relaxing and pain-free. The energy delivered by the LEDs does not rely on heat and hence it safely and gently treats all types of skin. The skin becomes smoother and softer in 4–8 sittings. The red and brown spots fades away and one can carry on with their normal activities after the treatment. Another advantage of LED photomodualtion is that it can be used alone or in combination with any other rejuvenation techniques to enhance the slow down process of skin aging and ensure a true and full face rejuvenation.

4.26.2 Intense Photofacial Treatment

Intense pulsed light (IPL) phototherapy is an innovative and effective treatment to eradicate red facial veins and flushing, improve acne rosacea, treat irregular pigmentation and reduce fine facial lines. IPL system delivers light energy through the skin removing facial redness, erasing pigment spots, reducing pore size and improving fine lines. Typically 4 – 6 sittings are required in 3 – 4 weeks time. This procedure is associated with mild discomfort and postoperative facial pinkness. The persons undergoing this procedure can attend to their normal duties after the treatment. Added to this, IPL can also be used to treat aging, photo-damaged skin on the neck, chest and hands safely. That is, this procedure is safe and successful in treating rosacea, red flushed faces secondary to acne rosacea, facial blood vessels and capillaries, sun damaged skin, pigmented facial spots and enlarged pores.

4.27 COSMETIC LASERS ARE AT THE THRESHOLD OF A NEW ERA

In the past, doctors used dye lasers to treat varicose veins. Now they can choose the frequency-doubled Nd:YAG to perform the treatment. The pulsed dye laser was used for many years to treat port wine stains. Although the results are acceptable, they are far from perfect. Multiple procedures are often required and port wine stains become darker before they fade away.

These lasers can selectively damage larger, abnormal veins while leaving smaller veins intact. This means that port wine stains and spider and varicose veins can be treated successfully.

In the past, medical lasers required manual adjustments but today they represent a sophisticated hardware and interactive databases. The system allows physicians to command a pre-programmed treatment modality at the push of the button. Laser manufacturers also have become more attuned to the needs of their customers. In the past, laser systems were designed for a single application. Today many laser systems can be started with just the capability needed to operate them and upgraded when necessary. Combination of a KTP, a Nd:YAG and an alexandrite is a versatile dermatology laser used for tattoo removal and scar minimization. This is because no single laser can match the absorption wavelengths of all tattoo pigments and skin colours. Combination of CO_2 and Er:YAGs in a single system is targeted for dermatologists. More recently, KTP lasers have met with great success because the 532 nm wavelength ablates tissue instead of coagulating them.

Fibres can be either side-firing or end-firing. Side-firing configurations are used to reach areas that are not in the line of sight of the fibre. These configurations find use in urology for the treatment of ureteral strictures, bladder tumours and enlarged prostates.

Matching the pulse length of a frequency-doubled Nd:YAG to thermal relaxation time of enlarged varicose veins improves the outcome of treatment. Light can also be delivered via scanners to surface tissues. Scanners expand and shape the laser beam so that it delivers a precise amount of energy in a fairly large spot size. Scanners eliminate the accumulation of thermal energy in any given area and minimize the discomfort that it would cause. They find application in hair removal and skin resurfacing where large areas have to be reproducibly covered in a short time.

Lasers in biotech research are becoming indispensable. New spectroscopic methods coupled with an increased knowledge base are making the early diagnosis of disease a reality. Medical practice has not yet caught up with this capability. But with continued improvements in lasing materials and delivery methods plus accumulated experience in their use and suitable selection of surgical parameters, this imbalance surely will be corrected with time.

Laser treatments cure sun damage, enlarged pores, wrinkles, skin discolorations, melasma and acne scars effectively. It repairs aging and sun damaged skin, pixel by pixel and spot by spot. Further, it provides a safer and more effective treatment with shorter treatment time. There is no need for blue dye to be applied to the patient's face.

4.28 Q-SWITCHED ND:YAG REMOVE TRAUMATIC TATTOOS

Tattooing is an ancient art. Lasers have long been used to remove unwanted decorative, cosmetic and traumatic tattoos and benign pigmented skin marks. In earlier days, those who removed tattoos were left with significant scar. The non-laser methods for removal of tattoos have disadvantages such as incomplete removal, non-selective tissue destruction and unsatisfactory cosmetic results such as atrophic or hypertrophic scarring. These methods are associated with a high incidence of scarring and pigmentation disturbances. The other methods of tattoo removal involve the abrasion with salt (salabrasion), cryosurgery, dermabrasion, electrocoagulation and the use of infrared coagulator. Conventional surgical methods are limited to the removal of small tattoos only. A surgical method of large tattoo removal is disastrous. Hence the use of lasers to remove tattoos began in the early 90s. The first successful tattoo removal was done with Q-switched ruby lasers. Even today this laser finds its importance in tattoo removal. However, it should be carefully used in dark skin individuals.

With the advent of Q-switched laser systems, tattoos are easily removed with little or no scarring. The Q-switched laser with a wave length 1064 nm allows deep penetration and at the same time exhibits less melanin absorption. This laser is very effective in removing dark blue-black ink in tattoos. Further, it is especially useful in removing dark ink from cosmetic eyeliner tattoos. The second harmonic generation of Nd:YAG laser of wave length 532 nm (green light) is used to remove tattoos containing red and orange ink. The decorative tattoos as well as traumatic tattoos caused from accidents have been treated with outstanding results. Cosmetic tattoos including eyebrow and lip liner can also be removed using lasers. Removal of accidents, gunshots or explosives marks with Q-switched Nd:YAG laser is possible.

Q-switched Nd:YAG, ruby, and alexandrite lasers are widely used for complex multicoloured tattoo removal. Each of these lasers emits a specific wavelength of light which targets specific tattoo colour for removal. A combination of erbium laser/Q-switch laser treatment is used for tattoos which are unresponsive to traditional laser treatment. The Figure 4.19 shows professional tattoo (left) and its removal using a Nd:YAG Q-Switched 1064 nm laser.

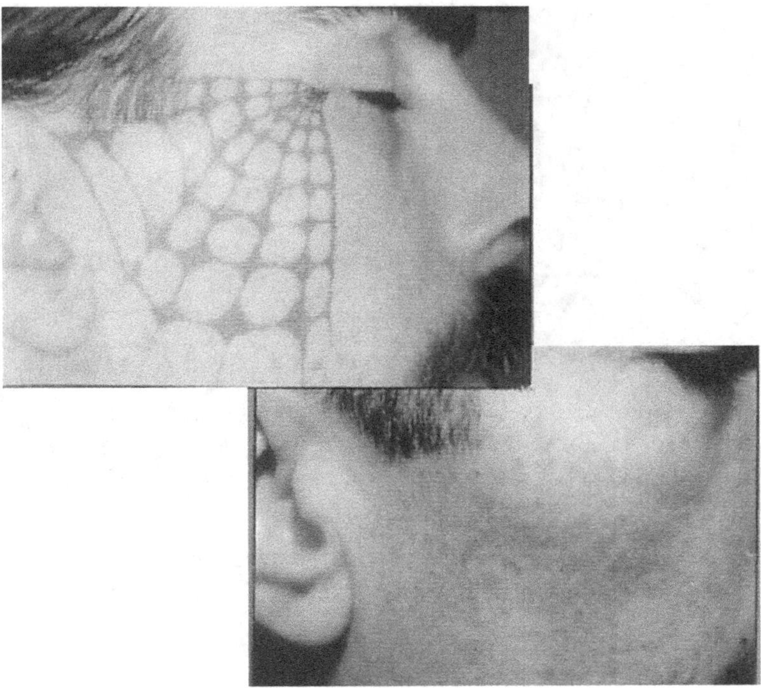

Figure 4.19 Professional tattoo (left) was removed after 15 sittings using a Q-Switched 1064 nm Nd:YAG laser (Courtesy: Biophotonics)

Scientists suggest the use of 1064 nm Nd:YAG laser, emitting a 10 ns pulses at 10 Hz for the removal of 3 mm tattoo spot. The fluence can be varied between 5 and 7 J/cm^2. The ideal laser for treatment of these conditions would be a laser with a cooling system, so that one could use a higher fluence and at the same time the epidermis could be saved from scarring and pigment changes. The possibility to vary wavelength and pulse duration also would be very valuable.

Other uses of tattoo lasers are removal of traumatic tattooing resulting from mechanical penetration of foreign particles into the body. In addition, unwanted cosmetic tattoos such as eyeliner and lip liner tattoos can be removed by means of Q-switching lasers. Today, the treatment of choice and standard of care for tattoo removal are lasers and this branch is appropriately called as **Cosmetic Photonics.** The moon-bat tattoo removal with Q-switched frequency-doubled Nd:YAG laser in four sittings is shown in Figure 4.20.

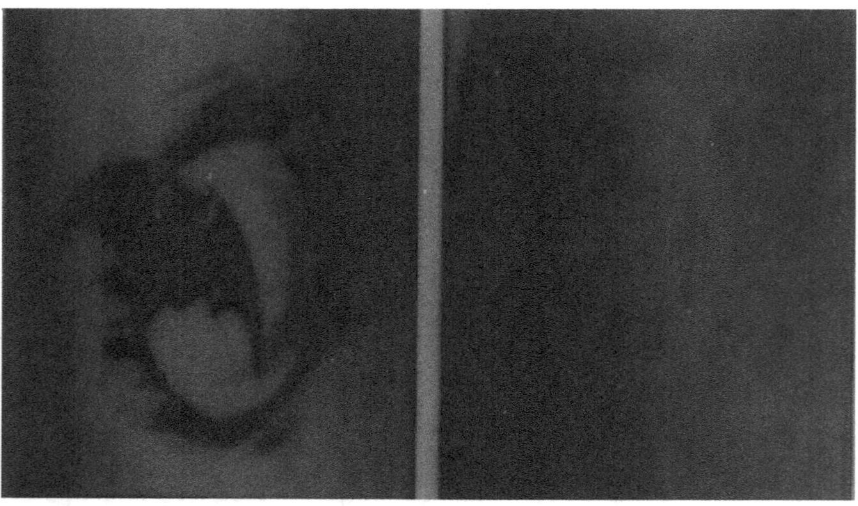

Figure 4.20   Four sittings with Q-switched frequency-doubled Nd:YAG laser removed "moon-bat" tattoo (Courtesy: Biophotonics)

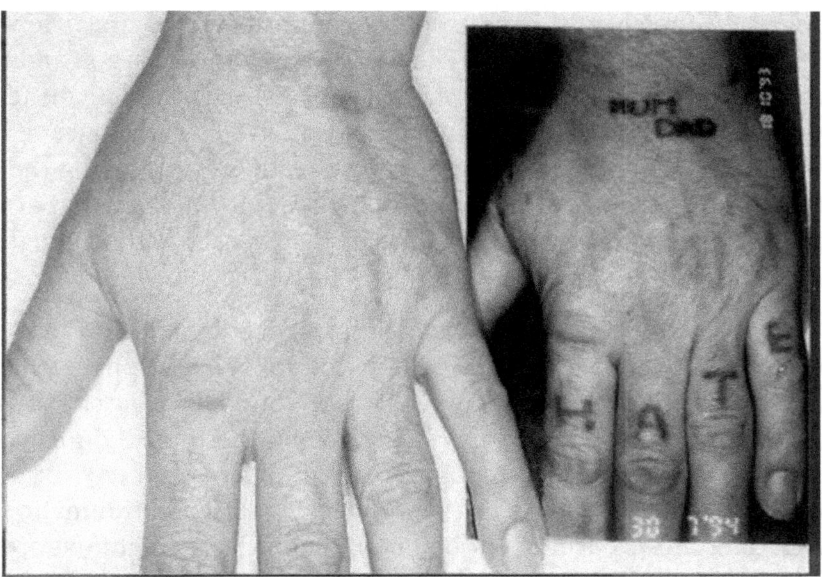

Figure 4.21 Mafia group tattoo removal (Courtesy: Biophotonics)

The mafia group tattoo removal is shown in Figure 4.21. The Q-switched Nd:YAG laser (pulse repetition frequency up to 10 Hz) from Candela is smallest, affordable and a high performance laser. This laser effectively treats a broad range of tattoo colours as well as epidermal pigmented lesions. The dual wavelengths of 1064 nm and 532 nm broaden treatment options, allowing for removal of red tattoos and tattoos in darker skin types.

4.29 LASER SCAR REMOVAL

i)   Acne Scars

Acne is a genetic, hormonal disease characterized by overproduction of oil by the sebaceous glands, plugging of the sebaceous glands to form micro- and macro-comedones (blackheads) and finally action of skin bacteria. The oil produced is trapped underneath the skin to produce red inflammatory cystic lesions. Acne scars can appear as depressed or uneven areas of the face, small holes in the skin called 'ice pick' scars or raised red or pink scars.

The treatment of acne scars has been limited to various resurfacing procedures such as dermabrasion and chemical peels. Unfortunately, prolonged erythema and hypertrophic scar formation or recurrence after these procedures is common. The CW carbon dioxide, argon and Nd:YAG lasers have also been utilized to vapourise scar tissue but recurrence is frequent. The 585 nm flash-pumped pulsed dye laser (fluence 6.5 J/cm^2; 7 mm spot size) has been shown to be effective in improving the clinical appearance of a variety of hypertrophic scars including facial acne scars and keloids without scar worsening or recurrence. A good progress was noticed after one sitting.

The conventional therapies involving antiseptics and antibiotics have their benefits but they also have limitations of being inconvenient and occasionally toxic. Acne scar removal was traditionally treated with erbium and carbon dioxide laser resurfacing. While these procedures can yield excellent results, they do require post-care and several days of post-procedure down time. Laser treatment for acne, facial and traumatic scarring is successful. Acne treatment before and after laser treatment are shown in Figures 4.22 and 4.23.

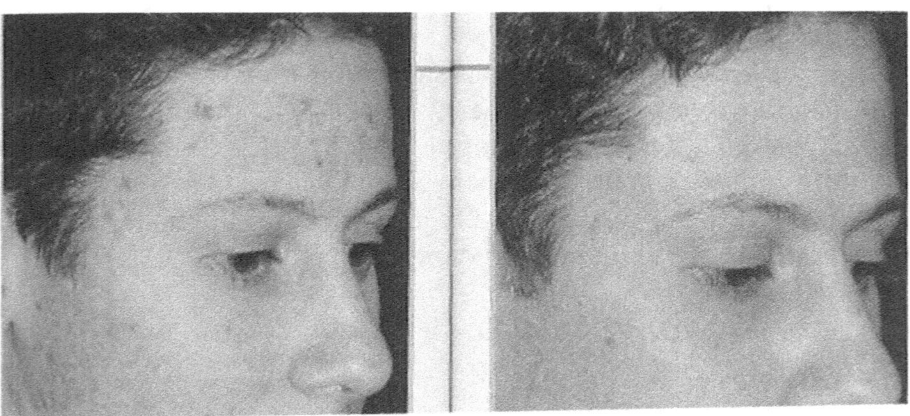

Figure 4.22 Acne treatment using lasers (Courtesy: Biophotonics)

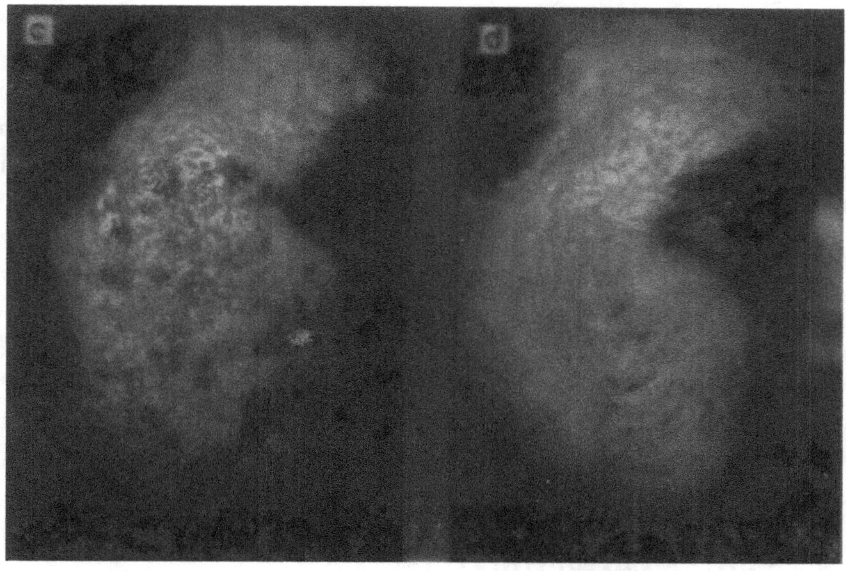

Figure 4.23 Acne treatment using lasers (Courtesy: Biophotonics)

Photodynamic therapy is a new emerging technique for treating acne and it appears to be well-tolerated, best for mild, moderate and even severe acne.

4.30 LASERS IN LESIONS AND VARICOSE VEINS

Longer wavelengths in the 590 nm to 600 nm range generally are used to treat older patients with older lesions caused by larger and deeper vessels. Other lasers that treat port wine and other small vessel vascular lesion include long pulse 582 nm, CW 532 nm, CW argon – dye and copper vapour (which emit at 511 or 578 nm) lasers. Large veins such as varicose veins commonly seen on the legs require a different approach. Doctors use longer laser wavelength pulses to penetrate more deeply to heat larger areas to shrink blood veins in the leg without scarring. They also employ dye alexandrite and frequency-doubled Nd:YAG lasers with long pulses, as well as pulsed and CW near-infrared diode lasers.

4.30.1   *Surgical and Traumatic Scars*

Surgical scars often present themselves as keloids, hypertrophic or depressed areas with or without associated erythema (redness). Depending on the type and severity of these scars, these can be treated with pulsed dye, erbium and carbon dioxide lasers.

4.30.2   **Facial blood vessel treatment**

Green laser proved to be of tremendous advance in removing facial vessels in a single treatment in an effective manner. After treatment patients may return to their normal activities without any significant cosmetic inconvenience. Earlier patients experienced the severe postoperative bruising with the older pulsed dye lasers.

4.30.3   *Skin imperfection*

Laser treatment produces thousands of tiny but deep columns of treatment in skin known as microthermal treatment zones. This treatment eliminates old epidermal pigmented cells. It also penetrates deep into the dermis. For every microthermal zone that the laser targets and treats intensively, it leaves the surrounding tissue unaffected and intact. This fractional treatment allows the skin to heal much faster than if the entire area were treated at once, using the body's natural healing process to create new, healthy tighter tissue to replace skin imperfections. Laser shows significant success in treating skin around eyes, skin texture, wrinkles and skin discolorations such as age spots and sun spots. It is important to note laser treatment spares healthy tissues and it is effective on delicate skin areas such as neck, chest and hands. Laser treatment can be performed using topical anaesthetics. The treatment area will be thoroughly cleansed prior to the procedure. In this treatment, one will experience a mild sunburn sensation for about an hour and then virtually no discomfort. The skin will have a pinkish tone for five to seven days. New epidermal skin develops within 24 hours. This process of skin repair involves:

1.   Bronzing (skin gives bronze appearance after laser exposure).

2.   Flaking (something like minor sunburn without pain. Moisture can mask the appearance of flaking).

3.   Sunscreen (avoid sun exposure during healing process).

4.31   HAIR REMOVAL

Laser treatment for hair removal currently represents one of the most exciting areas within laser medicine and surgery. Hair removal is one of the largest potential markets for aesthetic laser equipment and treatments. The center for laser surgery was one of the first in the world to use the 800 nm diode laser from Lumenis (Coherent medical group) for laser removal. Long pulse ruby lasers, long pulse alexandrite lasers, long pulse Nd:YAG lasers, long pulse diode lasers and quasi CW pulsed diode laser systems are employed for this purpose. Long pulse 100 msec diode laser and long pulse Nd:YAG laser are safe for dark skin patients including African Americans.

4.31.1   Biology of hair growth

Hair growth cycles are divided into three phases. The anagen follicle or growing hair is the major target for laser energy and represents the most vulnerable phases of the hair growth cycle. Telogen or resting hairs are not actively growing and appear to be more resistant to the laser energy. The transitional phase between anagen and telogen phases known as the catagen phase is brief but also relatively resistant to laser removal.

Depending on the body site, various percentages of hairs are in the anagen, catagen and telogen phase. As a result, it is necessary to treat a given anatomic area more than once in order to attempt to achieve a permanent hair removal. Since the anagen phase is most vulnerable, a period of one to three months between treatments is necessary to allow the resting of telogen phase hairs to once again enter the anagen cycle and become more sensitive to the laser energy.

4.31.2   Role of lasers in hair removal

At present, four laser wavelengths are available for the treatment of unwanted body hair. In essence, these wavelengths target pigment granules in the hair (melanin) in an effort to destroy hair follicles. Hair follicles are capable of producing hairs of various thickness and colours. Dark hair contains the pigment melanin which serves as the target for energy at these wavelengths. Four wavelengths of 694 nm, 755 nm, 800 nm, and 1064 nm produced by the ruby laser, alexandrite laser, diode laser and Nd:YAG laser respectively have been shown to be effective in the removal of pigmented hair. The pulsed laser energy absorbed by the pigmented hair shaft is transferred to the surrounding follicle.

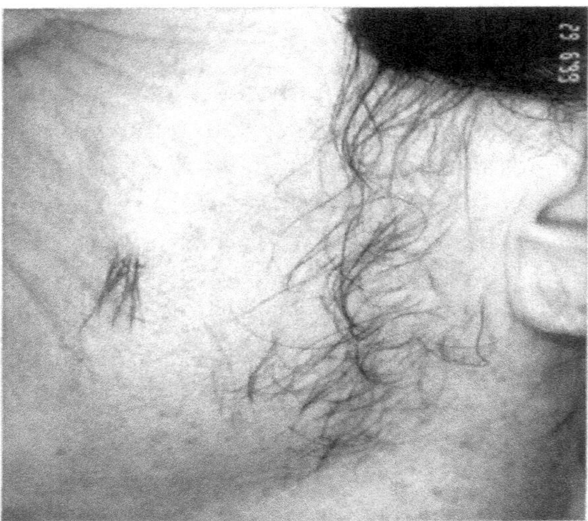

Figure 4.24 Unwanted hair growth

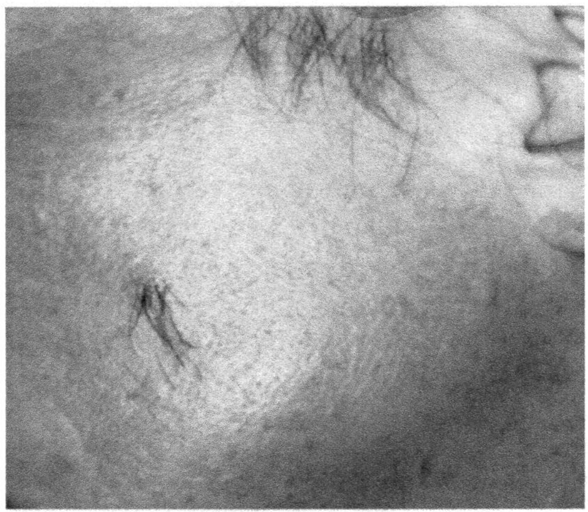

Figure 4.25 Removal of hair after laser treatment

The heat build-up caused by the absorption energy by the hair itself is capable of creating follicular damage and retard or prevent future hair production by that follicle. The application of these laser energies to the skin results in almost complete removal of all actively growing hairs. The difficulty in eradication of unwanted hair or excess hair lies in the fact that the follicle has tremendous regenerative capabilities and that these recuperative powers are highly variable from individual to individual and from one anatomic site to another. The unwanted hair growth and their removal by lasers are depicted in the Figures 4.24 and 4.25.

4.31.3   *Procedure of laser hair removal*

Laser hair removal is a time consuming but relatively straightforward process. One has to apply topical anaesthetic cream before treatment. The cream greatly reduces the discomfort associated with the laser hair removal process. Prior to the treatment the hairs will be shaved and the laser treatment will proceed. Treatment times vary from a few minutes for areas such as the chin and neck to a few hours for extensive areas of the legs, back and chest. After the procedure, cool compresses and soothing gels are applied to the treated area and the patients spend time relaxing before being discharged.

Laser hair removal methods rely on selective photothermolysis interaction with the hair follicles. Although the underlying mechanisms are not completely understood, they probably depend upon the type of laser and specific methods employed. In one method, a carbon-based ointment is rubbed into hair follicles, with the carbon particles serving as primary absorbers of laser energy. In other "ointment free" methods, melanin particles resting the hair follicles are thought to absorb the laser energy.

4.31.4   **PRECAUTIONS**

Blood tests are necessary to uncover any hormone-related causes which may be associated with the excess production of body hair. Patients who are dark-skinned type may use a bleaching cream (Hydroquinone 4% or Rojic acid) for three to four weeks prior to treatment in order to lessen the effects of brown melanin pigment in the skin surrounding the hair follicle. Laser hair removal has proven to be a very safe procedure.

4.32   **HAIR TRANSPLANTATION**

Hair transplantation is nothing but grafting healthy follicles from the back and sides of the head into the bald areas. These follicles retain their anatomical and physiological properties for almost the entire life of the individual. This is proven by the fact that bald men almost always have hair remaining in the nape of the neck and the temples. So, hair transplantation means the relocating of follicles from one site (where there are plenty) to another (where there are no longer any follicles). Following transplantation, these follicles continue to function normally and grow healthily. These transplanted hairs after growth can be cut or trimmed regularly. These can be shampooed or dyed if required. These hairs do not require any medicines to maintain the growth as it occurs naturally and permanently. Even after complete shaving or tonsuring, these hairs will grow back and tend to do so for the rest of the life.

In laser-assisted hair transplantation, a laser creates skin pockets that can accept hair follicle transplants. A char-free laser vaporizes a slit-type pocket only several millimeters deep. Char-free lasers, usually CO_2 laser, cause minimal thermal necrosis and charming at edges of pockets as is required for the transplanted hair follicle to grow successfully. Figure 4.26 shows hair transplantation.

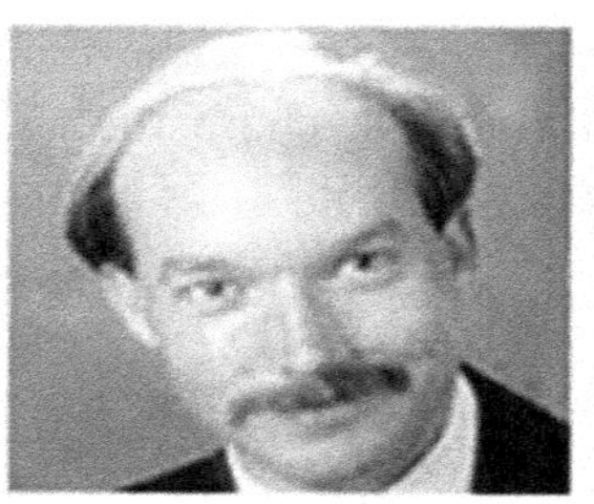

Before Hair Restoration

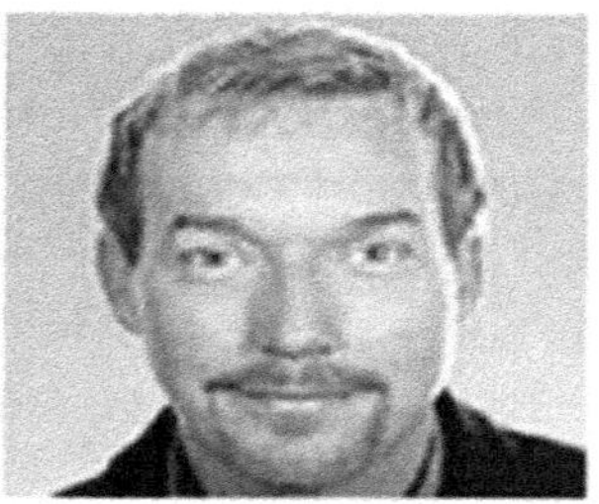

After Hair Restoration

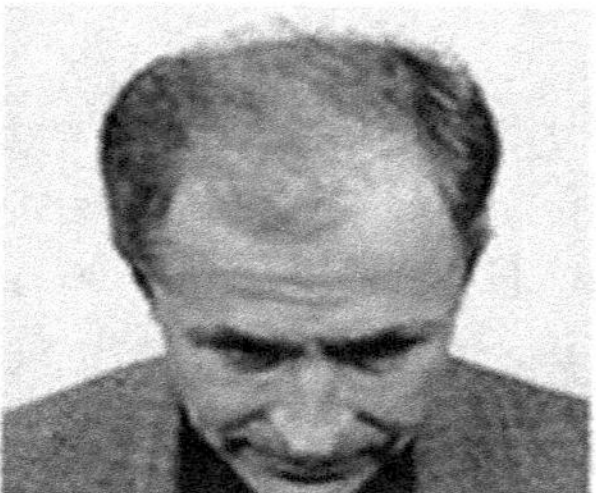

Before Hair Restoration

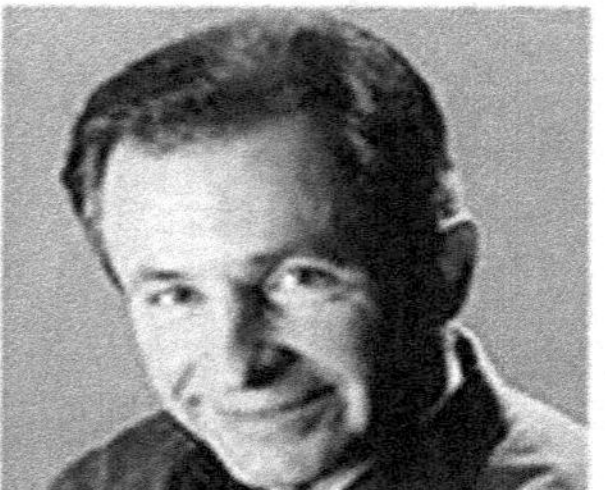

After Hair Restoration

Figure 4.26 Hair transplantation

4.33 LASER TREATMENT ON VITILIGO

White patches of skin on face, eyelashes, eye brows, lips, hands, arms or other parts of the body are called as vitiligo. It is a rare skin condition and they neither produce pain or discomfort nor are they medically harmful. But the patches do not go away without treatment. It causes great emotional distress and mental tension. The etiology of vitiligo is unknown. It is believed that it is caused by one's own immune system. Pigment cells in the skin produce melanin, the substance responsible for unique and individual skin tone. When these cells are attacked and destroyed by the body's own defence system they stop making melanin, resulting in the skin becoming lighter or even completely white.

Vitiligo is treated using topical steroids or creams to stimulate pigmentation. In recent times, phototherapy has proven to be one of the most effective vitiligo treatments as it is free from side effects. Phototherapy helps in repigmentation of the pale skin patches by stimulating neighbouring pigmentation cells (melanocytes) into producing skin colour again. These neighbouring cells are often located towards the edges of the affected areas, near the base of hair follicles, or possibly within the patch itself. The excimer lasers which emit ultraviolet radiation play a vital role in treating vitiligo successfully. Ultraviolet-A (UVA) light combined with the drug psoralen or narrowband Ultraviolet-B (UVB) light is used for the purpose. This treatment is safe and repigmentation is possible within a year. The narrowband UVB light therapy is often administered three times a week on non-consecutive days. Once 75% repigmentation is achieved, the vitiligo treatment is usually reduced to twice a week or less.

With an excellent success rate, narrowband UVB light therapy is the best choice for vitiligo treatment. It is done without drugs, without injections and without side effects. Since the therapy is well-tolerated, it is quite often the best option for children and long-term care.

4.34 LASER REMOVAL OF MOLES (NEVI) AND STRETCH MARKS

Moles are a nevocellular skin occurrence located in the skin's various layers. Everybody has moles which appear as a dark brown spot. Moles have a wide range of size and shape. Sometimes moles protrude from the skin and some of them may be dangerous. Most moles come out during the first twenty years of a person's life. They become darker on the exposure to sun.

Moles are easily removed with the Er:YAG laser that remove moles effectively for a clear skin complexion. A combination of high and low intensity lasers are used to break up the pigment and erase imperfections. However, results vary from patient to patient. Results from laser mole treatment are generally progressive and may require multiple treatments. When one responds to the first treatment, second treatment will usually be as good as the first and the third treatment will be almost good. Newer and shallower moles respond better than older and deeper moles.

The patients that respond the best to laser treatment for moles are those with:

1.   Fair complexion and light pigmentation

2.   Shallow scars or moles

Pulsed lasers (pulses hundreds of times per second) are used for mole removal. This pulsing action prevents heat damage to the skin and minimises the risk of scarring. Laser treatment for mole removal usually gives great cosmetic results. Laser treatment is a valuable alternative to traditional surgical excision procedure. Lasers are particularly valuable in treating lesions in anatomic areas which are difficult to approach surgically such as the face, lips, nose, and ears. In addition, lasers are quite useful for removing multiple benign facial growths during a single treatment session. Figure 4.27 illustrates the mole removal using laser.

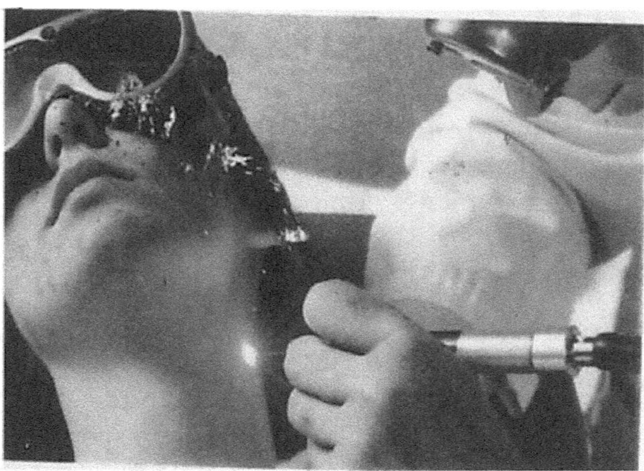

Figure 4.27   Mole removal using laser (Courtesy: Biophotonics)

4.35   LASER REMOVAL OF STRETCH MARKS

Striae distensae (SD) are stretch marks that are common in many healthy women and men and often occur during puberty and pregnancy. They can be seen following a rapid weight gain or loss in weight lifters as well as in Cushing's disease or debilitating infections. Striae distensae are often seen over the thighs, buttocks, breasts, shoulders and lower back. A possible etiology is endocrine imbalance, rapid stretching of the skin and mast cell degranulation with elastolysis. Striae distensae may be a form of dermal scarring in which the dermal collagen ruptures possibly under the influence of steroids. The intervening gap is filled with newly synthesised collagen which becomes aligned horizontally in response to local stress forces. Early striae are flat and have a faint pink colour. As they mature, they widen, elongate and take a purple hue. After months or years, the lesions become thin, atrophic white-yellow streaks. Flash lamp pulsed dye vascular laser (585 nm) with a pulse duration of 450 microseconds at fluencies of 3–3.5 joules/cm^2 responds well for the treatment of striae distensae. This laser effectively treats striae distensae which presents a challenge to the dermatologists interested in cosmetic dermatology.

Stretch marks present as unsightly red to white areas which commonly occur on the abdomen, arms, chest and thighs. The cause of stretch marks is basically unknown but it can result from pregnancy, weight gain, trauma and hormonal influence. The stretch mark represents a dermal scar in which connective tissue (collagen and elastin) within the dermis is disrupted. Pulsed dye laser therapy for removal of stretch marks is safe and can be effective.

4.36   LASER REMOVAL OF WARTS

Most of us have had a wart on a part of our body at some time in our lives. Warts are one of the most common infections caused by a microscopic virus that infects the skin. Most warts are harmless and can disappear on their own without a warts removal treatment. However, warts on parts of the body that are bumped or touched frequently can be painful and cause bleeding. Warts can also be embarrassing if they occur on the face or appear in noticeable clusters on the hands and feet. Carbon dioxide or erbium YAG laser for warts removal treatment is effective and permanent on fingers, finger nails, face, feet, hands, elbows and knees. Figure 4.28 shows warts on the big toe.

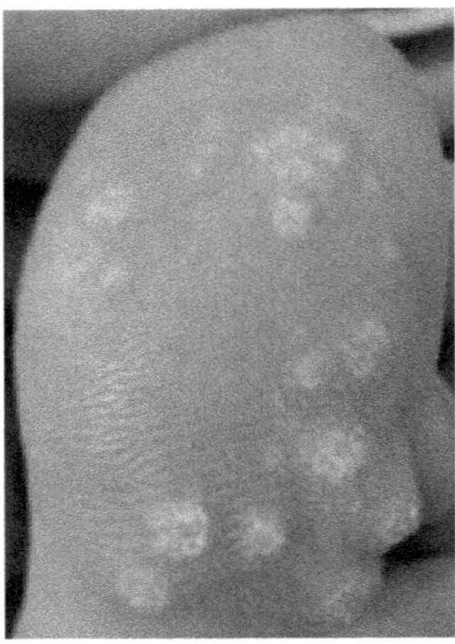

Figure 4.28 Warts on the big toe

Flash lamp excited pulse dye laser is the most versatile laser for treating leg telangiectasia, facial spider veins, port wine stains, hemangiomas, rosacea, stretch marks, vulvodynia, scars, warts and other vascular abnormalities. The tuning capability of this laser enhances the clinical response when treating veins and lesions of different size, shapes, location and depth. The multiple wavelengths (585, 590, 595 and 600 nm) enable the physician to control the depth of laser penetration and vessel coagulation. The ScleroPLUS from Candela (1500 microseconds) delivers laser energy to vessels over longer periods of time, resulting in gentle, uniform heating/coagulation across the entire vessel diameter.

4.36.1 *Sclerotherapy*

The scleroplus laser (1500 microsecond pulse duration) from Candela provides a clinically effective alternative to sclerotherapy for leg telangiectasia up to one millimeter in size. This results in gentle, uniform coagulation across the entire vessel. The system incorporates two wavelengths that enable the physician to enhance the depth of laser penetration and vessel coagulation.

4.37 LASERS DELIVER DRUGS WITHOUT INJECTION

The drugs administered with needles may cause infection and pain. Hence there has long been an interest in delivering drugs without injection. The stratum corneum, outermost skin layer (10 to 100 micrometre) protects the interior of our body from the outside elements and organisms in the atmosphere. With the aid of a 694.3 nm Q-switched ruby laser it is possible to open a microcrack in this wall temporarily. A small reservoir of the drug is placed on the skin's surface and covered by a black plastic pouch. The absorbed laser energy creates a stress wave which opens a temporary pass in the stratum corneum and allows molecules as large as 40 kilodaltons to diffuse passively through it. The laser beam itself does not penetrate the skin. After the procedure, the stratum corneum remained permeable for as long as 15 minutes before returning to normal. This may also be extended to as much as an hour with the help of surfactants. This new approach is a great boon to diabetic patients who take insulin (which is only 6 kilodalton in size) periodically.

4.38 WHITER TEETH FOR BRIGHTER SMILES

Humans wish to keep their teeth whiter for cosmetic beauty. Lasers are used for this purpose. Toothpaste-like whitening agents are applied on teeth and low intensity argon or CO_2 lasers are then used to activate them. The teeth and gums are not exposed directly to the two lasers. The low intensity of lasers does not cause any problems on gums. This new method for teeth whitening using lasers has been widely accepted by dentists and the common man. More than 300 dental centers have already been established in the State of Utah, USA.

Lasers which started at laboratory level have extended their wings to industry, medical, entertainment, cosmetic, food, military, biology, veterinary science and to several other areas. The emerging new laser technologies help us in developing new mechanisms which control the delivery of laser energy. Manufacturers attempt to develop smaller, faster and more accurate delivery systems to keep up with the demands of the cosmetic market. Future scanners can have improved performance and can fit into smaller hand pieces that are more comfortable and easier for beauticians to use. Another application in clinical trials is the use of lasers for tissue-welding to improve cosmetic skin closure results after breast cancer surgery.

References

1. A. Einstein. (1917). *Zur Quantentheorie der Strahlung. Physikalische Zeitschrift* 18:121.

2. T.H. Maiman. (1960). "Stimulated optical radiation in ruby". *Nature.* 187:493.

3. R.H. Ossoff, J.A. Coleman, M.S. Courey, J.A. Duncavage, J.A. Werkhaven, Rein. Q. Peng et al. (2008). "Lasers in medicine". *Reports on Progress in Physics.* 71:056701.

4. J.L. Boulnois. (1986). "Photophysical Processes in Recent Medical Laser Developments: a Review". *Lasers in Medical Science.* 1:47–66.

5. A.L. McKenzie. (1990). "Review article: Physics of thermal processes in laser–tissue interaction". *Physics in Medicine and Biology.* 35:1175–1209.

6. M.H. Niemz. 2004. Laser–Tissue Interactions, Third revised edition. *Springer–Verlag.*

7. G. Paltauf and P.E. Dyer. (2003). "Photomechanical Processes and Effects in Ablation" *Chem. Rev.* 103:487–518.

8. P.N. Prasad. 2003. "Introduction to Biophotonics". *Wiley Inter–Science.*

9. J.L. Boulnois. (1986). "Photophysical processes in recent medical laser developments: A Review". *Lasers Med. Sci.* 1:47–66.

10. F. Cammarata and M. Wautelety. (1999). "Medical lasers and laser–tissue interactions". *Phys. Educ.* 34:156–61.

11. A. Vogel and V. Venugopalan. (2003). "Mechanisms of Pulsed Ablation of Biological Tissues". *Chem. Rev.* 103:577–644.

12. R.H. Ossoff and S.A. Matar. (1988). "The advantages of laser treatment of tumors of the larynx". *Oncology* (Williston Park) 2:58–61 & 64–65.

13. T.G. Polanyi, H.C. Bredemeier, T.W. Davis. (1970). "A CO_2 laser for surgical research". *Med. Biol. Eng.* 8:541–548.

14. S.M. Shapshay Jako. (1996). "Laser surgery of the vocal cords; an experimental study with carbon dioxide lasers on dogs". *Laryngoscope* (1972) 82:2204–2216; *Laryngoscope* 106:935–938.

15. R.T. Sataloff, J.R. Spiegel, M. Hawkshaw, A. Jones. (1992). "Laser surgery of the larynx: the case for caution". *Ear Nose Throat J.* 71:593–595.

16. M.H. Haug, P. Møller, J. Olofsson. (1993). "Laser surgery in otorhinolaryngology: A 10-year experience". *J. Otolaryngol.* 22:42–45.

17. L. Reinisch and R.H. Ossoff. (1996). "Laser applications in otolaryngology". *Otolaryngol Clin. North Am.* 29:891–892.

18. W. Xu, D. Han, L. Hou, L. Zhang, Z. Yu, Z. Huang. (2007). "Voice function following CO_2 laser microsurgery for precancerous and early stage glottic carcinoma". *Acta Oto-Laryngologica.* 127:637–641.

19. S.M. Zeitels and J.A. Burns. (2006). "Laser applications in laryngology: past, present, and future". *Otolaryngol. Clin. North Am.* 39:159–172.

20. K. McMillan, S.M. Shapshay, J.A. McGilligan, Z. Wang, E.E. Rebeiz. (1998). "A 585 nm pulsed dye laser treatment of laryngeal papillomas: Preliminary report". *Laryngoscope.* 108:968–972.

21. M.S. Strong, G.J. Jako. (1972). "Laser surgery in the larynx. Early clinical experience with continuous CO_2 laser". *Ann Otol. Rhinol. Laryngol.* 81:791–798.

22. S.M. Zeitels, J.A. Burns, L.M. Akst, R.E. Hillman, M.S. Broadhurst, R.R. Anderson. (2006). "Office-based and microlaryngeal applications of a fibre–based thulium laser". *Ann. Otol. Rhinol. Laryngol.* 115:891–896.

23. Z. Wang, A.K. Devaiah, L. Feng, U. Dasai, G. Shapira, O. Weisberg, D.S. Torres, S.M. Shapshay. (2006). "Fibre-guided CO_2 laser surgery in an animal model". *Photomed. Laser Surg.* 24:646–650.

24. S.M. Zeitels, J.B. Kobler, J.T. Heaton, W. Faquin. (2006). "Carbon dioxide laser fiber for laryngeal cancer surgery". *Ann. Otol. Rhinol. Laryngol.* 115:535–541.

25. A. Ferlito, J.G. Buckley, R. Ossoff, A. Rinaldo, N. Weir. (2001). "The Future of Laryngology". *Acta Oto-Laryngologica.* 121:859–867.

26. K.S. Lee, B.N. Chen, C.C. Yang, Y.C. Chen. (2007). "CO_2 laser supraglottoplasty for severe laryngomalacia: A study of symptomatic improvement". *Int. J. Pediatr. Otorhinolaryngol.* 71:889–895.

27. F. DeLeon and M. Baggish, 2008. *Glob. libr. women's med.* (ISSN: 1756–2228) ; DOI 10.3843/GLOWM.10023.

28. Z. Huang. (2005). "A review of progress in clinical photodynamic therapy". *Technol. Cancer Res. Treat.* 4:283–293.

29. J.D. Luketich, N.A. Christie, P.O. Buenaventura, et al. (2000). "Endoscopic photodynamic therapy for obstructing esophageal cancer: 77 cases over a 2-year period". *Surg. Endosc.* 14:653–657.

30. B. Ortel, C.R. Shea, P. Calzavara–Pinton. (2009). "Molecular mechanisms of photodynamic therapy". *Frontiers in Bioscience.* 14:4157–4172.

31. N.R. Rigual, K. Thankappan, M. Cooper, et al. (2009). "Photodynamic therapy for head and neck dysplasia and cancer". *Arch Otolaryngol. Head Neck Surg.* 135:784–788.

32. M. Triesscheijn, P. Baas, and J.H.M. Schellens. (2006). Photodynamic therapy in oncology. *Oncologist.* 11 1034–1044.

33. M. Fujimura, T. Kumabe, T. Tominaga, et al. (2004). Routine clinical adoption of magnetic resonance imaging was associated with a better outcome after surgery in elderly patients with a malignant astrocytic tumour: A retrospective review. *Acta Neurochir.* (Wien) 146:251–255.

34. F. Sala, and P. Lanteri. (2003). "Brain surgery in motor areas: the invaluable assistance of intraoperative neurophysiological monitoring". *J.Neurosurg. Sci.* 47:79–88.

35. P.J. Kelly. (2000). "Stereotactic surgery: What is past is progogue". *Neurosurg.* 46:16–27.

36. W. Stummer, U. Pichlmeier,T. Meinel, et al. "Fluorescence-Guided Surgery with 5-Aminolevulinic Acid for Resection of Malignant Glioma: An Aandomised Controlled Multicentre Phase III Trial". (2006). *Lancet Oncology.* Early online publication April 13,. DOI: 10.1016/S1470–2045 (06) 70665–9.

37. S.M. Zeitels, J.B. Kobler, J.T. Heaton, and W. Faquin. (2006). "Carbon dioxide laser fiber for laryngeal cancer surgery". *Ann. Otol. Rhinol. Laryngol.* 115:535–541.

38. W. Robert Bastian. (2014). "Early Vocal Fold Cancer: Remove with a Laser, or Radiate?". *J. Observational Laryngol.*

39. (2010). "Annals of Otology, Rhinology & Laryngology; Massachusetts General Hospital." *J. Voice.* 24:102–109.

40. S.M. Zeitels, J.A. Burns, L.M. Akst, R.E. Hillman, M.S. Broadhurst, R.R. Anderson. (2006). "Office-based and microlaryngeal applications of a fiber-based thulium laser". *Ann. Otol. Rhinol Laryngol.*

41. I. Kaplan, J. Goldman, and R. Ger. (1953). "The treatment of erosions of the uterine cervix by means of the CO_2 laser". *Obstet. Gynecol.* 41:1973.

42. J.H. Bellina. (1974). "Gynecology and the laser". *Contemp. Obstet. Gynecol.* 4:24.

43. J.H. Bellina. (1973). "Microsurgery of the fallopian tube with the carbon dioxide laser: Analysis of 230 cases with a two year follow-up". *Lasers Surg. Med.* 3:255.

44. M.C. Anderson, and R.B. Hartley. (1980). "Cervical crypt involvement by intraepithelial neoplasia". *Obstet. Gynecol.* 55:546–50.

45. H. De Vuyst, G.M. Clifford, M.C. Nascimento, M.M. Madeleine, S. Franceschi. (2009). "Prevalence and type distribution of human papillomavirus in carcinoma and intraepithelial neoplasia of the vulva, vagina and anus: A meta-analysis". *Int. J. Cancer.* 124:1626–36.

46. J.H. Dorsey. (1991). "Laser surgery for cervical intraepithelial neoplasia". N. Chohan, H.A. Barron, (eds.) Obstetrics and Gynecology Clinics of North America. Philadelphia, Pa: WB Saunders Company, pp. 429–489.

47. W.R. Keye Jr, L.W. Hansen, M. Astin. (1987). "Argon laser therapy: A review of 92 consecutive patients". *Fertil. Steril.* 47:208.

48. M.S. Baggish. (1979). "Management of cervical intraepithelial neoplasia by carbon dioxide laser". *Obstet. Gynecol.* 54:565.

49. M.S. Baggish, J.H. Dorsey, M. Adelson. (1989). "A ten year experience treating intraepithelial neoplasia with the CO_2 laser". *Am. J. Obstet. Gynecol.* 161:60.

50. P.D. Indman, B.C. Arndt. (1985). "Laser treatment of cervical intraepithelial neoplasia in an office setting". *Am. J. Obstet. Gynecol.* 152:674.

51. J. Buscema, D. Woodruff, T.H. Parmley et al. (1980). "Carcinoma *in situ* of the vulva". *Obstet. Gynecol.* 55:225.

52. H.D. Wolcott, D.G. Gallup. (1984). "Wide local excision in the treatment of vulvar carcinoma *in situ*: A reappraisal". *Am. J. Obstet. Gynecol.* 150:695.

53. M.S. Baggish. (1985). "Carbon dioxide laser treatment of vulvar intraepithelial neoplasia". In M.S. Baggish (ed): *Basic and Advanced Laser Surgery in Gynecology*. Norwalk, CT, Appleton–Century–Crofts.

54. M.S. Baggish, E.H. Sze, M.D. Adelson et al. (1989). "Quantitative evaluation of the skin and accessory appendages in vulvar carcinoma *in-situ*". *Obstet. Gynecol.* 74:169.

55. M.S. Baggish, J.H. Dorsey. (1985). "Carbon dioxide laser for combination excisional vaporization conisation". *Am. J. Obstet. Gynecol.* 151:23.

56. V.C. Wright, and E. Davies. (1987). "Laser surgery for vulvar intraepithelial neoplasia: Principles and results". *Am. J. Obstet. Gynecol.* 156:374.

57. M.S. Baggish. (1980). "Carbon dioxide laser treatment for condylomata acuminata venereal infections". *Obstet. Gynecol.* 55:711.

58. H.B. Krebs. (1989). "Prophylactic topical 5-fluorouracil for the treatment of human papilloma virus associated lesions of the vulva and vagina". *Obstet. Gynecol.* 68:837.

59. R. Reid. (1992). Superficial laser vulvectomy III. Am. J. Obstet. Gynecol. 166 815.

60. D.N. Kramer, S.J. Cutler, (1976) Incidence and histo–pathology of malignancies of the female genital organs in the US. Am. J. Obstet. Gynecol. 118 443.

61. D.E. Townsend, R.U. Levin, C.P. Crun, R.M. Richart, (1982) Treatment of vaginal carcinoma in situ with carbon dioxide laser. Am. J. Obstet. Gynecol. 143 101.

62. J.H. Dorsey, M.S. Baggish, 1986 Multifocal vaginal intraepithelial neoplasia with uterus in situ. In F. Sharp, J. Jordan (eds.): Gynecological Laser Surgery. Proceedings of the Fifteenth Study Group of the Royal College of Obstetricians and Gynecologists. Ithaca, New York, Perinatology Press,.

63. J.H. Bellina, A.C. Fick, J.D. Jackson, (1984) Application of the CO_2 laser to infertility surgery. Surg. Clin. North Am. 64 899.

64. W.R. Keye, J.A. Dixon, (1983) Photocoagulation of endometriosis by the argon laser through the laparoscope. Obstet. Gynecol. 62 383.

65. E.C. Lotze, G.M. Grunert, (1989) The use of lasers in infertility surgery. Clin. Obstet. Gynecol. 323 79.

66. D.C. Martin (ed): 1990 Laparoscopic Appearance of Endometriosis, second edn., Memphis, Resurge Press, , p. 38.

67. C.J. Sutton, K.D. Jones, (2002) Laser laparoscopy for endometriosis and endometriotic cysts. Surg. Endosc. 16 1513–17.

68. E.M. Lichten, J. Bombard, (1987) Surgical treatment of primary dysmenorrhea with laparoscopic uterine nerve ablation. J. Reprod. Med. 32 37.

69. D.C. Martin, M.P. Diamond, (1986) Operative laparoscopy: Comparison of lasers with other techniques. Curr. Probl. Obstet. Gynecol. Fertil. 9 563.

70. A.M. Siegler, 1975 Tubal surgery for infertility. In J.J. Sciarra (ed.): Gynecology and Obstetrics, Hagerstown, MD, Harper & Row. p. 123.

71. M.E. Boer–Meisl, E.R. te Velde, J.D. Habbema et al., (1986) Predicting the pregnancy outcome in patients treated for hydrosalpinx: A prospective study. Fertil. Steril. 45 23.

72. B.G. Bateman, W.C. Nunley Jr, J.D. Kitchin III: (1987) Surgical management of distal tubal obstruction: Are we making progress? Fertil. Steril. 48 523.

73. W.B. Stromme, Salpingostomy for tubal pregnancy. Obstet. Gynecol. 1 (1953) 472.

74. A.H. De Cherney, R. Romero, F. Naffolin, (1980) Surgical management of unruptured ectopic pregnancy. Fertil. Steril. 33 411.

75. D.A. Johns, R.P. Hardie, (1986) Management of unruptured ectopic pregnancy with laparoscopic CO_2 laser. Fertil. Steril. 46 703.

76. J.D. Paulson: (1992) The use of carbon dioxide laser laparoscopy in the treatment of tubal ectopic pregnancies. Am. J. Obstet. Gynecol. 167 382.

77. G. Bandieramonte, F. Chiesa, M. Lupi, R. Marchesini, (1987) Lasers Surg. Med. 7 478–86.

78. S.K. Powers, (1992) Semin. Surg. Oncol. 8 226–32.

79. W. Jerjes, Z. Hamdoon, C. Hopper, (2012) Head & Neck Oncol. 4 17. doi:10.1186/ 1758-3284–4–17; (http://www.headandneckoncology.org/content/4/1/17)

80. J.M. White, S.I. Chaudhry, J.J. Kudler, N. Sekandari, M.L. Schoelch, S. Silverman, (1998) Nd:YAG and CO_2 laser therapy of oral mucosal lesions. J. Clin. Laser Med. Surg. 16 299–304.

81. P.M. Villarreal Renedo, F. Monje Gil, L.M. Junquera Gutiérrez, J.C. De Vicente Rodríguez, A.J. Morillo Sánchez, (2004) Treatment of oral and oropharyngeal epidermoid carcinomas by means of CO_2 laser. Med. Oral. 9 172–175.

82. O. Pradier, H. Christiansen, H. Schmidberger, A. Martin, M.C. Jäckel, W. Steiner, P. Ambrosch, E. Kahler, C.F. Hess, (2005) Adjuvant radiotherapy after transoral laser microsurgery for advanced squamous carcinoma of the head and neck. Int. J. Radiat. Oncol. Biol. Phys. 63 1368.

83. http://www.headandneckoncology.org/content/4/1/17.

84. J. Cobb, D. Claremont, (2001) Medical Engineering & Physics 23 417–425.

85. Laser applications in medicine and Biology, M.L. Wolbarsht (ed.), 1971 Plenum press, New York,.

86. Laser medicine and surgery, G.T. Absten (ed.), 2004 The Laser training institute, Marathon Shores.

Review Questions

1. What is laser therapy? List the laser therapy procedures

2. What is the importance of lasers in medical applications?

3. Explain the advantages of solid-state lasers over carbon dioxide laser in open surgery.

4. What is advantage of laser in medicine over classical methods?

5. Discuss the role of Nd:YAG and Er:YAG lasers for medicine

6. What is photodynamic therapy? Explain with examples.

7. Explain the role of optical fibres in surgery.

8. Explain in detail the removal of tumour of vocal cords using laser.

9. Explain in detail the surgery for brain tumours using laser.

10. What is endoscope? What are its uses? Explain with examples.

11. 'Destroying cancer cells with laser directed light'. Justify with examples.

12. List the procedure for the image-guided technology for neurosurgery.

13. What is meant by ablative lasers? Where are they used?

14. Distinguish between ablative and non-ablative lasers along with their uses.

15. Explain in detail laser therapy in gynaecology.

16. What are the advantages of gynaecological CO_2 laser microsurgery?

17. Write a note on cervix–cervical intraepithelial neoplasia.

18. Explain colposcopy, laparoscopy and hysteroscopy.

19. Discuss and explain the diagnosis and treatment of endometriosis using laser.

20. Discuss and explain cervical dysplasia.

21. Explain the role of lasers in oncology.

22. Write a note on lasers in oncology.

23. Write a note on radiation oncology.

24. Write a note on gynaecological oncology.

25. Write a note on laser oncosurgery.

26. Write in detail on cosmetic lasers emphasising on:

27. (i) skin resurfacing

28. (ii) skin wrinkles

29. (iii) tattoo removal

30. (iv) hair removal

31. (v) hair transplantation

32. (vi) port wine stain removal

33. (vii) whitening teeth

Chapter 5

Laser Safety

INTRODUCTION

Laser is a wonderful and unique radiation. Apart from its wider use in ophthalmology and ENT, the number of doctors and nurses in our country who actually use lasers is few. But very soon, lasers are going to be a standard tool in our medical and surgical wards. Hence one has to learn to manage this exciting dynamic technology.

Traditional medical service, whether in a hospital or private practice, requires a wide range of technical and administrative skills to employ lasers. When lasers are introduced, the skills have to be modified with a new knowledge based on biophysics, high-tech instrumentation and safety. Although lasers are not new to medicine, it has taken quite a long time to gain widespread acceptance. Recently, lasers are rapidly accepted in medical practices, surgery and at treatment centres.

In the last several years, technological changes have made a variety of lasers available in health care. With the increased use of lasers and multiple wavelengths in medicine and surgery, laser safety requires specific guidelines. This demands an urgent need for doctors and nurses to learn about lasers. The inclusion of a laser to a patient's treatment plan takes a considerable amount of the doctor's time in addition to their responsibility to educate, counsel patients and to provide physical and emotional support.

It is essential for doctors working with lasers to have an understanding of the fundamentals of the technology and its integration into current practice. In the earlier chapters we have already seen about lasers and their different types. To know, more about lasers uses, one has to look at an important question, viz., how do I protect myself and my patient from laser radiation? Since lasers are considered a high risk source, all personal who work with laser should be exposed to biophysics and safety.

LASER DELIVERY SYSTEMS

All lasers regardless of their properties and biophysical effects can cut, coagulate and vaporize tissue to some degree. The wavelength determines the typical delivery system to be used. Carbon dioxide laser energy must be delivered by means of hollow tubular system with mirrors to reflect the beam down to the output device.

Equipment to deliver carbon dioxide laser radiation include handpieces, microscope adaptors, rigid endoscopes and both flexible and semi-rigid waveguides. All other wavelengths can be transmitted across fibre optics. Laser fibres and flexible quartz with various coatings to protect the core and create purge channels for coaxial cooling. Today's fibres are disposable, durable and reliable and come in a wide variety of sizes and configurations. Fibres make the use of flexible endoscopes. It opens up new horizons where the areas unreachable with either the carbon dioxide laser or conventional instrumentation, can be reached with this technology.

Contact tips and sculptured fibres are used in contact with the tissue and deliver a thermal effect. This technique converts the Nd:YAG laser from a coagulation device to a device that can cut and coagulate simultaneously.

Regardless of the delivery system, the surgical use of laser energy requires a focusing device to produce a small spot of energy that can be carefully and controllably directed to the operative site. Focusing lenses built into the delivery system (handpiece, fibre and microscope connector, etc.) can be short or long, allowing the beam to focus at varying distance from the tissue. As the distance from tissue changes, so does the size of the laser beam. That is, when the beam is focused to a very small spot, the energy is concentrated into a high power density beam which cuts or vaporizes tissue rapidly and precisely. As the beam moves away from tissue, the spot size increases and lowers energy concentration so that with low power density, only a shallow surface effect is created.

Irradiation time affects the depth of penetration and hence we should take care of tissue damage. Time exposure is usually measured in terms of joules or watts multiplied by time. The total dosimetry is expressed in terms of energy density (Watts × time × area or spot size). This determines the complete picture of tissue effect regardless of wavelength.

LASER HAZARDS

A laser can be considered as a high source of extremely intense electromagnetic radiation that is defined by three basic characteristics, viz., monochromatic, directional and coherent. Due to the temporal and spatial coherence of the laser beam, it can be considered as a point source with the brightness exceeding that of sun. Lasers are more directional light sources than any other radiation. The higher the optical output power of the laser, the greater the potential hazard.

The hazards from lasers can be divided into four categories, viz.,

1. Eye hazards such as retinal or corneal burns,

2. Skin hazards such as burns,

3. Electrical hazards from high-voltage equipment and

4. Fire and flood hazards.

Eye hazard is the major hazard from laser radiation which enters the eye since eye is the most sensitive organ to light. The lens in the human eye focuses the laser beam into a tiny spot that can burn the retina. The visible and near-infrared range of the spectrum have the greatest potential for retinal injury, as the cornea and lens are transparent to these wavelengths and the lens can thus focus the laser energy onto the retina. The maximum transmission by the cornea and lens, and the maximum absorption of laser energy in the retina falls in the range of 550 nm to 400 nm. Argon and YAG lasers emit radiation in this range and hence they are the most hazardous lasers. Wavelengths of less than 550 nm can cause a photochemical injury similar to sunburn. Photochemical effects are cumulative and result from exposures over 10 seconds to diffuse or scatter light. When a laser beam enters the human eye retinal burns can occur. Laser beams are almost parallel, thus the lens of the human eye will focus them down to a small spot. A laser beam with low divergence entering the eye, can be focused down to a spot 10 to 20 microns in diameter. The energy density (energy per unit area) of the laser beam increases as the spot size decreases. That is, the energy of a laser beam can be intensified up to 100,000 times by the focusing action of the eye. A one-watt laser beam when focused down to a small spot can produce temperatures higher than the surface temperature of the sun. Thus even a low-power laser in the milliwatt range can cause a burn if focused directly onto the retina.

Skin hazard is the exposure of the skin to high-power laser beams (1 or more watts) which can cause burns. The heat from the laser beam under five watt level will cause a flinch reaction before any serious damage occurs. The sensation is similar to touching any hot object. With higher power lasers, a burn can occur even though the flinch reaction may rapidly pull the affected skin out of the beam. These burns can be quite painful as the affected skin is burnt and forms a hard lesion that takes ages to heal.

Electrical hazards are due to the laser operating voltage. Most medium-and high-power lasers operate on 220 or even higher AC voltages which draw lots of current and frequently use multi-phase electrical connections. The power supply (exciter) for the laser typically doubles or even triples the line voltages before feeding them to the laser head where lethal voltages can be present. An additional electrical hazard exists where water-cooling of the power supply (exciter) is used. Minor leaks in the water-cooling pipes can cause high voltages to short to the water or case of the unit both of which are usually at ground potential.

Fire and flood hazards occur unexpectedly while using lasers. High-power laser beams deflected onto flammable materials can cause ignition and fires. A 10 watt laser will drill a hole in cinder block when focused. Almost any material except metal is a potential fire hazard, especially wood and drapes. Nylon or rayon clothing is especially bad for burns as the plastic fabric melts and clings to skin increasing the burn duration and intensity. Hose connections at the water feed and the hoses themselves can leak. Water cooling system can also leak in unexpected places inside the equipment causing flooding and water damage. A further hazard exists if there is a pool of water or a damp area on the floor as it provides a good ground for an electrical discharge through your body. When working around laser, it is best to wear shoes that have insulated soles.

Safety Precautions

Eye safety—laser safety glasses/goggles with specially coated lenses should be used. The coatings on the lenses are designed to absorb or attenuate certain wavelengths so that if one is accidentally struck in the eye by the beam, damage is minimized. Unfortunately, these glasses often make it difficult if not impossible to see the beam. A pair of welder's goggles will work as they reduce the light to the eyes by a factor of 10 X to 50 X. While welding goggles will not give total protection, they may reduce the beam power down to levels where damage is less likely.

Electrical safety—One should follow the same kinds of safety precautions around lasers as with any other power tool or electrical device.

Sign boards — In laser-operating areas, always sign boards such as "**Caution:** Laser in use" or "danger laser radiation" should always be used. This sign contains an area at the bottom where the details of the laser type (Argon Laser) and output power (100 mW) are inscribed.

LASER HAZARD CLASSIFICATION

The classification of laser based on the level of hazards caused depends upon the intensity of the emitted beam. It describes the ability of the laser to injure personnel. The higher the number, the greater the possible hazard. These are not to be confused with FDA classification, levels, which relate to the type of medical device.

Essentially all of the surgical lasers (those that by definition are used to vaporize or burn tissues) are all classified as class 4 lasers. These lasers present potential burn hazards from even diffuse reflections of the beam, if close enough to the reflecting surface. The lower classes of lasers present potential eye hazards, varying in chance and severity with the class of hazard.

Class 1 lasers   These lasers are exempt from general controls because they present no hazards when used under ordinary circumstances. These include lasers like small semiconductor gallium-arsenide (GaAs) lasers used in low-level light therapy.

Class 2a lasers   These are very-low-power visible lasers which will not present hazards, even if viewed directly, for short periods of time. They are not intended for prolonged viewing—in the range not to exceed 1000 seconds (over 15 minutes of direct viewing). Common experience will reveal that one cannot even stare directly into a 100 watt light bulb for that length of time without any discomfort. This should put laser hazards into some perspective.

Class 2b lasers   These are low-power visible lasers which normally do not present a viewing hazard, but only result in the normal human aversion response, (blinking and/or turning away within 0.25 seconds). They could present a problem if viewed for extended periods of time. It is interesting to note that this level of hazard also applies to many conventional light sources (like endoscopic light sources). They include low-power lasers such as He–Ne laser pointers or the grocery store scanners. The only way to be hurt is to intentionally overcome one's natural aversion and stare directly into the beam (This is about as hard as intentionally staring into the sun).

Class 3a lasers   These lasers are safe if viewed only momentarily with the unaided eye, but the use of collecting optics may create hazard.

Class 3b lasers   These are lasers that can definitely produce a hazard when viewed directly, including the intrabeam viewing of specular reflections (acutely reflected beams such as from a mirror-like surface). Only the higher powered 3b lasers present hazards from diffuse reflections.

Class 4 lasers   These include most of the surgical laser systems, which produce hazards from both specular and diffuse reflections. They may also present fire and skin burn hazards.

SAFETY MEASURES

When laser light falls on the tissue, scattering occurs below the surface of the tissue (forward scatter) or on the tissue surface (backscatter). Each wavelength creates different amounts of scattering, with different consequences.

Carbon dioxide laser has no backscatter because it is absorbed immediately in the surface water, allowing visibility of each plane of tissue as vaporization occurs. This controls depths and prevents deep tissue damage leading to scarring and other complications.

Nd:YAG produces deep forward scattering radiation and a large amount of backscattering. As the portion of the laser beam scattered off the surface of the tissue, the energy efficiency creates an ocular hazard which requires careful monitoring and protective lenses.

Visible laser usually penetrates not more than 3 mm but does produce backscattering. But Nd:YAG laser wavelength react to light coloured tissues due to increased backscattering. Darker tissues with large amounts of pigments or vasculature reduce backscattering due to increasing absorption. This can lead to unwanted tissue damage and scarring. Surface areas adjacent to the operative site must be protected to avoid this complication when using a laser such as argon or KTP laser.

Reflection can occur whenever a laser beam strikes a specular surface. Even though the intensity of the energy may be decreased in the reflected beam, it is still a hazard. Black instruments can still be reflective, if they do not have a dull or roughened surface to diffuse the energy. All instruments to be used in the direct path of the laser beam should be anodized to prevent reflection hazards.

The high energy of the laser and the potential for promoting combustion pose special problems when the surgical field is in close proximity to the airway. An endotracheal tube can be converted into a flaming blowtorch with catastrophic injury to the patient. To minimize the incidence of such complication, anaesthesiologists who are involved in laser airway surgery should be familiar with the elements of laser operation, the type of lasers and special anaesthetic considerations for safe laser surgery.

Laser surgery hazards can be broadly classified as follows.

	Operation theatre	**Human**
a. Fire	a. Fire	a. UV, plasma, free radical generation
b. Electric shock	b.Smoke	b.Shock wave, heat and light
	c.Environmental gas pollution	c.Medical/paramedical personnel
	d.Explosion of anaesthetic agent	

Unless safety measures are followed completely (without compromise) the use of lasers put the safety of both the patient and personnel in danger.

In USA, the American National Standards Institute (ANSI) document z-136.3 is the only nationally accepted, non-regulatory guideline for laser safety. This document is increasingly referenced by regulatory agencies, the military, professional organizations, and institutional accreditation agencies.

The Australian / New Zealand Standard 4173:1994 serves as the national guidelines in those countries as well as for some Pacific Rim countries. This document was published in 1994 and is comprehensive and understandable.

Some issues addressed in most standards include administrative control or laser services (laser committee, policies/procedures), the role and responsibility of the laser safety officer, hazard identification, control measures, selection of eyewear, airborne contaminants, terminology, service and testing and an appendix of recommendations for many surgical specialties.

Before a laser is used clinically, a program should be established according to standards and guided by written policies and procedures, documentation forms and appropriate quality management systems.

Though the revised ANSI standard is no longer mandatory, a laser committee can serve to monitor an institution's safety program. Representation should include hospital administration, laser safety officer, operating room supervisor, biomedical engineer, continuing education managers, physicians from each specialty, anaesthesia, marketing and risk management. Meetings should be scheduled frequently during the first year of a new laser program. A physician is usually appointed to chair the committee, with the laser safety officer appointed as co-chair. Agenda items can include education, technology assessment, new applications, equipment acquisition, documentation and statistics review, marketing, budget, policy updates, and expansion strategies.

The laser safety officer (LSO), laser scientist or laser engineer supervises the clinical, technical and administrative components of the laser programme. The position may be filled by a laser-trained personnel, biomedical engineer or other properly trained person who will be available in the operating theatre whenever lasers are in use. The LSO must have both responsibility and authority to monitor and enforce compliance with standards and policies. In hospitals having minimal laser usage, the LSO can be a laser-trained staff nurse or laser-trained nursing supervisor with other duties. However, in large programmes having multiple laser systems and multiple users, it is necessary for this position to be filled in by a more qualified person.

Some of the LSO's responsibilities include hazard evaluation and control of all laser systems and rooms, implementation of policies and procedures, education and training of staff, documentation review, laser committee functions, audits of safety equipment, evaluation of new instrumentation, revision of policies, patient education, marketing, research and supporting the laser team.

Physician education should be complete for the development of safe practices in the operating room. By providing continuing education for physicians which includes updating specific characteristics and safety of new wavelengths, the laser safety can be greatly improved. Lasers are considered high-risk equipment. Educating all persons involved with laser utilization is of utmost importance to prevent accidental injuries.

Educational programmes for both medical and nursing staffs should be conducted by a credible institution, taught by recognized experts in the field. Attendance at such a course should be required prior to operational or commercial in-service. Validation through written exams, completion of a skills checklist or return demonstrations, should be a component of every certification policy. An annual in-service is usually required in order to keep staff inline with current development.

In hospitals using multiwavelength lasers, there is an increased chance for an error to occur. For example, the different eye wears with different lasers becomes important. Violation can lead to inadequate protection safety. As the number of lasers used increases and lasers of several wavelengths are used, non-compliance commonly creeps in hospitals. Hence, the institution can colour code eyewear, provide a pocket resource for personnel and implement continuous quality improvement activities in order to improve safety practices.

Some laser procedures (patient under general anaesthesia, high-acuity extensive instrumentation, new operators, etc.) require a third person staffed as the designated laser operator. This person can be nurse, technician, biomedical or other properly trained person. Laser operator responsibilities are to set up, test, operate and repair laser equipment, monitor safety, document procedures and to communicate with the LSO.

When a local or regional anaesthetic is used, it may be unnecessary to staff a third person. Patient safety, physician preference and staff skill level, may help the LSO to determine whether or not to assign a dedicated operator.

Baseline eye examination is usually required for all personnel who may have access to a laser treatment room, prior to beginning work with lasers.

Safety is everyone's responsibility. Physicians operating with laser must be familiar with the hospital policies and insist on compliance by all personnel in the room.

Very strict safety is necessary for high-intensity laser and its potential for tissue damage and combustion. The laser should not be aimed at highly polished or mirror-like surfaces. Tracheal laceration leading to late complications, tooth damage, injury to soft tissue and continuous burns to operating room personnel have been reported during laser surgery. The eye can be easily damaged by the laser, and careful protection is mandatory. Unless safety measures are followed completely (without compromise), the use of laser energy is not safe for to both patient and personnel. The carbon dioxide laser is absorbed by ordinary eyeglasses and hence adequate protection should be provided. The use of eyeglasses with side guards is suggested. Special glasses or goggles are required for all other lasers. In surgical theatres, the appropriate laser and an opaque covering of the operating room windows should be used. A warning sign should be placed on the operating room door to alert personnel to the use of the laser. A smoke evacuator should be used to eliminate the products of combustion. The patient should be draped with wet towels that are periodically moistened to keep them wet. Disposable operating room drapes can be flammable and difficult to extinguish since they are water-repellent.

Patient safety depends on knowledgeable personnel and consistent application of known safety practices. Should anyone refuse to comply, an incident report should be written and a report made to the laser committee.

The LSO has the authority to evaluate an incident of non-compliance, and make a decision to either terminate or continue a laser procedure. This decision is usually based on several factors.

Laser hazards can also be divided into two categories, viz., beam hazards and flame hazards.

Beam hazards include flammability, reflection, skin burns, and ocular damage. These hazards are present whenever the laser is activated. For this reason, the laser operator should always be at the control of laser when it is in the operate mode and should always place the laser in the standby mode (disabling the shutter) when the beam is not focused on the target. It is important to keep the entire path of the beam free of obstruction and watch the operative site for interference.

Flammability hazards represent most of the accidents occurring with lasers. Dry disposable materials such as cotton, gauze, tongue blades, drapes, lap sponges and towels can ignite when a laser beam strikes. To prevent fire, place only wet materials in the operative field and remove all excess draping from the impact site. An open basin of water should be kept near the laser operator in case of fire in the surgical field. A fire extinguisher should be in the room or immediately available, in case of equipment fire. If non-woven drapes are used, a fire blanket should be in the room, to smother the material if such a fire occur, since water cannot be used.

Another hazardous material is alcohol. Any compound or solution containing alcohol (including Hibitane, tape removers, skin degreasers and benzoin, etc.,) can ignite if it comes in contact with the heat from the laser beam. Flash fires can also occur if the indoors in pooled or aerosolized betadine are heated by a focused laser beam. Nurses should evaluate each case for sterile, clean status and for potential risk to the patient and prepare the patient accordingly.

Another flammability risk is expulsion of methane gas during lasing of the perianal area. To prevent the possibility of a serious burn to either patient or surgeon, protect the anus by covering the area with a wet towel, or a wet section of the under-buttocks drape.

Whenever external areas of tissue are being vaporized with a carbon dioxide laser, a layer of carbon can build up. If carbon is allowed to remain, the beam will overheat it, causing extensive tissue damage, resulting in carbon sparking. If this occurs at the surface of the skin, it can cause fire, skin burns and injury to the surgeon. When this condition develops, stop lasing, irrigate the operative site and remove the carbon layer from the surface.

If treating a lesion along a hairline, be sure that the hair is completely free of alcohol containing preparations such as commonly used hair sprays, gels and mousses. A thorough cleaning of the area should be required as part of nursing assessment and admission.

Biophysics explains that each wavelength interacts differently with tissue and therefore can produce different types of ocular injuries. Carbon dioxide absorbed in water will cause a corneal or surface burn of the eye, but depending on power density, the burns can go as deeply as 7–9 microns. Nd:YAG, KTP, and dye wavelengths can pass thorough water, clear structures, and be refocused by the human lens to strike the retina, causing damage to central vision.

Ocular damage is entirely preventable by wearing appropriate safety eyewear whenever a laser is in use. All eyewear is labelled with optical density and wavelength of protection afforded and it is essential that each individual read the labels before putting on protective eyewear, assuring that it is the correct pair.

Safety eyewear should be worn by all personnel in the room, when the laser is in the operative mode. Eyewear must be used during endoscopy or video procedures because of the potential for fibre breakage or mechanical accident, releasing uncontrolled and often invisible laser energy into the room. Wavelength-specific safety lenses or filters are available for endoscopes and microscopes, and must be used over the viewing port to protect the surgeon.

Patients should receive the same eye protection as personnel, if they are awake during the procedure. It is ensured that the goggles fit properly and do not slide away when the patient lies down or changes position. For patients under general anaesthesia, a wet cloth towel can be draped over the eyes for protection. Never use oil-based eye lubricant, dry eye pads, or metal or plastic masks to cover patient's eyes. Safety goggles can be placed over the eyes, if they can be held in place easily and safely and do not interface with anaesthesia.

Optical density can be calculated by the LSO, according to published formulae for maximum permissible exposure or can be set at a level not less than 4.5 for most lasers in the clinical setting.

Non-beam hazards include mechanical accident, electrical hazards, failure to maintain controlled access and exposure to laser plume. Crowded operating rooms full of tangled power cords and poorly positional equipment are the leading cause of mechanical "laser" accidents. Equipment should be positioned away from doorways and the number of cords minimized. The footswitch should be given only to the credentialed laser surgeon, separated from all other pedal-operated devices, to avoid mistaken activation of laser.

The laser is a high-voltage electrical device and appropriate electrical safety precautions should always be taken. The laser operator should be sure that inflammable solutions and containers of fluids are not placed near lasers and all cords, footswitches, and circuit breakers should be checked periodically. Only properly trained and approved service technicians should be allowed to work on a laser, to remove the outside covers and to handle the electrical components.

Controlled access is the responsibility of the laser operator. Doors to a laser room should be cooled whenever the laser is in use and posted with the regulation DANGER signs. Safety goggles should be hung on the door sign, for the protection of anyone entering during laser operation. Signs should be removed when the laser is not in use.

Only those who are trained in laser safety should be allowed in the room when the laser is in use. Risk for accident increases when a room is crowded with people who do not understand the potential hazards.

All windows must be covered with shades or other filters, to prevent accidental transmission of a beam through the windows. But the carbon dioxide beam is blocked by glass or plastic windows only and therefore does not require additional window coverings.

The most effective way of limiting access to the laser is to keep the key in a secured place, allowing access only to those who are authorized to operate the equipment.

Laser-generated airborne contaminants are the subject of widespread debate. Research has shown that when human cells are heated to the point of disruption through the application of laser or electro-surgical devices, the cellular content ejected contains harmful particulates, including DNA carbonaceous carcinogens and viral strands.

Gynaecological, neurosurgical and other types of laser surgery not in proximity to the patient's airway, do not require the modification of conventional anaesthetic techniques since the possibility of an airway fire is small. The use of the laser near the airway, however, necessitates that anaesthetic techniques to be modified for patient safety because the laser's high energy density can easily perforate ordinary endotracheal tubes and the anaesthetic gases passing through the endotracheal tube may readily support and enhance its combustion. This may result in a torch fire which is an apt description of the flames streaming from an endotracheal tube after laser ignition. Severe patient injury or even death is possible from these fires.

Airways fires can cause severe burns and make ventilation of the patient impossible. In a survey of the complications of laser carbon dioxide laryngeal surgery, it was found that endotracheal explosions were the most frequent complication.

It is known that the noxious odour and thick smoke can cause airway and eye irritation, as well as bronchial and pulmonary congestion, similar to excessive exposure to cigarette smoke. The plume is potentially hazardous and should be evacuated properly. Studies comparing the combustibility of red rubber and PVC endotracheal tubes have produced conflicting results. The question as to whether a red rubber or PVC endotracheal tube should be used for laser surgery in proximity to the airway can be answered on the basis of the products of combustion. It has been noted that the combustion products of PVC namely hydrochloric acid and other toxic compounds cause severe respiratory symptoms.

The use of metal foil tapes has been advocated to protect combustible endotracheal tubes from laser impact. The tape should be wrapped in an overlapping fashion so that bending of the tube will not expose uncovered areas.

Once the appropriate noncombustible tape is applied to an endotracheal tube, the wrapped portion of the tube is considered to be protected from a direct hit by a carbon dioxide laser. The endotracheal tube is still subject to indirect combustion. This may be caused by a high temperature in proximity to the tube or hot sparks which can cause the combustion of even a foil-wrapped tube.

The wrapping of endotracheal tubes with foil leaves the cuff unprotected. The cuffs on PVC and red rubber endotracheal tubes can be punctured when struck by a carbon dioxide laser with a power of only 10 W in 0.1 s. Normal saline should be used to fill the endotracheal tube cuffs. Using this technique, a carbon dioxide laser impact on the cuff will produce a fine spray that will serve as a "built-in automatic sprinkler system". The saline will serve as a heat sink that will absorb the laser's energy, thus preventing combustion of the cuff. A small quantity of methylene blue or indigo carmine should be added to the saline in the cuff to make perforation more obvious. So far, our discussion of the prevention of laser combustion of endotracheal tubes has centred on decreasing the combustibility of the endotracheal tubes by modifying them. The gases flowing within the endotracheal tube, however, can increase the intensity of tube combustion. Nitrous oxide, although often considered inert, supports combustion by its decomposition into oxygen and energy.

$$2NO \rightarrow 2N + O_2 + energy$$

A glowing splinter introduced thrust into a container containing nitrous oxide will burn vigorously with oxygen. It should be avoided during laser endoscopic surgery. In its place, a mixture of oxygen and air, oxygen and nitrogen or oxygen and helium should be used. Helium has a higher thermal conductivity than nitrogen and may decrease combustion to a greater extent. An anaesthesia machine equipped to provide these gas mixtures and incorporating an oxygen analyser should be available in operating rooms where laser surgery is performed. Pulse oximetry should be used so that the lowest inspired concentration of oxygen to achieve satisfactory oxygen saturation can be used.

Should potent inhalation agents be used for laser surgery? It has been determined that the minimum flammable concentrations of halothane, enflurane and isoflurane are 4.75%, 5.75% and 7.0% respectively. Thus, in the concentrations clinically used, halothane, enflurane, and isoflurane can be used without problems of combustion.

Management of an Airway Fire

The possibility of a fire in the airway during laser surgery makes it necessary that a plan of action be developed before this catastrophe occurs (Table 5.1). The endotracheal tube used should be secured with a minimal amount of tape so that easy extubation can be readily accomplished. Saline should be available to douse any flames. At the first sign of an airway fire, the anaesthesiologist should stop all ventilation and terminate the flow of all anaesthetic gases, including oxygen, since they promote combustion. After extinguishing any flames, the endotracheal tube should be quickly removed, since even brief combustion will damage the tube, making it unsuitable as an airway. The patient should be ventilated with a mask and the airway should be thoroughly examined. If the fire is quickly extinguished, little or no damage may occur. In such a case, the decision can be made to proceed with surgery. Extensive airway burns may necessitate mechanical ventilation, positive and expiratory pressure, antibiotics and steroids.

The Venturi Jet ventilation technique was devised by Sanders as a means of artificial ventilation without the presence of an endotracheal tube. A catheter was clamped inside an operating bronchoscope or laryngoscope and was connected to a source of oxygen at 50 1b-per-square-inch pressure. With the use of a toggle switch, a jet of oxygen was directed down the bronchoscope. The result was adequate ventilation of an anaesthetized patient. Using this technique, room air is entrained with the oxygen jet. When used with an operating laryngoscope, laser surgery of the vocal cords can be accomplished even in the posterior or interarytenoid areas normally obscured by the endotracheal tube. The absence of an endotracheal tube makes laser surgery easy and this technique produces no fire in the airway. The adequacy of ventilation and oxygen delivery by this technique has been demonstrated by measurement of arterial blood gas tensions. These steps should be taken simultaneously by the anaesthesiologist and surgeon.

Table 5.1 Airway fire protocol

---

1. Cease ventilation and turn off all anaesthetic gases including oxygen.
2. Extinguish flames with saline.
3. Remove endotracheal tube.
4. Ventilate by mask.
5. Evaluate airway for burns.

Pure oxygen is generally administered during jet ventilation because the entertainment of air will reduce the faction of oxygen that the patient receives. Inhalation anaesthetics should be avoided, since they pollute the operating room. A totally intravenous anaesthetic technique should be used.

Venturi jet ventilation uses a very high-pressure source in the airway. The 50–1b–square-inch pressure commonly used is equivalent to 3,500 cm water pressure. This is greatly in excess of normal airway pressures. These pressures may cause barotraumas such as pneumothorax or pneumomediastinum. No battier to the passage of vomitus, blood, or debris into the trachea exists with this technique, since no cuffed endotracheal tube is used. The venturi jet must be kept in perfect alignment with the trachea, or gastric dilatation with possible regurgitation may occur. An immobile field may be difficult to maintain because of the movement of the vocal cords by the jet.

The anaesthesiologist should watch vigilantly for bilateral chest excursions to ensure adequate ventilation during jet ventilation. A precordial stethoscope should be used as well as the usual anaesthetic monitoring devices described previously. The special endotracheal tubes such as Bivona "fome-cuff" nalli-nick-rodt. Xomed and Norton laser endotracheal tubes are available at present.

Smoke evacuation systems are recommended for all plume-producing procedures. Tubing should be held no more than 2 cm from the impact site and instruments with collection ports may be necessary.

Wall suction can become clogged and lose its efficiency, if used without in-line filters placed between the wall and the suction canister. All filtration materials should be rated at levels of 0.1 micron or below, in order to remove known plume particulates.

Laser masks can provide added protection if worn properly. Plume cannot be filtered if it is drawn into gaps along the sides or under the nosepieces of tie-on masks. Laser masks should be worn during all plume-producing procedures. It is important to remember to change laser masks after each case and discard them properly.

All plumes filtering equipment should be handled according to infection control procedures in the operating room. Used suction equipment is contaminated and universal precautions should be worn during handling and changing of tubing and filter canisters.

Safety education for patients helps to reduce their anxiety levels. Protective eyewear limits eye contact and can interfere with patient–nurse communication and so patients should prepare ahead of time, by showing them photographs, perhaps bound in a brief booklet, demonstrating patients and staff wearing goggles, the equipment to be used and what a laser looks like as it strikes tissue.

Don't forget to show them a photo of the DANGER signs on the door and explain the reason for the warning. Seeing that sign on the way into the treatment room, can scare the patient if they are not explained earlier.

Patients should be instructed to tell the nurse or doctor when they experience discomfort, so that the procedure can be managed without danger which may cause accidental burns. For laser safety, precaution team work and good communication are the most important.

Although we currently have lasers for use in virtually all surgical specialties, the future promises many exciting changes in the technology, as we move into the next century. Holographic imaging, virtual reality, minimally invasive instrumentation, tissue welding, biostimulation, multiwavelength systems, new wavelengths, diodes, and the dynamics of photobiology will change medicine and surgery in the near future.

Lasers and the professional members of clinical laser teams, partnered with industry, research centres, the government, and the international community, will make it all possible. Pre-operative nurses are vital members of these teams, with unlimited opportunities for new careers, professional growth and exciting challenges, as future technology becomes today's reality.

Nearly every laser currently used in medical applications is a class IV system and by definition they have potential for eye injury or fire hazard either by their direct or reflected beam. It is therefore necessary to identify these potential hazards and the various conditions that tend to influence these hazards in the normal use of laser energy. The regulations, hazards evaluation and analysis are an important part of laser curriculum. Thus, safety measures are atmost important in laser surgery and hence our nation needs more laser personal, laser scientists and laser engineers.

In summary, the following points.

1. As CO_2 ($\lambda = 10.6\mu m$) lasers are frequently used in laser surgery, CO_2 laser goggles of 2 mm thick, optical density (O.D)—0.35 can protect the eye.

2. Various types of burns develop according to direct or indirect (reflected) laser beam. Hence exposures to lasers should be avoided.

3. Non-inflammable and non-explosive anaesthetic agents should be used.

4. For patients, non-flammable drape should be used. Non-operative field should be covered with normal saline-soaked gauze. With intra-oral lesions, appropriate care should be taken with orthodontic appliances and gold dentures, etc.

5. All the shining operative instruments should be coated with black or chrome electrical coating.

6. Suction tip should be covered with rubber tube.

7. The operation table and other instruments in light should be non-reflecting, non-shining and heat-tolerant.

8. Control of power is checked at the focusing head by calorimeter.

9. He–Ne (3 mW) should be used as light guide.

10. Lighting in the operation theatre should be proper.

11. The power of the laser for the operation of various organs depends on the size and the age of the person. The approximate power chart is as follows. The chart just gives an idea and the doctors are advised to start with low power from that mentioned in the chart.

Tissue	Power	Tissue	Power
Skin	5–15 W	Cartilage	15–20 W
Subcutaneous tissue	10–15 W	Bone	20–35 W
Fat	10–20 W	Kidney	25–35 W
Fascia	5–10 W	Liver	35–40 W
Muscle	10–20 W	Lung	25–35 W
Mucosa	5–10 W	Brain	20–35 W
		Peritoneum	5–10 W

Apart from power chart the other factors to keep in mind in performing laser surgery are:

1. At high power, tissue is cut more deeply.

2. With slow speed, the tissue is cut more deeply.

3. With low water content in the tissue, the cut is very deep.

4. With pressure, the cutting surface will separate more easily.

By keeping these points in mind, one can easily control the depth of cutting and can perform laser surgery safely.

Review Questions

1. List the methods by which CO_2 radiation can be delivered safely.

2. What is the importance of focusing system in laser delivery?

3. How are the time exposure and total dosimetry expressed?

4. Discuss the four categories of laser hazards.

5. Explain the safety precautions to be adopted while using lasers for biological applications.

6. Classify laser hazards for various types of lasers.

7. Discuss on the safety measures to be adopted while using lasers in biological applications.

8. What is the role of Laser Safety Officer in laser programs?

9. What are flammability hazards?

10. What is the importance of safety eye-water?

11. What are non-beam hazards? Explain.

12. List the airway fire protocol.

Ablation Removal of tissue using a laser. The corneal tissue is evaporated by the energy of the laser. An average of 0.25 microns of corneal tissue can be ablated per laser pulse.

Absorption (electromagnetic radiation) Transformation of radiant energy to a different form of energy by the interaction of matter, depending on temperature and wavelength.

Accessible emission limit (AEL) Maximum accessible emission level which is permissible in the appropriate class of laser.

Accessible radiation Laser radiation that can expose human eye or skin in normal usage.

Acne Localized skin inflammation as a result of overactivity of the oil glands at the base of hair follicles.

Acoustic effect Laser beams are capable of causing a localized vaporization of tissue which in turn can create a mechanical shock wave to be propagated through the tissue.

Active medium Collection of atoms or molecules capable of undergoing stimulated emission at a given wavelength.

Administrative controls Administrative controls consist of procedures and information provided to personnel for the purpose of reducing laser hazards. Examples of administrative controls include warning signs and labels, standard operating procedures, and safety training.

Alexandrite A rare oxide mineral and is a colour changing variety of the mineral chrysoberyl, $BeAl2O4$.

Amplification The growth of the radiation field in the laser resonator cavity. As the light wave bounces back and forth between the cavity mirrors, it is amplified by stimulated emission on each pass through the active medium.

Anaesthesia Loss of feeling or awareness. A general anaesthetic puts the person to sleep. A local anaesthetic causes loss of feeling in a part of the body such as a tooth or an area of skin without affecting consciousness. Regional anaesthesia numbs a larger part of the body such as a leg or arm, also without affecting consciousness.

Anaesthetic A substance that causes lack of feeling or awareness. A local anaesthetic causes loss of feeling in a part of the body. A general anesthetic puts the person to sleep.

Argon (Ar) A gas used as a laser medium. It emits blue/green light primarily at 448 and 515 nm.

Articulated arm CO_2 laser beam delivery device consisting of a series of hollow tubes and mirrors interconnected in such a manner as to maintain alignment of the laser beam along the path of the arm.

Attenuation The decrease in energy (or power) as a beam passes through an absorbing or scattering medium.

Average power Total energy of an exposure divided by the duration of the exposure.

Beam A collection of rays that may be parallel, convergent, or divergent.

Biostimulation treatments It uses a laser to deliver healing heat to the patient's skin. Biostimulation treatments can be used to treat scars, inflammatory processes of the skin or to regenerate and oxidize the skin. The procedure is non-invasive and painless.

Cancer An abnormal growth of cells which tend to proliferate in an uncontrolled way and, in some cases, to metastasize (spread).

Carbon dioxide Molecule used as a laser medium. Emits far infrared energy at 10,600 nm (10.6 micrometers).

Cardiology A medical specialty dealing with disorders of the heart (specifically the human heart).

Cavity The laser resonator, or tube, in which the lasing process occurs.

Chromium-doped gain media Laser gain media doped with chromium ions.

CO_2 laser A widely used laser in which the primary lasing medium is carbon dioxide gas. The output wavelength is 10.6 micrometers in the far infrared spectrum. It can be operated in either CW or pulsed.

Coherent light light waves that are "in phase" with one another. Monochromaticity and low divergence are two properties of coherent light.

Collagen Protein within the skin that adds youthful volume and elasticity. As the aging process progresses, the amount of collagen produced and maintained by the body decreases and results in the appearance of wrinkles. Collagen production can be increased through laser skin resurfacing, chemical peels, and microderm abrasion.

Continuous wave (CW) Constant, steady-state delivery of laser power.

Copper vapour laser (CVL) Uses vapours of copper as the lasing medium in a 3-level laser. It produces green laser light at 510.6 nm and yellow laser light at 578.2 nm.

Cornea The cornea is the transparent layer of tissue covering the surface of the eye.

Cryogenic lasers Lasers where the gain medium is operated at cryogenic temperatures.

Crystal A solid with a regular array of atoms. Sapphire (Ruby Laser) and YAG (Nd:YAG laser) are two crystalline materials used as laser sources.

CW Abbreviation for continuous wave; the continuous-emission mode of a laser as opposed to pulsed operation.

Dentistry The branch of medicine that is involved in the study, diagnosis, prevention, and treatment of diseases, disorders and conditions of the oral cavity.

Dermatology The branch of medicine concerned with the diagnosis, treatment, and prevention of diseases of the skin, hair, nails, oral cavity and genitals.

Dermis The layers of the skin between the epidermis and the deeper layers of tissue.

Diffraction Deviation of part of a beam, determined by the wave nature of radiation and occurring when the radiation passes the edge of an opaque obstacle.

Diode An electronic device that conducts a current in only one direction.

Diode laser A laser that emits coherent light through the injection of electric current into a semiconductor diode.

Directional Lasers emit light that is highly directional, that is, laser light is emitted as a relatively narrow beam in a specific direction.

Divergence The increase in the diameter of the laser beam with distance from the exit aperture. The value gives the full angle at the point where the laser radiant exposure or irradiance is 1/e or 1/e2 of the maximum value, depending upon which criteria are used.

Dosimetry Measurement of the power, energy, irradiance, or radiant exposure of light delivered to tissue.

DPSSL Diode pumped solid-state lasers.

Dye lasers Lasers based on liquid or solid dyes as gain media.

Electromagnetic spectrum The range of all possible frequencies of electromagnetic radiation.

Electrical pumping Can be achieved by keeping the laser medium in the electron beam so that the electrons create a population inversion by transferring the energy to the atoms or molecules under collision.

Emission Act of giving off radiant energy by an atom or molecule.

Emissivity The ratio of the radiant energy emitted by any source to that emitted by a blackbody at the same temperature.

Energy The capacity for doing work. Energy is commonly used to express the output from pulsed lasers and it is generally measured in Joules (J). Energy is the product of power (Watts) and duration (seconds). One Watt second = one Joule.

Engineering controls Engineering controls are design features or devices that are applied to a laser or its environment for the purpose of reducing laser hazards. Engineering controls are considered to be the most effective types of control.

Epidermis The outermost layer of the skin, the epidermis acts as a barrier between the body's important structures and the outside environment.

Erbium (Er) The fluorescence properties of erbium in various host materials and the stimulated emission around 1.6 μm is of interest to ophthalmologists because the eye is subjected to less retinal damage by laser radiation.

Erbium Laser Cosmetic laser treatment used to reduce the appearance of bags and dark circles under the eyes. Unlike the stronger Fraxel laser, the Erbium laser only penetrates the first few layers of delicate skin to increase collagen production and reduce the dark circles.

Erbium-doped gain media Laser gain media doped with erbium ions.

Excimer "Excited Dimer"—A gas mixture used as the active medium in a family of lasers emitting ultraviolet light.

Excitation mechanism The excitation mechanism of a laser is the source of energy used to excite the lasing medium. Excitation mechanisms typically used are electricity from a power supply, a flashtube, lamp, or the energy from another laser.

Excitation Energizing a material into a state of population inversion.

Excited State Atom with an electron in a higher energy level than it normally occupies.

Facelift A surgical procedure designed to make the face appear younger by pulling loose facial skin taut.

Facial enhancements Any cosmetic facial rejuvenation procedure which addresses a cosmetic issue. Common facial enhancements include facial cosmetic surgery, peels and facials, and dermal injections.

Facial hair removal Cosmetic process which removes unwanted hair on the beard, neck, sideburns, or upper lip of men and women. Common facial hair removal procedures include laser hair removal, electrology and waxing.

Facial resurfacing Cosmetic skin procedure which utilizes lasers, chemicals, or manual instruments to strip the dead layers of skin from the face and reveal rejuvenated layers beneath. Resurfacing is often performed to combat the appearance of wrinkles, dull skin, hyperpigmentation, and acne.

Feedback mechanism A laser's feedback mechanism is used to reflect light from the lasing medium back into itself and typically consists of two mirrors at each end of the lasing medium.

Femtoseconds 10^{-15} seconds.

Fibre optic cable Flexible glass or plastic strands made into a cable, used to carry light from one place to another.

Flashlamp A tube typically filled with krypton or xenon. Produces a high intensity white light in short duration pulses.

Fluence The effects of laser radiation on biological tissue. Fluence = (Watt × time)/Spot size.

Fluorescence The emission of light of a particular wavelength resulting from absorption of energy typically from light of shorter wavelengths.

Folded resonator Construction in which the interior optical path is bent by mirrors; permit compact packaging of a long laser cavity.

Frequency doubling The phenomenon that an input wave in a non-linear material can generate a wave with twice the optical frequency.

Frequency The number of light waves passing a fixed point in a given unit of time, or the number of complete vibrations in that period of time.

Full width half maximum (FWHM) A pulse duration is usually defined at full width half maximum (FWHM).

GaAlAs laser The most common DPSS laser in use is the 532 nm wavelength green laser pointer. A powerful (>200 mW) 808 nm wavelength infrared GaAlAs laser diode pumps a neodymium-doped yttrium aluminium garnet (Nd:YAG).

Gain A measure of the strength of optical amplification.

Gain Another term for amplification.

Gas laser A type of laser in which the laser action takes place in a gas medium.

Gastroenterology Covers the diseases concerning ulcers and tumours of the oesophagus, stomach, liver, gall blader, ileum, colon and rectum.

Gold vapour laser (GVL) Uses vapours of gold as the lasing medium in a 3-level laser. It produces laser light at 627.8 nm. The main applications of gold vapour laser are in the experimental cancer treatment of photo-dynamic therapy (PDT).

Ground state Lowest energy level of an atom.

Gynaecology The medical practice dealing with the health of the female reproductive system (uterus, vagina, and ovaries).

Haze Also referred to as healing tissue or scar tissue. This can affect LASEK patients to varying degrees but it is usually mild and clears up within a few months. Patients sometimes complain of glare at night and vision that is similar to that when looking through frosted glass or dirty glasses.

HeCd Lasers Metal vapour lasers using helium in conjunction with cadmium metal which vaporizes at a relatively low temperature. It produces continuous-wave sources for violet (442 nm) and ultraviolet (325 nm) output.

Helium-Neon Laser (HeNe) A laser in which the active medium is a mixture of helium and neon. Its wavelength is usually in the visible range.

Holmium YAG (Ho:YAG) laser A solid-state diode pumped laser with 2.1 μm wavelength useful for tissue ablation, kidney stone removal and dentistry.

Hyperpigmentation Areas of skin that are darker in colour than surrounding tissue caused by sun exposure, genetics, medications, and some scarring.

Hypopigmentation Areas of skin void of any pigment. Often develops in response to trauma (i.e., skin cancer surgery, burn, or chemical peel).

Infrared radiation Electromagnetic radiation of wavelength from 700 nm to 1 mm.

Integrated radiance Product of the exposure duration and the radiance. Also known as pulsed radiance.

Intensity The magnitude of radiant energy.

Ion laser A type of laser employing a very high discharge current, passing down a small bore to ionize a noble gas such as argon or krypton.

Irradiance Power per unit area, expressed in watts per square centimeter.

Keratectomy Surgical excision of part of the cornea with a diamond knife. "Kera" means cornea and "tectomy" means cutting.

KTP (Potassium Titanyl Phosphate) A crystal used to change the wavelength of an Nd:YAG laser from 1060 nm (infrared) to 532 nm (green).

LASER An acronym for light amplification by stimulated emission of radiation. A laser is a cavity, with mirrors at the ends, filled with material such as crystal, glass, liquid, gas or dye. It is a device which produces an intense beam of light with the unique properties of coherence, collimation and monochromaticity.

Laser crystals Crystals used as solid-state lasers active media.

Laser device Either a laser or a laser system.

Laser hair removal Cosmetic laser treatment used to remove unwanted face and body hair. Laser light is attracted to the pigment within the follicles of unwanted hair, permanently impairing future hair growth with several regular applications to the desired area(s).

Laser medium (Active Medium) Material used to emit the laser light and for which the laser is named.

Laser pumping The act of energy transfer from an external source into the gain medium of a laser. The energy is absorbed in the medium, producing excited states in its atoms. When the number of particles in one excited state exceeds the number of particles in the ground state or a less-excited state, population inversion is achieved.

Laser resonators Optical resonators serving as basic building blocks of lasers.

Laser resurfacing It is a technique in which molecular bonds of a material are dissolved by a laser.

Laser rod A solid-state, rod-shaped lasing medium in which ion excitation is caused by a source of intense light, such as a flash lamp. Various materials are used for the rod, the earliest of which was synthetic ruby crystal.

Laser Safety Officer (LSO) One who has authority to monitor and enforce measures to the control of laser hazards and effect the knowledgeable evaluation and control of laser hazards.

Laser System An assembly of electrical, mechanical, and optical components which includes a laser.

LASIK or LASIK Eye Surgery A type of Laser Eye Surgery where a flap is created first, and a laser treatment is applied under the flap. The flap is then returned into its original position and allowed to seal. LASIK has a fairly quick recovery time, because all the surface cells are saved.

Lens The lens of the eye focuses light to form images in the eye.

MASER Microwave Amplification by Stimulated Emission of Radiation.

Melanin The biological pigment of skin. It is also found in hair, the pigmented tissue underlying the iris of the eye, and the stria vascularis of the inner ear.

Micrometer A unit of length in the International System of Units (SI) equal to one millionth of a meter. Often referred to as a 'micron'.

Microprocessor A digital chip (computer) that operates, controls, and monitors some lasers.

Milliamperes (mA) A unit of electrical current equal to one-thousandth of an ampere.

Milliwatt (mW) A unit of power equal to one-thousandth of a watt.

Mode locked A method of producing laser pulses in which short pulses (approximately 10–12 second) are produced and emitted in bursts or a continuous train.

Mode locking A group of techniques for generating ultrashort pulses in lasers.

Mode A term used to describe how the power of a laser beam is geometrically distributed across the cross section of the beam. Also used to describe the operating mode of a laser such as continuous or pulsed.

Mode-locked lasers Lasers which emit ultrashort pulses on the basis of the technique of mode locking.

Modulation The ability to superimpose an external signal on the output beam of the laser as a control.

Monochromatic The light emitted from a laser is monochromatic, that is, it is of one colour/wavelength.

MPE (Maximum Permissible Exposure) The maximum level of laser radiation to which a human can be exposed without adverse biological effects to the eye or skin.

Nanometer (nm) A unit of length in the International System of Units (SI) equal to one-billionth of a meter. It is abbreviated as nm, a measure of length. One nm equals 10^{-9} meter, and is the usual measure of light wavelengths.

Visible light ranges from about 400 nm in the purple to about 760 nm in the deep red.

Nanosecond One-billionth (10^{-9}) of a second. Longer than a picosecond or femtosecond, but shorter than a microsecond. Associated with Q-switched lasers.

Nd,Cr:GSGG Laser rods made of gadolinium scandium gallium garnet (GSGG) doped with neodymium and chromium, which is important for laser applications in high radiation environments.

Nd:Glass laser A solid-state laser of neodymium: glass offering high power in short pulses. A Nd-doped glass rod is used as a laser medium to produce 1064 nm light.

Nd:YAG Laser Neodymium:Yttrium Aluminium Garnet A synthetic crystal used as a laser medium to produce 1064 nm light.

Neodymium (Nd) Nd^{3+} was the first trivalent rare earth ions to be used in a laser. It is the active element in Nd:YAG lasers and Nd:Glass lasers.

Neodymium-doped yttrium orthovanadate ($Nd:YVO_4$) Crystal which produces 1064 nm wavelength light from the main spectral transition of neodymium ion.

Neurosurgery (or neurological surgery) The medical specialty concerned with the prevention, diagnosis, treatment, and rehabilitation of disorders which affect any portion of the nervous system including the brain, spinal cord, peripheral nerves, and extra-cranial cerebrovascular system.

Nominal Hazard Zone (NHZ) The zone inside which laser radiation that is direct, reflected, or scattered exceeds the MPE for the laser. Control measures are not needed outside the NHZ.

Ocular Relating to the eye. "Oculus" is Latin for eye.

Opacity The condition of being non-transparent.

Operation The performance of the laser or laser system over the full range of its intended functions (normal operation). It does not include maintenance or services as defined in this glossary.

Ophthalmology The branch of medicine that deals with the anatomy, physiology and diseases of the eye.

Optical cavity (Resonator) Space between the laser mirrors where lasing action occurs.

Optical density A logarithmic expression for the attenuation produced by an attenuating medium, such as an eye protection filter.

Optical pumping The excitation of the lasing medium [to raise (or 'pump') electrons from a lower energy level in an atom or molecule to a higher one] by the application of light rather than electrical discharge.

Optically pumped lasers A type of laser that derives energy from another light source such as a xenon or krypton flashlamp or other laser source.

Orthopaedics The study of the human musculoskeletal system.

Otorhinolaryngology The branch of medicine and surgery that specializes in the diagnosis and treatment of disorders of the head and neck.

Output coupler The output coupler of a laser is usually a partially transparent mirror on one end of the lasing medium that allows some of the light to leave the lasing medium in order that the light is used for the production of the laser beam. The output coupler is usually part of the feedback mechanism.

Output power The energy per second emitted from the laser in the form of coherent light. Laser output power is measured in watts (W) or milliwatts (mW) for continuous wave laser operation.

Phase Waves are in phase with each other when all the troughs and peaks coincide and are 'locked' together. The result is a reinforced wave in increased amplitude (brightness).

Photoablation The cold process of tissue removal using laser radiation with incredibly precise cuts with no evidence of tissue burning in adjacent cells. Ultraviolet light is so powerful that the molecular bonds of the target tissue are broken apart causing ablation.

Photoablative effect A pure ablation of materials without thermal lesions. The molecular bonds are broken and the tissue components are vapourized without generation of any heat at the edges. Used in eye surgeries like band keratoplast, and endarterectomy of peripheral blood vessels.

Photochemical effect Laser radiations (low intensity) are used for photo excitation and hence the chemical energy breaks the chemical bonds or excite the molecules to reactive state, which can result in changes to tissue.

Photocoagulation Use of the laser beam to heat tissue below vaporization temperatures with the principal objective being to stop bleeding and coagulate tissue.

Photodissruptive The pulsed laser energy associated with acoustic energy (Photoacoustic high pressure acoustic wave) cause mechanical interaction with the tissue.

Photodynamic therapy (PDT) A treatment that utilizes a specific wavelength of light and a photosensitizing agent that reacts to that light by generating a form of oxygen to kill specific cells. It can be used to treat acne, pre-cancerous cells, cancer, and other skin conditions.

Photon In quantum theory, the elemental unit of light, having both wave and particle behavior. It has motion, but no mass or charge. The photon energy (E) is proportional to the EM wave frequency (v) by the relationship $E = hv$; where h is Planck's constant (6.63×10^{-34} Joule sec).

Photonics The science and technology of light. It is nothing but the generation and harnessing laser radiations.

Photosensitizers Chemical substances or medications which increase the sensitivity of the skin or eye to irradiation by optical radiation, usually to UV.

Phototherapy Any skin treatment which uses the power of light to treat skin conditions and cosmetic skin issues of the face and body.

Photothermal effect Laser light above threshold intensity falling on tissue produces heat and hence there is a rise in temperature. This property is used for endoscopic control of bleeding, e.g., bleeding peptic ulcers, oesophageal varices.

Picosecond A period of time equal to 10^{-12} seconds.

Pigment A substance that gives colour to tissue. Pigments are responsible for the colour of skin, eyes, and hair.

Pigment epithelium A layer of cells at the back of the retina containing pigment granules, i.e., a cloud of charged particles surrounding a laser impact.

Pigmentation The coloring of the skin, hair, mucous membranes, and retina of the eye.

Plastic surgery A medical specialty concerned with the correction or restoration of form and function. The cosmetic or aesthetic surgery is the best-known kind of plastic surgery.

Pockel's Cell An electro-optical crystal used as a Q-switch for building modulators.

Population inversion A state in which a substance has been energized, or excited, so that more atoms or molecules are in a higher excited state than in a lower resting state. This is a necessary prerequisite for laser action.

Power density Laser output per unit area, such as watts per square centimetre (W/cm2).

Power meter An accessory used to measure laser beam power.

Power The rate of energy delivery expressed in watts (joules per second). Thus 1 Watt = 1 Joule/1 sec.

Personal protective equipment (PPE) The instruments used to reduce laser hazards are eyewear, gloves and special clothing.

PRK or Photorefractive keratectomy A type of laser eye surgery where the surface cells are first removed and the laser treatment is applied to the surface of the eye.

Pulmonology The medical specialty dealing with disease involving the respiratory tract.

Pulse Duration The 'on' time of a pulsed laser. It may be measured in terms of millisecond, microsecond, or nanosecond as defined by half-peak-power points on the leading and trailing edges of the pulse.

Pulse pickers Electrically controlled optical switches used for extracting single pulses from a pulse train.

Pulse repetition frequency (PRF) The number of pulses produced per second by a laser.

Pulse repetition rate The number of pulses emitted per second, e.g., by a mode-locked or Q-switched laser.

Pulse A discontinuous burst of laser, light or energy, as opposed to a continuous beam. A true pulse achieves higher peak powers than that attainable in a CW output.

Pulsed laser Laser which delivers energy in the form of a single or train of pulses rather than continuously.

Pump To excite the lasing medium. (**See** Optical pumping or pumping.)

Pumping Addition of energy (thermal, electrical, or optical) into the atomic population of the laser medium, necessary to produce a state of population inversion.

Pupil/iris The pupil of the eye is the aperture through which light is directed into the eye. The iris is a layer of muscle tissue which can contract and expand around the circumference of the pupil in order to determine pupil size.

Q-switch Optical switches that has the effect of a shutter to control the laser resonator's ability to oscillate. These are typically used for generating nanosecond pulses in lasers.

Q-switching A method for obtaining energetic pulses from lasers by modulating the intracavity losses.

Q-factor A measure of the damping of resonator modes.

Q-switched laser A laser which stores energy in the laser media to produce extremely short, extremely high intensity bursts of energy.

Radial keratotomy (RK) A surgical treatment for myopia. A myopic eye has a cornea which is too steep, refracting light rays too much, so they land in front of the retina, instead of on it, for clear vision. To make the cornea slightly flatter, tiny incisions are placed around the pupil, angled from the pupil out to the edge of the cornea. The number of incisions and their exact location depends on the degree of myopia.

Radiant energy Laser energy emitted, expressed in joules (J).

Radiant exposure Radiant energy per unit area, expressed in joules per square centimeter.

Radiant power Laser power emitted, expressed in watts (W).

Refractive surgery Any surgical procedure that attempts to decrease or remove the patient's need for glasses. Usually the surgeon alters the shape of the cornea in order to change the focussing power of the eye.

Repetition rate Number of pulses per second produced by a pulsed laser.

Resonator The mirrors (or reflectors) making up the laser cavity including the laser rod or tube. The mirrors reflect light back and forth to build up amplification.

Retina The retina is made up of layers of nerve cells and is used for reception of the light in the eye. Damage to cells in the retina can result in loss of vision.

Ruby The first laser type; a crystal of sapphire (aluminum oxide) containing trace amounts of chromium oxide.

Sclera The firm white fibrous membrane that forms the white part of the eye.

Sclerotherapy Vein reduction/elimination technique in which sclerosing agents are injected into unsightly, unwanted vessels of the face and legs to minimize their appearance.

Semiconductor laser Lasers based on semiconductor gain media which produces its output from semiconductor materials such as GaAs.

Solid-state laser A laser where the lasing medium is a solid material such as a ruby rod. These can be optically pumped by a flash lamp or diodes. Solid-state lasers also include diode lasers as they use electrically pumped solids to produce light.

Spot size The mathematical measurement of the radius of the laser beam.

Stimulated emission Emission of multiphoton of precisely the same wavelength whose wave patterns are perfectly in phase.

Stratum corneum The stratum corneum is the outermost layer and consists of dead epithelial cells. The stratum corneum is capable of filtering some ultraviolet and far-IR wavelengths of light and prevents the light from penetrating to the deeper layers of the skin.

Superficial In anatomy, "superficial" means on the surface or shallow, as opposed to deep. The skin is super-ficial to the muscles. The cornea is on the superficial surface of the eye.

Tattoo removal Cosmetic laser procedure in which laser light is used to target and eliminate all colours of tattoo ink from within the skin.

Thermal effects Thermal effects are the major cause of tissue dam-age by lasers. Energy from the laser is absorbed by the tissue in the form of heat, which can cause localized, in-tense heating of sensitive tissues.

Threshold The input level at which lasing begins during excitation of the laser medium.

Transmission Passage of electro-magnetic radiation through a medium.

Transmittance The ratio of trans-mitted radiant energy to incident ra-diant energy, or the fraction of light that passes through a medium.

Tunable dye laser A laser whose active medium is a liquid dye, pumped by another laser or flashlamps, to produce various colours of light. The colour of light may be tuned by ad-justing optical tuning elements and/ or changing the dye used.

Tunable laser A laser system that can be 'tuned' to emit laser light over a continuous range of wavelengths or frequencies.

Ultraviolet radiation (UV) Electromagnetic radiation with wave-lengths between soft X-rays and visi-ble violet light.

Urology The medical and surgical specialty that focuses on the urinary tracts of males and females, and on the reproductive system of males.

Vanadate lasers Lasers based on rare-earth-doped yttrium, gadolinium or lutetium vanadate crystals, usually Nd:YVO4.

Vertical-cavity surface-emitting laser (VCSELs) A type of semi-conductor laser diode with the optical cavity axis along the direction of cur-rent flow rather than perpendicular to the current flow as in conventional laser diodes.

Vibronic lasers Lasers based on gain media with a large gain band-width, caused by a strong interaction of electronic transitions with phonons.

W/cm² – A unit of power density (ra-diant exposure) used in measuring the amount of energy incident upon a unit area.

Watt A unit of power (equivalent to one Joule per second) used to express laser power.

Watt/cm² A unit of irradiance used in measuring the amount of power per area of absorbing surface, or per area of CW laser beam.

Waveguide lasers Lasers with a waveguide structure in the gain medium.

Waveguides Spatially inhomogeneous transparent structures for guiding light.

Wavelength The length of the light wave, usually measured from crest to crest, which determines its colour. Common units of measurement are the micrometer (micron), the nanometer, and (earlier) the Angstrom unit.

Wrinkle treatments Range of cosmetic skin treatments used to diminish the appearance of facial wrinkles. Common wrinkle treatments include chemical peels, laser skin resurfacing, and facial filler injections.

Wrinkles Depressions or folds of the skin that develop in response to decreased collagen and skin elasticity.

YAG (Yttrium Aluminum Garnet) A widely used solid-state crystal which is composed of yttrium and aluminum oxides which is doped with a small amount of the rare-earth neodymium.

YAG lasers Lasers based on YAG (yttrium aluminum garnet) crystals, usually Nd:YAG.

YLF lasers Lasers based on YLF (yttrium lithium fluoride) crystals, usually Nd:YLF.

Ytterbium YAG (Yb:YAG) laser A solid-state diode/flash lamp pumped laser with 1.03 μm wavelength mainly used for optical refrigeration and materials processing.

Ytterbium-doped gain media Laser gain media containing laser-active ytterbium ions.

YVO$_4$ laser A laser created by exciting a YVO$_4$ crystal doped with an Nd ion using an LD or lamp. Produces a laser beam that has the same wavelength as YAG.

Z-cavity A term referring to the shape of the optical layout of the tubes and resonator inside a laser.

References

- Alexander A. Kaminskii. (1996). *Crystalline Lasers: Physical processes and Operating schemes.* CRC Press, Boca Raton.

- Arecchi, F.T. and E.O. Schulz–Dubois, (ed.). (1972). *Laser Handbook.* North–Holland Pub. Co.

- Bertolotti, M. and Adam Hilger. (1983). *Masers and Lasers : An Historical Approach.*

- Benjamin Chu. (1991). *Laser Light Scattering : Basic Principles and Practice.* Academic Press, New York.

- David Sliney and Myron Wolbarsht. (1980). *Safety with Lasers and other Optical sources : A Comprehensive Handbook.* Plenum Press, New York.

- Donald C. O'Shea, Russell Callen, W. and William T. Rhodes. (1977). *Introduction to Lasers and their Applications.* Addison–Wesley Pub. Co.

- Dainty, J.C. (ed.). (1984). *Laser Speckle and Related Phenomena.* Springer–Verlag, Berlin.

- Das. P. (1991). *Lasers and Optical Engineering.* Springer–Verlag, New York.

- Francis. A. L'Esperance, Jr. (1989). *Ophthalmic Lasers.* St. Louis:Mosby.

- Gabriel Laufer. (1996). *Introduction to Optics and Lasers in Engineering.* Cambridge University Press.

- John C. Miller, (ed.). (1994). *Laser Ablation : Principles and Applications.* Springer Verlag, Berlin.

- Kay A. Ball. (1995). *Lasers : The Perioperative Challenge.* St. Louis:Mosby.

- Kenichi Iga, and Richard B. Miles, (ed.). (1994). *Fundamentals of Laser Optics.* Plenum Press, New York.

- Koichi Shimoda. (1986). *Introduction to Laser Physics*. Springer–Verlag. New York.

- Larryl Matthews and Gabe Garcia. (1995). *Laser and Eye safety in the Laboratory*. SPIE Optical Engineering Press, New York.

- Martin von Allmen. (1987). *Laser Beam Interactions with Materials: Physical Principles and Applications*. Springer–Verlag, New York.

- Matt Young. (1992). *Optics and Lasers : Including Fibres and Optical Waveguides*. Springer–Verlag, Berlin.

- Orazio Svelto and David C. Hanna, (ed.). (1989). *Principles of Lasers,* Plenum Press, New York.

- Robert Ginsburg, (ed.). (1989). *Primer on Laser Angioplasty*. Futura Pub. Co., New York.

- Siegman. A.E. (1971). *An Introduction to Lasers and Masers*. McGraw–Hill, New York.

- Wolbarsht, M.L. (ed.). (1971). *Laser Applications in Medicine and Biology.* Plenum press, New York.

- Winston E. Kock. (1975). Engineering Applications of Lasers and Holography. *Plenum Press, New York.*

- Freeman, W.H. (1969). *Lasers and Light, readings from Scientific American,* San Francisco, U.S.A.

- Yariv, Amnon, Holt, Rinehart and Winston. (1971). *Introduction to Optical Electronics*.